Pediatric Drug Directory

FIFTH DECADE OF PUBLICATION

Pediatric Drug Directory

10th Edition

Suraj Gupte

MD (PGIMER, Chandigarh) FIAP FSAMS (Sweden) FRSTMH (London)
Professor and Head (Emeritus)
Postgraduate Department of Pediatrics
Mamata Medical College and General and Super Specialty Hospitals
Khammam, Telangana, India
E-mail: drsurajgupte@gmail.com
Website: www.drsurajgupte.com

Chairperson: Pediatric Education Network—A Worldwide Pediatric Community

Editor: The Short Textbook of Pediatrics; Recent Advances in Pediatrics (Series), Textbooks of Pediatric Emergencies, Neonatal Emergencies, Pediatric Nutrition, and Pediatric Gastroenterology, Hepatology and Nutrition (Indo-American Venture); Pediatric Infectious Diseases; Influenza; Influenza: Complete Spectrum; Case-based Reviews in Pediatric Emergencies, Clinical Problem Solving in Neonatal Emergencies, and Intensive Care, etc.

Author: Differential Diagnosis in Pediatrics, Instructive Case Studies in Pediatrics, Influenza, Perspectives in Influenza, Nutrition in Neonatal ICU, Speaking of Childcare, etc.

Chief Editor (Gastroenterology Section): International Journal of Gastroenterology, Hepatology, Transplant and Nutrition.

Co-editor: Asian Journal of Maternity and Child Health (Manila, Philippines).

Section and Guest Editor: Pediatric Today (New Delhi).

Editorial Advisor: Asian Journal of Pediatric Practice (New Delhi).

Editorial Advisory Board Member/Reviewer: Indian Journal of Pediatrics (New Delhi), Indian Pediatrics (New Delhi), Indian Journal of Child Health (Gwalior), Synopsis (Detroit, USA), Maternal and Child Nutrition (Preston, UK), Journal of Infectious Diseases (Turkey), EC Pediatrics (London), Journal of Clinical Pediatrics (Patna), EC Pediatrics (London), Acta Scientific Gastrointestinal Disorders, etc.

Examiner: Several Universities, including National Board of Examinations (NBE) for DNB, New Delhi; All India Institute of Medical Sciences (AIIMS), New Delhi; Postgraduate Institute of Medical Education and Research (PGIMER), Chandigarh; Sher-I-Kashmir Institute of Medical Sciences (SKIMS), Srinagar; Indira Gandhi Open University (IGNOU), New Delhi, India.

Pediatric Faculty Selection Expert: All India Institute of Medical Sciences (AIIMS), Punjab Public Service Commission, Jammu and Kashmir Public Service Commission, and Union Public Service Commission.

Novy Gupte MD
Associate Professor
Department of Pharmacology
Army College of Medical Sciences
New Delhi, India
E-mail: drnovyguptemd@gmail.com

Foreword
Upendra Kinjawadekar

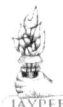

JAYPEE BROTHERS MEDICAL PUBLISHERS
The Health Sciences Publisher
New Delhi | London

Jaypee Brothers Medical Publishers (P) Ltd.

Headquarters

Jaypee Brothers Medical Publishers (P) Ltd
EMCA House, 23/23-B
Ansari Road, Daryaganj
New Delhi 110 002, India
Landline: +91-11-23272143, +91-11-23272703
+91-11-23282021, +91-11-23245672
Email: jaypee@jaypeebrothers.com

Corporate Office

Jaypee Brothers Medical Publishers (P) Ltd
4838/24, Ansari Road, Daryaganj
New Delhi 110 002, India
Phone: +91-11-43574357
Fax: +91-11-43574314
Email: jaypee@jaypeebrothers.com

Overseas Office

JP Medical Ltd.
83, Victoria Street, London
SW1H 0HW (UK)
Phone: +44 20 3170 8910
Fax: +44 (0)20 3008 6180
Email: info@jpmedpub.com

Website: www.jaypeebrothers.com
Website: www.jaypeedigital.com

© 2024, Jaypee Brothers Medical Publishers

The views and opinions expressed in this book are solely those of the original contributor(s)/author(s) and do not necessarily represent those of editor(s) or publisher of the book.

All rights reserved. No part of this publication may be reproduced, stored or transmitted in any form or by any means, electronic, mechanical, photocopying, recording or otherwise, without the prior permission in writing of the publishers.

All brand names and product names used in this book are trade names, service marks, trademarks or registered trademarks of their respective owners. The publisher is not associated with any product or vendor mentioned in this book.

Medical knowledge and practice change constantly. This book is designed to provide accurate, authoritative information about the subject matter in question. However, readers are advised to check the most current information available on procedures included and check information from the manufacturer of each product to be administered, to verify the recommended dose, formula, method and duration of administration, adverse effects and contraindications. It is the responsibility of the practitioner to take all appropriate safety precautions. Neither the publisher nor the author(s)/editor(s) assume any liability for any injury and/or damage to persons or property arising from or related to use of material in this book.

This book is sold on the understanding that the publisher is not engaged in providing professional medical services. If such advice or services are required, the services of a competent medical professional should be sought.

Every effort has been made where necessary to contact holders of copyright to obtain permission to reproduce copyright material. If any have been inadvertently overlooked, the publisher will be pleased to make the necessary arrangements at the first opportunity.

Inquiries for bulk sales may be solicited at: jaypee@jaypeebrothers.com

Pediatric Drug Directory

First Edition: May 1979; Second Edition: Jan. 1980; Third Edition: May 1982; Fourth Edition: Sept. 1984; Fifth Edition: Sept. 1986; Sixth Edition: Jan. 1991; Seventh Edition: 2001; Eighth: Edition 2014; Ninth Edition: 2019

Tenth Edition: **2024**

ISBN: 978-93-5696-314-6

Dedicated to
Everybody striving to contribute to child health and welfare for a brighter future globally.

Foreword

The time-honored manual, *Pediatric Drug Directory*, first launched in 1979, has achieved the distinction of being in the midst of fifth decade of its publication. I am delighted to be invited to write the foreword for its 10th edition.

I have critically reviewed the drafts of the new edition of the *Pediatric Drug Directory* by the noted pediatric educationist, researcher, innovator and author, Dr Suraj Gupte and Dr Novy Gupte—a pharmacologist with special interest in pediatric pharmacotherapy. The overall feeling is that the 10th edition of this popular handbook provides a yet better, updated, state-of-the-art and expanded plethora of handy information eagerly sought by all those involved in the pharmacotherapy of sick children, including neonates and adolescents. New incorporations include recently introduced molecules and updating and expansion of all sections, especially the section on pediatric emergencies. What is equally remarkable is that the contents are skillfully compiled in a very crisp, catchy, and easy-to-understand format and are downright reader-friendly.

On top of the excellent contents, the presentation in this manual continues to be simple, lucid and to-the-point. Rational categorization of the 60 chapters in 9 sections and listing of the drugs of various groups in alphabetic order are of great help to the reader. Furthermore, a comprehensive index facilitates easy and speedy access to and retrieval of the requisite information.

All-in-all, the 10th edition of Dr Suraj Gupte and Dr Novy Gupte's *Pediatric Drug Directory* is a warmly recommended title for the undergraduates, pediatric postgraduates/scholars, and practitioners of child health and disease on account of the wealth of information the book provides on pediatric drug therapy.

Upendra Kinjawadekar
National President (2023)
Indian Academy of Pediatrics (IAP)
E-mail:upen228@gmail.com

Preface to the Tenth Edition

With its 10th edition, the *Pediatric Drug Directory* enters the fifth decade of its publication. The new edition stands further revised, somewhat modified, and updated in keeping with the changing concerns, concepts, and advances in the field as also to meet the growing needs of the readers, who include not only the medical students, residents, and pediatricians, but also general practitioners and family physicians.

Section 1 deals with an overview of the basics of pediatric drug therapy, including principles, pharmacodynamics, pharmacokinetics, drug monitoring, etc.

Section 2 specifically provides salient information about general medications, beginning with analgesics, antipyretics, and anti-inflammatory drugs through antihypertensives to vitamins.

Section 3 embarks on antimicrobials including antibiotics and antiviral, antifungal and antiparasitic drugs.

Section 4 embarks on unclassified drugs.

Section 5 focuses on drugs employed in neonatology.

Section 6 gives guidelines on standard therapeutic approach to neonatal and pediatric emergencies.

Section 7 provides useful information on vaccines (both conventional and new), including combination vaccines. Also provided are the national and Indian Academy of Pediatrics (IAP) immunization schedules and adverse events following immunization.

Section 8 deals with drugs for neutralizing toxicity/poisoning of chemical agents.

Section 9 is a spotlight on common adverse reaction and the causative drugs.

A plethora of Appendices provide valuable information related to different aspects of pediatric drug therapy. Fresh entries include newer molecules applicable in pediatric practice.

Furthermore, a detailed Glossary of Abbreviations and Index are incorporated.

Over and above the essential details of the drugs, adverse drug reactions (ADRs), drug interactions, contraindications and cautions are particularly included, as and when warranted, in the interest of safety of the sick children.

We are confident that the 10th revised, updated, and enlarged edition of the *Pediatric Drug Directory* will provide the readers with yet more fruitful reading material in the larger interest of the child patients in need of medication.

Suraj Gupte
Novy Gupte

Preface to the First Edition

Drugs, says Professor Harry C Shirkey, are our fine servants and awful masters. This holds nowhere as good as in pediatric practice. Their injudicious use in infants and children can indeed prove disastrous.

Yet, the most troublesome to the freshers in the field of pediatrics, as also to the general practitioners who care for children as well, is the pediatric drug therapy. Which drug to give to a particular patient? The brand name? How available? How much to give? Side effects? The young doctors—many not-so-young also—sure feel puzzled.

Pediatric Drug Directory aims to be the answer. It provides the much-needed information as pointed out above plus much more. Section 1—the largest—deals with the brand names, availability, dosage and side effect of the important drugs. As a rule, drugs are arranged alphabetically according to the generic names. Section 2 deals with drugs excreted into the breast milk, Section 3 with drugs that discolor the stools and Section 4 with drugs that discolor the urine. Drugs likely to cause hemolysis in G6PD deficient individuals are listed in Section 5. Sections 6 and 7 deal with the WHOs urban and rural immunization schedules. The important patent formulary and surface area chart are the other highlights.

Dr (Mrs) VV Gujral has been gracious enough to advance highly useful criticism and to write the Foreword to the book.

While thanking all those who helped us in compiling this directory, we sincerely look forward to constructive criticism and suggestions from the readers. That will be a vital contribution to the subsequent editions.

Suraj Gupte
Rita Smith

Acknowledgments

Our gratitudes are due to:
- Dr Upendra Kinjawadekar, National President (2023), Indian Academy of Pediatrics (IAP) for his graciousness in reviewing the drafts and writing the *Foreword* for the 10th edition of the book.
- The Indian Academy of Pediatrics, American Academy of Pediatrics (AAP) and Ministry of Health and Family Welfare, Government of India, for access to their publications/websites.
- The international series, *Recent Advances in Pediatrics*, for using some state-of-the-art material published in its various volumes.
- *Nelson Textbook of Pediatrics*, 22nd edition, for using some state-of-the-art material.
- Dr Rita Smith, who actively shared the editorship from the inception through the seventh edition of the book, for continuing her association with the book as Advisor Emeritus in spite of her overwhelming commitments in other academic endeavors, including pharmacovigilance initiative globally.
- Dr Gagan Hans, Associate Professor, Department of Psychiatry, All India Institute of Medical Sciences, New Delhi, India, for voluntary help at various stages of development of this book, including inputs concerning neuropsychiatric drugs.
- Our readers for providing us a much-needed feedback from time to time to enhance the utility of the book.

Finally, we warmly appreciate the efforts of the concerned staff of M/s Jaypee Brothers Medical Publishers (P) Ltd, New Delhi, India, for the highly skillful production qualities of the book.

Contents

SECTION 1: Basics of Pharmacotherapy in Neonates, Infants, and Children

1. Principles *3*
2. Rational Drug Therapy *21*
3. Therapeutic Drug Monitoring *25*
4. Certain Golden Rules of Safe Pediatric Drug Therapy *28*

SECTION 2: General and Systemic Medications

5. Analgesics/Antipyretics/Nonsteroidal Anti-inflammatory Drugs *33*
6. Antacids *44*
7. Anti-acne Drugs *46*
8. Antiasthma Drugs/Bronchodilators *48*
9. Anticancer (Antineoplastic) Drugs *60*
10. Anticoagulants *68*
11. Anticonvulsants *73*
12. Antidiarrheals *89*
13. Antiemetics *95*
14. Antifibrillatory Drugs *100*
15. Antihistaminic Drugs *108*
16. Antihypertensive Drugs *119*
17. Antimyasthenic Drugs *132*
18. Antireflux Drugs *135*
19. Antipsychotic Drugs *141*
20. Antispasmodics/Antiflatulence Drugs *146*
21. Antitoxins *151*
22. Antitussives and Cough Expectorants *154*
23. Cardiotonic Drugs *157*
24. Chelating Agents *164*

25.	Colony-stimulating Factors	168
26.	Diuretics	171
27.	Drugs for Attention-deficit Hyperactivity Disorder	177
28.	Drugs for Apnea of Prematurity	180
29.	Drugs for Bleeding Control	182
30.	Drugs for Endocrinal Disorders/Hormones/Enzymes	185
31.	Drugs for Gout	198
32.	Drugs for Vertigo	201
33.	Hematinics	203
34.	Immunoglobulins	209
35.	Macrominerals	217
36.	Micronutrients	221
37.	Muscle Relaxants	224
38.	Nasal Decongestants	227
39.	Nutritional Supplements	229
40.	Plasma Volume Expanders	231
41.	Stool Softeners/Laxatives	235
42.	Vasodilators	238
43.	Vitamins	241

SECTION 3: Drugs for Infectious Diseases

44.	Antibacterial Drugs (Antibiotics)	251
45.	Antimycobacterial Drugs	314
46.	Antiviral Drugs	332
47.	Antifungal Drugs	352
48.	Antiparasitic (Intestinal) Drugs	359
49.	Antiparasitic (Extraintestinal) Drugs	373

SECTION 4: Unclassified Drugs

50.	Miscellaneous Drugs	391

SECTION 5: Drug Therapy in Neonates

51. Drug Dosage in Neonates **407**
52. Emergency Drugs in Neonates **424**

SECTION 6: Pharmacotherapy in Pediatric Emergencies

53. Important Emergency Drugs... **429**
54. Pharmacotherapy of Common Pediatric Emergencies..... **432**

SECTION 7: Immunization and Vaccines

55. Conventional and New Vaccines for Routine Use............ **459**
56. Combination Vaccines **491**
57. Immunization Schedules in India **495**
58. Adverse Events Following Immunization **502**

SECTION 8: Drugs for Neutralizing Toxicity/Poisoning of Chemical Agents

59. Specific Antidotes.. **507**

SECTION 9: Adverse Drug Reactions

60. Adverse Drug Reactions Specific to Certain Drugs **513**

APPENDICES: Useful Information Related to Pediatric Drug Therapy

Appendix 1: Principles of Drug Administration in Infants and Young Children **541**
Appendix 2: Various Solutions Used in the Treatment of Dehydration and Dyselectrolytemia **543**
Appendix 3: Drugs in Treatment/Prevention of Fetal Disease **544**
Appendix 4: Therapeutic Range of Some Drugs........................ **545**
Appendix 5: Drugs Excreted into Breast Milk............................. **547**
Appendix 6: Drugs that Discolor the Stools **550**

Appendix 7:	Drugs that Discolor the Urine	*551*
Appendix 8:	Drugs Likely to Cause Hemolysis in G6PD Deficiency	*553*
Appendix 9:	Drugs that may Cause Peculiar Side Effects	*555*
Appendix 10:	Drug Groups with Adverse Effects on Vitamin Status	*556*
Appendix 11:	Potential Drug Interaction with Chemotherapy	*558*
Appendix 12:	Banned Single-dose Drug Combinations (in India)	*560*
Appendix 13:	Banned Fixed Dose Drug Combinations with Other Agents (in India)	*563*
Appendix 14:	Nomogram for Estimation of Surface Area	*564*
Appendix 15:	Weight to Surface Area Conversion Chart	*566*
Index		*567*

Abbreviations

ABC	–	Airway, breathing, and circulation
ABG	–	Arterial blood gases
ACE	–	Angiotensin-converting enzyme
ACTH	–	Adrenocorticotropic hormone
ADE	–	Adverse drug events
ADHD	–	Attention-deficit hyperactivity disorder
ADR	–	Adverse drug reaction
AED	–	Antiepileptic drug
AEFI	–	Adverse events following immunization
AIDS	–	Acquired immune deficiency syndrome
ARF	–	Acute renal failure
ATT	–	Antituberculous therapy
BCG	–	Bacillus Calmette–Guérin
BD	–	Twice a day
BMI	–	Body mass index
BP	–	Blood pressure
BPD	–	Bronchopulmonary dysplasia
BUN	–	Blood urea nitrogen
BW	–	Body weight
CCF	–	Congestive cardiac failure
Cap	–	Capsule
CLD	–	Chronic lung disease
CMV	–	Cytomegalic virus
CNS	–	Central nervous system
CP	–	Cerebral palsy
CSF	–	Cerebrospinal fluid
DIC	–	Disseminated intravascular coagulopathy
Div	–	Divided
DTP	–	Diphtheria, tetanus, and pertussis
ECG	–	Electrocardiograph

ET	–	Endotracheal
G6PD	–	Glucose-6-phosphate dehydrogenase
GERD	–	Gastroesophageal reflux disease
g	–	Gram
Hib	–	*Haemophilus influenzae* type b
HIV	–	Human immunodeficiency virus
Hr	–	Hour, hourly
HSV	–	Herpes simplex virus/vaccine
HZV	–	Herpes zoster virus
ICP	–	Intracranial pressure
ID	–	Intradermal
IgG	–	Immunoglobulin G
IM	–	Intramuscular
IPV	–	Inactivated polio virus
IT	–	Intratracheal
ITP	–	Idiopathic (immune) thrombocytopenic purpura
IV	–	Intravenous
IVH	–	Intraventricular hemorrhage
IVIG	–	Intravenous immunoglobulins
JIA	–	Juvenile idiopathic arthritis
LBW	–	Low-birth weight
MDR	–	Multidrugs resistant
Mg	–	Milligram
Min	–	Minute
MMR	–	Measles, mumps, and rubella
MRSA	–	Methicillin-resistant *Staphylococcus aureus*
Ng	–	Nanogram
NG	–	Nasogastric
NSAID	–	Nonsteroidal anti-inflammatory drug
OD	–	Once a day

Abbreviations

OPV	–	Oral polio vaccine
PCM	–	Paracetamol
PEM	–	Protein-energy malnutrition
PDA	–	Patent ductus arteriosus
PO	–	Per os/oral (by mouth)
PR	–	Per rectum
q	–	Every
RDS	–	Respiratory distress syndrome
ROP	–	Retinopathy of prematurity
SAM	–	Severe acute malnutrition
SC	–	Subcutaneous
Sec	–	Seconds
Susp	–	Suspension
Syr	–	Syrup
Tab	–	Tablet
TDS	–	Thrice a day
VRSA	–	Vancomycin-resistant *Staphylococcus aureus*
Wk	–	Week
Wt	–	Weight
Yr	–	Year

Section 1

Basics of Pharmacotherapy in Neonates, Infants, and Children

1. Principles
2. Rational Drug Therapy
3. Therapeutic Drug Monitoring
4. Certain Golden Rules of Safe Pediatric Drug Therapy

Chapter 1

Principles

INTRODUCTION

According to a famous dictum, "the child is not a mini adult". Likewise, the neonate is not a mini child. This holds good at least from the angle of drug therapy and dosages that are based on not only the indication but also on the pharmacokinetics and pharmacodynamics.

PHARMACOKINETICS IN PEDIATRIC AGE GROUPS

Age-based grouping of pediatric population is given in **Box 1**. As a result of studies related to developmental pharmacokinetics, today we know that:

- Pharmacokinetics are quite immature in the neonates, especially in the preterm, low birthweight (lbw) infants and infants suffering from intrauterine growth restriction/retardation (IUGR)
- During age 1–12 months, the pharmacokinetics show an improvement in maturity.

BOX 1: Age-based grouping of the pediatric population based on age.

- Preterm newborn (<37 weeks' gestation)
- Newborn (0–28 days)
- Infant (>28 days–12 months)
- Toddler (>12 months–23 months)
- Preschool child (2–5 years)
- School age child (6–11 years)
- Adolescents (12–18 years)

- During age 1–4 years, these are nearly stabilized.
- During age 5–11 years, these are even somewhat above the status in adults.
- During adolescence, these are fully matured.

The old practice of drug prescribing in neonates, infants, and children just by arbitrary modification of the adult dose was by all means erroneous and ill-founded.

As a rule, most of the factors influencing the drug disposition are unique in neonates and infants who represent the most fragile group due to physiological instabilities and increased potentials for toxic effects as compared to children and adults. However, only limited work has been done in these areas in pediatric age group, leaving quite a few gray areas for elucidation. This age group should, therefore, receive special attention for pharmacokinetic, pharmacodynamics, and toxicologic research.

SEVEN "RIGHTS" OF SAFE DRUG THERAPY

1. Right child
2. Right drug
3. Right dose
4. Right time (frequency and duration)
5. Right route
6. Right reason (indication)
7. Right documentation

Frequently, there is a mention of only "five rights". Here the last two above-mentioned rights are skipped.

CERTAIN DEFINITIONS

The term, *pharmacokinetics,* refers to what the body does to the drug. It is, thus, a mathematical expression of the time course of movements in the body. A drug's pharmacologic effects, toxic effects or both correlate best with its concentration in blood or some other biologic fluid rather than the administered absolute dose. The dose and dose interval to attain a defined target concentration for the desired pharmacological effect is based on pharmacokinetics.

The term, *pharmacodynamics*, denotes the correlation of pharmacological response to a measured drug concentration in blood or some other body fluid that reflects the drug concentration at the receptor site. In short, pharmacokinetics refers to "What the drug does to the body?"

Rational prescribing is dictated by the pharmacokinetics and pharmacodynamics of the drug. An additional factor of paramount importance is age of the subject.

APPLIED CLINICAL PHARMACOKINETICS AND DRUG THERAPY

The drug's pharmacologic effects, toxic effects or both correlate well with its concentration in a biologic fluid rather than the absolute dose administered.

As a rule, amount of drug in the body (usually measured in terms of serum concentration) is determined by the dose administered. This is called *principle of linear or first-order pharmacokinetics.*

Some such drugs as phenytoin, salicylates and alcohol do not follow this principle. Though they exhibit first order or linear principle at low dose, with increasing dose, their elimination pathway becomes saturated and the drug concentration in blood changes disproportionately to the dose administered. Such drugs are, therefore, said to follow the *principle of zero order* (the so-called *Michaelis–Menten kinetics*).

Drug Absorption and Bioavailability

The drug's bioavailability is the fraction of the amount absorbed following extravascular drug administration relative to intravenous (IV) administration, the drug administered by latter route being considered as 100% bioavailable. It is calculated as the ratio of the area under drug concentration time curve (AUC) determined after extravascular drug administration to the drug AUC obtained after IV administration as shown below:

$$\text{Bioavailability} = \frac{\text{AUC (oral)}}{\text{AUC (IV)}}$$

Volume of Distribution

The distribution of drugs in blood depends mainly on its lipid solubility, ionization, pH of blood, available protein-binding capacity and difference in the regional blood flow.

Whereas lipid-soluble drugs are, as a rule, distributed throughout the extracellular and intracellular spaces, the water-soluble drugs are distributed mainly in the extracellular space and hardly in the cerebrospinal fluid (CSF) or other body fluids.

As far as the selective distribution of drugs is concerned, it occurs as a result of protein-binding in blood (penicillins) and in tissues (mepacrine). In case of such drugs as are not bound to proteins (insulin), distribution remains confined to the extracellular space. Obviously, these drugs can be utilized to measure extracellular space.

The drugs which get speedily absorbed from the gastrointestinal tract on account of their lipid solubility readily diffuse into the CSF and brain tissue.

The drugs which get poorly absorbed from the gastrointestinal tract (streptomycin and neostigmine), demonstrate poor penetration into various body fluids.

A noteworthy point is that, in case of inflamed meninges, there is a remarkable elevation in the penetration of all drugs into the CSF.

The initial dose or loading dose is not influenced by the drug clearance or elimination from the body. Thus, the initial dose remains the same for subjects with normal renal function as for those with compromised renal function.

Metabolism

Once the drug has performed its action (effectively or otherwise), it has got to be metabolized and finally excreted. Liver is the major site of drug metabolism which occurs in two phases:
1. Conversion to pharmacologically-inactive substances.
2. Conversion to pharmacologically-active substances (prednisone, cortisone, imipramine, and cyclophosphamide).

Drugs are chiefly metabolized by enzymes in hepatic microsomes and to some extent, by the enzymes in blood and elsewhere in the body. In the nonsynthetic reaction, the molecule is changed by oxidation, reduction or hydrolysis. In the synthetic reaction, the molecule is conjugated with other substances such as glucuronic acid (glucuronidation), acetic acid (acetylation), sulfate (ethereal sulfate formation), etc.

Just a word about enzyme induction. Such drugs as phenobarbital, phenytoin, alcohol, dichlorodiphenyltrichloroethane (DDT) and phenylbutazone (often called "bute") are examples of enzyme-inducers. Enzyme induction by alcohol consumption causes excessive breakdown of phenobarbital. As a result alcoholics develop tolerance to it. On the other hand, isoniazid (INH), anticoagulants and phenylbutazone depress enzyme induction and, thus, the phenytoin metabolism. Phenytoin toxicity even with recommended doses may, therefore, occur in such subjects.

Elimination of Half-life

The term, *half-life*, denotes time required for half the amount of drug present in body fluid to be cleared. It is expressed as t½ and is frequently employed to determine a drug's dosage intervals. It may also be employed to find the time required to attain the steady-state concentration. By the latter term is meant the point at which the amount of drug dose is equivalent to the amount of drug cleared from the body. **Table 1** shows the relationship between different half-lives and steady-state concentration.

Clearance

It means the amount of drug removed from the body per unit of time. It is influenced by the integrity of blood flow and by the functional ability of the organs involved in removing the drug from the body.

Renal excretion: Plasma protein-binding of drug, glomerular filtration rate (GFR), back diffusion from glomerular filtration, active renal tubular reabsorption and active renal tubular secretion influence the renal excretion of drugs.

TABLE 1: Correlation between half-lives and steady-state concentrations.

Half-lives	Steady-state concentration (%)
Three	87.5
Four	93.8
Five	100

Chapter 1: Principles

Biliary excretion: Penicillin, rifampicin, erythromycin and tetracycline are examples of drugs excreted in bile. An important feature of such drugs is that they are often reabsorbed into circulation (the so-called "enterohepatic cycle"), thereby prolonging their half-life. Finally, they are excreted in urine.

Pulmonary excretion: The examples of drugs excreted through lungs are volatile lipid-soluble anesthetics and metabolites.

Excretion in breast milk: Drugs ingested by lactating mother and excreted in breast milk so as to harm the baby include antithyroid agents (propylthiouracil is an exception), cytotoxic agents, radioactive substances, lithium, bromocriptine and phenelzine.

Drug–drug Interaction

The term *drug–drug interaction* is applied when two or more drugs administered to a particular patient modify the pharmacokinetic and pharmacodynamics properties of each through combined interaction. The resultant effects may be unpredictable clinical responses or toxic effects. **Box 2** lists the different types of drug–drug interactions.

BOX 2: Various types of drug–drug interactions.

- Drug inactivation when compounds are mixed together physically before administration as in syringes, infusion tubing or parenteral fluid preparations
- Disposition characteristics of one compound are influenced by those of another, one drug reducing the rate but not the overall absorption, or a drug displacing the other drug from its protein-binding sites while concomitantly retarding its elimination from the body
- Metabolic-based drug–drug interaction as a result of competition by two compounds for the same metabolic site
- Competition by the drugs for the same receptor or physiologic system, thereby altering the patient's response to drug therapy

Therapeutic Drug Monitoring

Adjustment of the dose on the basis of clinical response and measurement of concentration of the drug in serum or plasma is called *therapeutic drug monitoring (TDM)*. Such an approach is termed *target concentration strategy*. In this strategy, a drug's pharmacologic or toxicologic response can be directly related to a specific serum concentration range. Major role of TDM is in knowing whether the dosage or dosage intervals require modification. The aim is optimizing the management of patients receiving drug therapy for the alleviation or prevention of illnesses.

TDM is a relatively new approach in the clinical pharmacology laboratory. It has moved a long way since the time it was considered a luxury. Today, it has evolved to be a necessity in certain hard situations such as an unsatisfactory seizure control despite a recommended drug in recommended dose and dosage interval.

Yet, mind you, TDM is neither necessary nor feasible for all drugs.

For more details, *see* Chapter 3.

CHARACTERISTICS OF VARIOUS ROUTES OF DRUG ADMINISTRATION

Intravenous Route

Absorption: Effect is large immediate.

Special indication: Excellent for emergency situations, for administering large amounts and for irritating agents that can be given in a diluted form.

Limitations: Expensive, requiring assistance of an expert for administration; unsuitable for oily preparations; boosts vulnerability to superimposed infection.

TABLE 2: Factors having a bearing on oral absorption of drugs.

Physiologic factor	Newborn	Infant	Child/adolescent
Gastric acid secretion	Reduced	Normal	Normal
Gastric emptying time	Reduced	Increased	Increased
Gastrointestinal motility	Reduced	Normal	Normal
Biliary function	Reduced	Normal	Normal
Microbial flora	Acquiring	Adult pattern	Adult pattern

Oral Route

Absorption: Most drugs are absorbed by passive diffusion, only some by active transport or facilitated diffusion; preferred route; influenced by a number of factors **(Table 2)**.

Special indication: Most natural, convenient, economical and safe route.

Limitations: There usually is a considerable lag period before action at the target level starts; it cannot be employed in uncooperative subjects; bioavailability is somewhat erroneous since some drugs may be inactivated by gastric juices whereas most drugs are metabolized in the liver after absorption.

Intramuscular Route

Absorption: Quite fast for aqueous solutions.

Special indication: Most suitable for oily preparations (vitamin A) and some irritating substances (iron-dextran complex).

Limitations: May cause local necrosis, induration or even abscess; may precipitate otherwise abortive poliomyelitis;

not advisable in bleeding diathesis and for such drugs as phenytoin and chloramphenicol which have erratic absorption.

Subcutaneous Route

Absorption: Quite fast for aqueous solutions.

Special indication: Appropriate for certain insoluble suspensions and implantation of solid pellets.

Limitations: Not appropriate when large volumes are to be administered; local pain and induration may occur.

Sublingual Route

Absorption: Quite fast absorption of lipid-soluble agents.

Specific indication: When it is desirable to bypass liver.

Limitations: Utility limited to drugs requiring direct effect on heart (nitroglycerine).

Rectal Route

Absorption: Quite prompt absorption.

Specific indication: Appropriate for subjects with persistent vomiting and in unconscious state; very effective for controlling acute seizures (rectal diazepam).

Intrathecal

Absorption: Prompt action at targeted site central nervous system (CNS).

Special indication: For prompt local effect in meningitis and other CNS infections.

Limitations: Not practicable for administering large doses of drugs; may cause chemical or iatrogenic meningitis.

Pulmonary (Aerosol and Nebulization)

Absorption: Quite prompt local as well as systemic effect.

Special indication: For direct absorption and action, bypassing the liver.

Limitations: Particle size has got to vary between 1 and 7 μ (<1 μ is likely to be exhaled whereas >7 μ is unlikely to reach small bronchi); poor ability to regulate dose; not always practicable in small children.

DRUG DOSAGE AND ITS CALCULATION

The best way of calculating drug dose is in terms of surface area employing the nomogram. However, it is quite cumbersome and not always practicable. Therefore, in practice, drug dose is usually calculated according to bodyweight in children. This approach is practical but not ideal because even within a population of similar age and weight, drug requirement may differ on account of maturational differences in absorption, metabolism and elimination.

According to the famous Clark's rule, pediatric drug dose can be calculated if we know the adult dose and child's weight. Fred's rule is similar, in place of weight in pounds, age in months employed. Now, both are infrequently employed because of their limitations. **Box 3** lists pediatric dose and the surface area formulas.

NEONATAL PHARMACOTHERAPY

Notwithstanding the advances in the basic science research that have improved our understanding of use of

BOX 3: Calculation of pediatric dose.

1. Nomogram (surface area) method:
   (a) Child's dose = Surface area (m^2)/1.73 × adult dose
   (b) Child's dose as percentage of adult dose =
       Surface area in m^2 × 60
2. Bodyweight method: mg/kg/day or mg/kg/dose
3. Clark's rule:
   Child's dose = Weight (lbs)/150 × adult dose
4. Fred's rule:
   Dose = Age (months)/150 × adult dose
5. Young's rule:
   Child's dose = Age/(age + 12) × adult dose

pharmacological agents in the neonate, neonatal pharmacotherapy remains an area that has not received the attention that it indeed deserves. Today, several drugs are used in the newborn in spite of the lack of specific clinical research in this vulnerable age group. In fact, present day pharmacotherapy in neonates is mainly based on the individual clinical expertise of specialized neonatologists and pediatricians. Around 60–70% drugs used in neonates and infants are unlicensed, the so-called "off-label drugs". These continue to be employed in neonatal drug therapy without the recommended regulatory phases of drug development.

Let us have some idea about the peculiarities of the neonate in relation to drug therapy.

- In the newborn, the individual response to a drug in terms of efficacy and safety is highly variable. Predicting drug dosing is complex since rapid physiological changes occurring during the perinatal and early postnatal periods affect the pharmacokinetic profile of several drugs.

Chapter 1: Principles

- Neonatal disorders such as renal and hepatic diseases may also have significant implications for drug pharmacokinetics.
- Pharmacotherapy in the newborn poses difficulties in accurate drug delivery and, consequent upon that a high risk of adverse drug reactions.
- The neonates, especially in neonatal intensive care unit (NICU), are highly exposed to the risk of medication errors with potentially serious adverse events.

In other words, the extensive variability in pharmacokinetics and pharmacodynamics because of its fast maturation is a glaring feature of the newborn. This together with the newly-evolving treatment modalities, environmental issues, and pharmacogenetics renders clinical pharmacological research in neonates utmost important though cumbersome.

Obviously, all this is challenging too. Why? This is understandable on account of quite a few reasons. First and foremost, the pharmacological trial in neonates is more difficult to perform. Secondly, appropriate dosing is hampered by the rapid physiological changes occurring at this stage of development and the selection of proper endpoints. Thirdly, biomarkers are complicated by the limited knowledge of the pathophysiology of the specific neonatal diseases. Fourthly, there are many ethical challenges in planning and conducting drug studies in the newborns.

These "pharmacological" challenges add to the ethical challenges that are always present in planning and conducting clinical studies in neonates. These challenges justify that clinical research in neonatology should be evaluated by ad hoc ethical committees with specific expertise.

How to overcome the challenges? Tailored tools and legal initiatives, combined with clever trial design are likely to result in more robust information on neonatal pharmacotherapy. This necessitates collaborative efforts between clinical researchers, sponsors, and regulatory authorities. Additionally, patient representatives and society need to make their contribution.

The regulatory framework for model-based neonatal medicinal development needs to be streamlined and initiated wherever it does not exist. In trials, success is assured by the implementation of specific pharmacokinetic assessments as a result of accurate drug dosing achieved with a combination of dose validation, population pharmacokinetics, and mathematical models of drug clearance and distribution.

Further, age-specific pharmacodynamics need to be considered via appropriate evaluations of drug efficacy with endpoints adapted to the peculiar pathophysiology of diseases in this age group.

Tailoring research tools are urgently needed. Development of dried blood spot techniques and the introduction of micro-dosing and tracer methodology in neonatal drug studies as well as building research networks and clinical research skills for neonates must take precedence and that too on priority. Both techniques can be combined with sparse sampling techniques through population modeling. Building the initiatives to build and integrate knowledge on neonatal pharmacotherapy through dedicated working groups, research networks and clinical research skills can go a long way in meeting the aims and objectives.

All in all, new innovations in pharmacokinetic research, such as population pharmacokinetic modeling, present opportunities to conduct clinical trials in neonates aimed at improving the safety and effectiveness of the drugs in this vulnerable population.

Untoward Effects of Drugs

- The term, *side effects,* denotes undesirable effects, e.g., drowsiness caused by antihistamines, dryness of mouth because of decongestant therapy or diarrhea secondary to ampicillin therapy.
- The term, *intolerance*, refers to the unwanted effects due to low threshold to normal pharmacologic action.
- The term, *idiosyncrasy,* means that a genetic abnormality [glucose-6-phosphate dehydrogenase (G6PD) deficiency, porphyria] predisposes an individual to a qualitative abnormal reaction to certain drug(s).
- The term, *secondary effects,* denotes indirect consequences following a prolonged use of certain drugs.
- The term, *hypersensitive,* relates to anaphylactoid shock (penicillin, serum), urticarial rash, angioneurotic edema, serum sickness syndrome and pulmonary reactions (antigen-antibody reaction).

Maternal Medication and Fetus

As a rule, the pregnant woman should receive no medication as all medications are potentially risky to the fetus, especially during the first trimester of pregnancy. A drug apparently safe for the mother may be harmful for her growing baby in utero. The golden rule is to prescribe for the pregnant woman only when its beneficial effect outweighs the risk for the fetus. Even in such a situation, attempt should be to prescribe a drug that has withstood the test of time or a drug which is likely to be least risky.

Table 3 provides a list of drugs that are likely to have a teratogenic effect on the fetus.

TABLE 3: Drugs likely to have adverse effects on the fetus when consumed during pregnancy.

Drug	Adverse effects (teratogenic)
Diazepam	Cleft lip, cleft palate, hypothermia, apnea deafness, thrombocytopenia, neurologic anomalies
Chloroquine (prolonged use)	Deafness
Sulfas	Hyperbilirubinemia
Streptomycin	Eighth nerve deafness, renal damage
Tetracyclines	Deposition in teeth, staining of teeth, enamel hypoplasia, retardation of bone growth, and congenital cataracts
Propranolol	Growth retardation and thrombocytopenia
Indomethacin	LBW, platelet dysfunction
Heroin	Intrauterine death, LBW, SIDS
Phenobarbital	Cleft lip, cleft palate, CHD, respiratory depression, withdrawal symptoms
Phenytoin	Various malformations in relation to limbs, heart, and face
Valproate	Facial anomalies, spina bifida, and developmental delay
Smoking	LBW and abnormal placentation
Alcoholism	IUGR, mental retardation, microcephaly, CHD, and flexion contractures
Diethylstilbestrol	Genitourinary anomalies in males and adenosis or carcinoma of vagina in females
Progesterone with testosterone	Masculinization of female fetus
Iodides (in third trimester)	Congenital goiter and hypothyroidism

Contd...

Contd...

Drug	Adverse effects (teratogenic)
Cyclophosphamide	Multiple deformities
Progesterone (in third trimester)	Malformations of external genitalia and postpubertal vaginal adenocarcinoma
Sulfonylurea (third trimester)	Neonatal hypoglycemia and brain damage
Thalidomide (in third trimester)	Limb deformities, defects of CVS, ears, and eyes
Radiation	Mental retardation and microcephaly

(CHD: coronary heart disease; CVS: cardiovascular system; IUGR: intrauterine growth restriction; LBW: low birthweight; SIDS: sudden infant death syndrome)

MATERNAL MEDICATION AND BREASTFEEDING

Many drugs are excreted to some extent into the breast milk and, naturally, ingested by the nursing infant. Some of them may have adverse effects on the neonate and the infant **(Table 4)**. The nursing mother must, therefore, never consume any medication without obtaining an approval of the pediatrician. In certain special situations, a sample of breast milk may be analyzed to get an idea about the amount of drug the infant is receiving or about the likely drug effects on the infant.

There is a fair consensus that breastfeeding should be continued in most cases even when the mother is receiving psychotropic drugs. Mind you, the benefits of breastfeeding outweigh the risk associated with small amount of drug that may be excreted in milk. The only contraindication is when mother is on chemotherapeutic agents or receiving radiation therapy.

TABLE 4: Maternal medication that may harm the baby who is on breastfeeding.

Agent	Adverse effect(s)
Antithyroids	Hypothyroidism
Phenobarbital	Drowsiness, rickets, rash, and methemoglobinemia
Diphenylhydantoin sodium	Rickets, rash, and methemoglobinemia
Diazepam	Drowsiness and rise in serum bilirubin
Laxatives (e.g., cascara)	Loose motions
Penicillin	Rash
Narcotics	Withdrawal symptoms
Theophylline	Irritability
Lithium	Hypotonia
Sulfas	Drug rash and hemolysis
Salicylates	Rash and interference in platelet function
Oral contraceptives	Failure to thrive and gynecomastia

2
Chapter

Rational Drug Therapy

INTRODUCTION

The phrase, "rational drug therapy", denotes drug treatment on sensible and sound reasoning. In other words, it denotes right drug, right child, right reason, right dose, right route, right time and right documentation. Some countries have a monitoring approach, *Rational Drug Therapy Program (RDTP)* that is dedicated to rational, safe, cost-effective, and patient outcome-oriented drug treatment. Understandably, irrationality in drug therapy may result from:
- Use of an unnecessary drug
- Wrong choice of drug
- Inappropriate dosage and route of administration
- Poor prescribing.

Factors contributing to irrational drug therapy include:
- Inappropriate model prescriber
- Undue pressures
- Unfair practices
- Personal ambitions and life goals
- Myths.

The irrational drug therapy is most dangerous when it comes to the abuse of antimicrobial agents leading to increasing antimicrobial resistance (AMR) of varying degrees and magnitudes. This trend was particularly observed during the years 2020–2022 [the era of peak waves of coronavirus disease 2019 (COVID-19)] when antibiotic misuse reached new heights. Currently, AMR ranks among the 10 top global public health problems. The seriousness of the problem compelled the World Health Organization (WHO) to declare 7th, April 2011 as the World Health Day with the theme "Antimicrobial Resistance: No Action Today, No Cure Tomorrow". On ongoing basis, the WHO observes worldwide the *World Antimicrobial Awareness Week* in November every year. The coordinated approach by all nations of the world is paramount to fight the AMR, especially that against multidrug resistant bacterial pathogens (superbugs). Antimicrobial stewardship and development of newer antibiotics are also important to fight the AMR and its morbid impacts on health and economy.

GENERAL

The following considerations are important in regard to rational antibiotic therapy:
- Variation in etiologic pathogens among age groups
- Microbiologic diagnosis (isolation of the pathogen from sterile body site) with sensitivity testing which should logically determine the choice of an antimicrobial agent. In its absence, clinical diagnosis with projection of the most likely pathogen(s) may determine the choice of antibiotic(s) which is, at beat, empirical
- Age-appropriate antibiotic dose, dosing frequency and route of administration
- Toxicity of the drug(s) likely to be effective
- Immunologic status since immunocompromised status may render the child more susceptible to microbes that are considered benign in immunocompetent children

- Likelihood of central nervous system (CNS) involvement in certain infections (e.g., *Haemophilus influenzae* type B, *Pneumococcus* and *Meningococcus*) pointing to more aggressive antimicrobial therapy
- Presence of a foreign body enhances the risk of bacterial infection
- Pattern of antimicrobial resistance in the community occurring through several modifications of the bacterial genome such as:
  - Enzyme inactivation of the antibiotic
  - Reduced cell membrane permeability to intracellularly active antibiotics
  - Efflux of antibiotic out of the bacteria
  - Protection or alteration of the antibiotic target site
  - Excessive production of the target site
  - Passing the antimicrobial site of action.

As a reflection of the route of administration, drug absorption, volume of distribution and drug elimination half-life and drug–drug interactions (altering enzymatic inactivation of an antibiotic or causing antimicrobial synergism or antagonism), serum levels of antibiotic. Target serum levels appropriate for different antibiotics are available.

SPECIAL SITUATIONS

Neonates

Empirical antimicrobial selection should take into consideration the fact that likely pathogens are typically acquired around the time of delivery and, therefore, from the maternal birth passage, e.g., *Escherichia coli*, Group B *Streptococcus (GBS), and Listeria monocytogenes.* Since these pathogens may cause meningitis, therapy must include antibiotic(s) that crosses (cross) the blood–brain barrier (BBB) and, thereby, covers CNS infection in case meningitis remains on the card.

Infants and Children

The pathogens relevant in infants and toddlers include *Haemophilus influenzae type B (Hib), Streptococcus pneumoniae, Meningococcus,* and *Staphylococcus aureus.*

Among older children, additional pathogens include *Moraxella catarrhalis,* nontypeable strains of *H. influenzae, Mycoplasma pneumoniae,* Group A *Streptococcus (GAS), Enterococcus,* and *Salmonella.*

Immunocompromised Subjects

In immunocompromised states or in situations of prolonged hospital stay, such pathogens as *Pseudomonas aeruginosa, Klebsiella pneumoniae, Enterobacter (E. faecalis* and *E. faecium), Serratia,* and *E. coli* assume particular importance as opportunistic pathogens. Treatment of these infections becomes extremely difficult on account of antimicrobial resistance, including resistance to vancomycin.

Medical Devices-associated Infections

Indwelling medical devices (venous catheter, ventriculoperitoneal shunt, and stent) predispose to infection with *S. aureus* and *coagulase-negative Staphylococcus.* Management warrants not only appropriate antibiotic therapy but also removal/replacement of the offending (colonized) prosthetic gadget.

Chapter 3

Therapeutic Drug Monitoring

INTRODUCTION

Therapeutic drug monitoring (TDM) is defined as a testing that measures the amount of certain *medicines* in patient's blood to make sure the amount of medicine he/she is taking is safe and effective. It is based on measuring the concentration of prescribed drugs in the serum or plasma in order to provide a rational basis for dosage adjustment in individual patients.

INDICATIONS

- Drugs with the following characteristics are commonly monitored
- Drugs with a good relationship between plasma concentration and clinical effects, e.g., theophylline
- Drugs with well-defined "therapeutic" and "toxic" levels for plasma drug concentrations, e.g., phenytoin
- Drugs with a narrow "therapeutic index" where toxic concentrations are very close to effective concentrations, e.g., digoxin
- Drugs for which there is no easily measured clinical response and/or failure of response is "all or nothing", e.g., anticonvulsants and antiarrhythmic drugs
- Drugs for which the pharmacological response is difficult to quantify, e.g., cyclosporin

- Drugs for which plasma concentration has prognostic significance in overdosage, e.g., paracetamol.

Drugs fulfilling some or all of the above criteria are listed in **Table 1**.

TABLE 1: Salient features of drugs commonly needing therapeutic monitoring.

Drugs	Sampling time(s) (micro-mole/L)[3]	Time to reach steady state[1]	Therapeutic plasma concentration range (mg/L)[2]	
			Minimum	Maximum
Aminoglycosides				
Amikacin	30 minutes after a dose and just prior of next dose		3–5	20–30
Gentamicin			1–2	5–10
Netilmicin			1–2	5–10
Tobramycin			1–2	5–10
Antiarrhythmics				
Amiodarone	Prior to next dose	1 month[3]	0.6–2.0	1.0–3.0
Disopyramide		24 hours	3–7	9–20
Flecainide		3 days	0.2–0.8	0.5–2.0
Lignocaine		12 hours	1.5–5	6–21
Mexiletine		2 days	0.7–2.3	4–13
Procainamide		16 hours	3–10	10–35
Quinidine		24 hours	3–6	10–18
Sotalol		48 hours	1.0–3.0	3.2–9.7
Anticonvulsants				
Carbamazepine	Prior to next dose	6 days	6–12	25–50
Clonazepam[4]		5 days	0.025–0.075	0.08–0.24
Ethosuximide		8 days	50–100	300–700
Phenytoin		5–7 days	10–20	40–80
Valproate[4]		40 hours	50–100	300–600

Contd...

Contd...

Drugs	Sampling time(s) (micro-mole/L)[3]	Time to reach steady state[1]	Therapeutic plasma concentration range (mg/L)[2]	
			Minimum	Maximum
Antidepressants				
Amitriptyline	Prior to next dose	3 days		
Imipramine		2 days	Varies if metabolites are measured; discuss with laboratory	
Nortriptyline		5 days		
Others				
Digoxin	6–8 hours after morning dose (nanomol/L)	7 days	1–2.5 (mg/L)	1.3–3.2
Lithium (mmol/L)	12 hours after last dose	3–4 days		0.8–1
Salicylate (mmol/L)	Prior to next dose	2–5 days	150–250	1–2
Theophylline		36 hours	10–20	55–110
Cyclosporin		2 days	Varies with method	

[1] Time (after starting drug or changing dose) to reach steady state during normal therapeutic use of the drug (given at usual dose intervals).
[2] Unless specified otherwise.
[3] Although the half-life of amiodarone is up to 10 weeks in some patients, the measured plasma concentration appears to reach a relatively constant value by 1 month.
[4] Therapeutic plasma concentration ranges for clonazepam and valproate are very approximate.

Chapter 4

Certain Golden Rules of Safe Pediatric Drug Therapy

INTRODUCTION

Appropriate drug administration, especially pertaining to drug safety, plays a pivotal role in child's health and well-being. In this behalf, it is imperative that certain well-meaning rules are not only respected but also followed:

- Remember the seven "Rights" of safe drug therapy: right child, right drug, right dose, right time, right route, and right documentation.
- Make sure not to overprescribe, keeping the number of drugs to the minimum.
- Aim at employing once or twice daily administration as far as possible.
- Never allow more than two intravenous infusion lines running at a time unless, of course, it becomes absolutely essential in very critically-sick subjects. In the latter situation, label each IV line with the drug running through it.
- Ensure recording the amount of fluid administered by every syringe pump by inspecting the movement of the syringe and the administration site every hour or so.
- Avoid changing the IV fluid regimen beyond twice a day.

Chapter 4: Certain Golden Rules of Safe Pediatric Drug Therapy

- Avoid flushing drugs or fluid through an established IV line with a temporary charge of the setting of the infusion pump.
- Never put more than double the amount of the drug in the syringe meant for injection.
- Employ an extra precaution against giving excess sodium to the neonate.
- In neonates, in particular, administration of potentially lethal drugs like digoxin or chloramphenicol should be avoided.
- Consider therapeutic drug monitoring as and when outcome of a drug is not on expected lines notwithstanding right drug for the particular indication, right dose, and right-dosing interval.

Section 2

General and Systemic Medications

5. Analgesics/Antipyretics/Nonsteroidal Anti-inflammatory Drugs
6. Antacids
7. Anti-acne Drugs
8. Antiasthma Drugs/Bronchodilators
9. Anticancer (Antineoplastic) Drugs
10. Anticoagulants
11. Anticonvulsants
12. Antidiarrheals
13. Antiemetics
14. Antifibrillatory Drugs
15. Antihistaminic Drugs

16. Antihypertensive Drugs
17. Antimyasthenic Drugs
18. Antireflux Drugs
19. Antipsychotic Drugs
20. Antispasmodics/Antiflatulence Drugs
21. Antitoxins
22. Antitussives and Cough Expectorants
23. Cardiotonic Drugs
24. Chelating Agents
25. Colony-stimulating Factors
26. Diuretics
27. Drugs for Attention-deficit Hyperactivity Disorder
28. Drugs for Apnea of Prematurity
29. Drugs for Bleeding Control
30. Drugs for Endocrine Disorders/Hormones/Enzymes
31. Drugs for Gout
32. Drugs for Vertigo
33. Hematinics
34. Immunoglobulins
35. Macrominerals
36. Micronutrients
37. Muscle Relaxants
38. Nasal Decongestants
39. Nutritional Supplements
40. Plasma Volume Expanders
41. Stool Softeners/Laxatives
42. Vasodilators
43. Vitamins

Chapter 5

Analgesics/Antipyretics/Nonsteroidal Anti-inflammatory Drugs

INTRODUCTION

Analgesics (painkillers) are drugs employed for achieving analgesia, i.e., relief from pain. Analgesics act in various ways on the peripheral and central nervous systems (CNS). Analgesics include paracetamol (acetaminophen), the nonsteroidal anti-inflammatory drugs (NSAIDs) such as the salicylates, ibuprofen, mefenamic acid, diclofenac sodium, etc. NSAIDs usually have anti-inflammatory action as well. Opioid drugs include morphine, codeine, etc. Severity and response to other medication and type of pain determines the choice of agent.

Acetaminophen (Paracetamol)

Brand names: Calpol, Crocin, Fibrinil, Metacin, Pyrigesic, and Tylenol

- *Available as:* Tablet 500 mg, 650 mg; Syrup 120 mg, 250 mg/5 mL; Drops 100 mg/dropperful (1 mL); Suppository 80 mg, 170 mg; Injection 150 mg/mL (Fibrinil).
  - *Fixed dose combination:* Calpol-T (paracetamol 325 mg + tramadol 7.5 mg). Combiflam (paracetamol 325 + ibuprofen 400 mg).

- *Indications:* Analgesic, antipyretic; anti-inflammatory action very mild.
- *Dose:*
  - 15 mg/kg/dose (PO); 25–50 mg/kg/day in four divided doses
  - 10–20 mg/kg/dose (R)
  - 5–7.5 mg/kg/dose [intramuscular (IM), intravenous (IV)] bolus in 15 minutes. IV paracetamol should be reserved for 15 minutes or only situations in which oral administration is not workable. Efficacy wise, it has no significant advantage over oral administration.
- *Adverse drug reactions (ADRs):* Infrequent, except for gastrointestinal (GI) upset; hypersensitivity reactions (skin rash), drowsiness, headache, hyperventilation, renal stone, methemoglobinemia, hemolysis, fever, neutropenia, and jaundice.
- *Caution:* Avoid in renal or hepatic impairment. Overdose may cause reversible icterus. Massive overdose produces a toxic metabolite which may lead to hepatic necrosis.

Acetylsalicylic Acid

Brand names: Aspirin, Delisprin, Disprin, Ecosprin, Micropyrin, Mejoral, and Zosprin

- *Available as:* Tablets 350 mg, 150 mg, 100 mg, and 75 mg.
- *Indications:* Analgesic, antipyretic, and anti-inflammatory.
- *Dose:*
  - 30–65 mg/kg/day (PO) in four to six divided doses as antipyretic; 65 mg/year of age/dose (PO) as analgesic.
  - 65–130 mg/kg/day (PO) in four divided doses for rheumatic fever (the initial dose should be toward the upper limit of the range).

Chapter 5: Analgesics/Antipyretics/Nonsteroidal Anti-inflammatory Drugs

- 30–60 mg/kg/day q 8 hours usually for the febrile period (often up to 2 weeks) for Kawasaki disease. Then the dose is reduced to 3–5 mg/kg once a day for 6–8 weeks.
- *Adverse drug reactions:* Deep and rapid respiration (air hunger), gastric irritation, hyperacidity, pain abdomen, nausea, vomiting, tinnitus, fever, cyanosis, pharyngo-conjunctival fever (PCF), twitching, convulsions, rigidity, coma, Reye syndrome (especially in children with chickenpox or other exanthemata).
- *Caution:* Avoid the drug on empty stomach and in children under 12 years, especially in viral exanthemata such as chickenpox, influenza, bleeding disorder, liver failure, erosive gastritis, and asthma.

In the event of development of tinnitus or hearing loss, it should be discontinued.

Auranofin

It is a gold complex, having pediatric use limited to adolescents.

Brand names: Goldar and Ridaura

- *Available as:* Tablet and capsule 3 mg.
- *Indications:* Rheumatoid arthritis and psoriatic arthritis.
- *Dose:* 0.1 mg/kg/day (PO) q 12 hours. Subsequently, this may be increased to 0.15 (maximum 0.2 mg/kg/day).
- *Adverse drug reactions:* Nausea, vomiting, diarrhea, pruritus, skin rash, and stomatitis.
- *Contraindications:* Bleeding disorder, congestive heart failure, systemic lupus erythematosus (SLE).
- *Caution:* Medication needs to be discontinued in case of fall of total leukocyte count (TLC) <4,000 mm^3 or platelet count <100,000 mm^3.

Codeine

It is a narcotic analgesic and cough suppressant.

Brand names: Codeine linctus, Codokuff, Lincotuss, and Phensedyl
- *Available as:* Syrup 10 or 15 mg/5 mL.
- *Indications:* Narcotic analgesic; also cough suppressant.
- *Dose:* 3 mg/kg/day for sedation or pain. 1–1.5 mg/kg/day in 4–6 divided doses for suppression of cough.
- *Adverse drug reactions:* Constipation, nausea, vomiting, anorexia, dizziness, sedation, excitement, convulsions, depression, and coma; addiction.
- *Contraindications:* Asthma, high intracranial pressure (ICP).

DEXTROPROPOXYPHENE HYDROCHLORIDE

Brand name: Proxyvon
- *Indications:* Moderate to severe pain.
- *Available as:* 65 mg in combination with other analgesics, such as paracetamol and ibuprofen.
- *Dose:* 2–4 mg/kg/day in two divided doses.
- *Adverse drug reactions:* Central nervous system (CNS) depression, nausea, vomiting, and mild addiction.
- *Contraindications:* Hepatic insufficiency.
- *Caution:* Avoid in infants, with alcohol and in pregnancy.

Diclofenac Sodium

Brand names: Voveran and Diclomax
- An aryl acetic acid derivative
- *Available as:*
  - Tablets 25 and 50 mg
  - Injection 25 mg/mL
  - Topical gel and transdermal patch

Chapter 5: Analgesics/Antipyretics/Nonsteroidal Anti-inflammatory Drugs

- *Indications:* As a strong anti-inflammatory analgesic, juvenile idiopathic arthritis.
- *Dose:* 25–50 mg/day in two divided doses. 2–3 mg/kg/day q 4 hours.
- *Adverse drug reactions:* GI upset and neurologic manifestations.
- *Contraindications:* Peptic ulcer, gastrointestinal bleeding, and aspirin-induced allergies.
- *Caution:* Avoid in dyspepsia, gastrointestinal disorders, liver disease, renal disease, congestive heart failure, blood coagulation disorders, dehydration, and fluid retention.

Fentanyl Citrate

A potent narcotic analgesic that binds to opium receptors; its 0.1 mg = 10 mg of morphine.

Brand names: Durasegic and Sublimaze

- *Available as:* Lozenges; transdermal (not yet in India); Injection (IV and IM).
- *Indications:* Narcotic analgesia; preoperative medication.
- *Dose:* For neonates/infants: 1–4 µg/kg/dose, may repeat q 2–4 hours; continuous infusion 0.5–5 µg/kg/h.
  - *Children:* 1–3 µg/kg/dose, may repeat every 30–60 minutes; continuous infusion 1–5 µg/kg/h.
- *Adverse drug reactions:* Nausea, vomiting, constipation, respiratory depression, CNS depression, hypotension, bradycardia, and urinary tract/biliary tract spasm.
- *Caution:* In case of infusion, be slow. Else, skeletal muscle and chest wall rigidity may cause poor ventilation and respiratory distress.

Ibuprofen

Brand names: Brufen, Ibugesic, Ibucon, Ibusynth, and Ibutab

- *Available as:* Tablets 200 mg, 400 mg, 600 mg; suspension 100 mg/5 mL.
  - Fixed dose combinations with paracetamol.
- *Indications:* As a strong anti-inflammatory, analgesic and anti-pyretic agent in rheumatic and nonrheumatic conditions. Also indicated in cystic fibrosis as high-dose long-term therapy and patent ductus arteriosus (PDA).
- *Dose:* 5–10 mg/kg/dose (PO) every 6–8 hours as antipyretic and analgesic. For juvenile idiopathic arthritis (JIA), 30–70 mg/kg/day every 4–6 hours.
  - For PDA 10 mg/kg (IV) stat; then 5 mg/kg (IV and PO) every 24 hours × 2 days.
  - For cystic fibrosis 20–30 mg/kg (PO).
- *Adverse drug reactions:* Gastrointestinal intolerance/bleeding, dyspepsia rash, and thrombocytopenia.
- *Contraindications:* Peptic ulcer, aspirin-induced allergy, and bronchial asthma.
- *Caution:* Avoid in subjects on anticoagulant and/or thiazide therapy.

Indomethacin

It is an indole derivative.

Brand names: Indocap, Indocin, and Indomethacin

- *Available as:*
  - *Capsule:* 25 mg, 50 mg, and 75 mg
  - *Injection:* 1 mg/vial
- *Indications:* As anti-inflammatory analgesic; in patent ductus arteriosus in preterms.

- *Dose:*
  - *For analgesis:* 3 mg/kg/day (PO) as analgesic in three divided doses. 0.2 mg/kg/dose (IV and PO) every 8 hours for three doses.
  - *For ductus closure:* 0.2 mg/kg/dose (IV) TDS × 3 days.
- *Adverse drugs reactions:* Nausea, vomiting, epigastric pain, gastrointestinal bleeding, icterus, headache, light headedness, leukopenia, thrombocytopenia, aplastic anemia, tinnitus, rash, pruritus, blurred vision, corneal deposits, and retinal disturbances.
- *Contraindications:* Gastrointestinal bleeding, peptic ulcer, aspirin-induced allergy/asthma.
- *Caution:* Avoid in psychiatric disorders, epilepsy, along with anticoagulant therapy.

Mefenamic Acid

It is an anthranilic acid derivative.

Brand names: Meftal and Ponstan

- *Available as:* Capsule 250 mg, 500 mg; Tablets 125 mg; Syrup 125 mg/5 mL.
- *Indications:* For relief of pain and as an antipyretic.
- *Dose:* 8 mg/kg/dose (PO); 20–25 mg/kg/day (PO) in three divided doses.
- *Adverse drug reactions:* Nausea, vomiting, diarrhea, dyspepsia, abdominal discomfort, rash, hemolysis, and leukopenia.
- *Caution:* Discontinue the medication in case of blood in vomitus or stools.

Morphine Sulfate

It is a powerful narcotic analgesic.

- *Available as:* Tablet 60 mg, 100 mg; Injection 60 mg.
- *Indications:* Severe pain; myocardial infarction.
- *Dose:* 0.1–0.2 mg/kg/dose (SC, IM, and IV).
- *Adverse drug reactions:* Nausea, vomiting, gross CNS depression, coma, miosis, cyanosis, tremors, convulsions, and slow and shallow respiration.
- *Caution:* In the event of respiratory depression, the specific antidote (naloxone), which should always be kept ready, needs to be administered. It is administered 0.1 mg/kg with a maximum of 2 mg (IV). If need be, a repeat shot may be given after 2–3 minutes.

Nimesulide

Brand names: Nimulid, Nise, Nimeril, Nimfast, and Zolandin

- *Available as:* Tablet 50 mg, 100 mg; Syrup 50 mg/5 mL.
- *Indications:* A NSAID, also useful as an antipyretic and analgesic agent.
- *Dose:* 5 mg/kg/day (PO) in two or three divided doses.
- *Adverse drug reactions:* Nausea, vomiting, diarrhea, heartburn, headache, rash, pruritus, dizziness, somnolence, and hepatic dysfunction (even acute hepatic failure). Moderate renal insufficiency.
- *Drug interaction:* Furosemide, valproic acid, methotrexate, and tolbutamide.
- *Contraindications:* Active peptic ulcer, moderate to severe hepatic insufficiency.
- *Caution:* In view of reported instances of acute liver failure as one of its adverse effects, routine use of nimesulide (especially in situations where a safer analgesic can be employed) should be discouraged.

Naproxen

Brand names: Artagen, Naxid, Naprosyn, and Nalyxan
- *Indications:* As a strong analgesic; juvenile rheumatoid arthritis (JRA).
- *Available as:* Tablets 250 and 500 mg.
- *Dose:* 10–20 mg/kg/day (PO) in two divided doses (higher dose is for JRA).
- *Adverse drug reactions:* Rash, constipation, tinnitus, headache, and drowsiness.
- *Contraindications:* Active peptic ulcer, aspirin allergy, NSAID allergy, and advanced renal insufficiency.
- *Caution:* Avoid in gastrointestinal lesions and in infants <6 months. Avoid concomitant administration of hydantoin and other anticonvulsants and anticoagulants.

Paracetamol

See acetaminophen.

Pentazocine HCl

Brand name: Fortwin
- *Available as:* Tablet 25 mg; Injection 30 mg/mL.
- *Indications:* A strong analgesic, only one-third to one-sixth as powerful as morphine and slightly more powerful than codeine.
- *Dose:* 0.5–1.0 mg/kg/day (PO, IM, and IV) q 4 hours.
- *Adverse drug reactions:* Nausea, vomiting, bloating, flushing, and vertigo.
- *Contraindications:* Head injury, respiratory depression, respiratory inductance plethysmography (RIP), and porphyria.

Pethidine Hydrochloride

A powerful narcotic (opioid) analgesic of the phenylpiperidine class.

Brand names: Demerol and Meperidine
- *Available as:* Injection 50–100 mg/mL.
- *Indications:* Severe pain, preoperative sedation, and adjunct to anesthesia.
- *Dose:*
  - 1–2 mg/kg/dose (IM and IV). May repeat q 3–4 hours in case of severe, persistent pain.
  - IV administration of the diluted drug (1–10 mg/mL) needs to be slow over 15–30 minutes time span.
- *Adverse drug reaction:* Nausea, vomiting, sedation, dizziness, diaphoresis, urinary retention, constipation; addiction.
- *Caution:* High ICP and head injury.

Piroxicam

Brand names: Dolonex, Piricam, and Pirox
- *Indications:* Juvenile idiopathic arthritis (JIA).
- *Dose:*
  - <15 kg 5 mg OD
  - 15–25 kg 10 mg OD
  - 26–45 kg 15 mg OD
  - 45 kg 20 mg OD.
- *Adverse drug reactions:* Nausea, anorexia, rash, pruritus, heartburn, edema, and CNS manifestations.
- *Contraindications:* Active peptic ulcer, aspirin, and other NSAID allergy.

Rofecoxib

A Cox-2 inhibitor that has less gastrointestinal side-effects and that does not inhibit platelet aggregation.

Brand names: Rodif, Rofetab, Roff, and Rofiz
- *Available as:* Tablets 12.5 mg, 25 mg, 50 mg
- *Indications:* Rheumatoid arthritis
- *Dose:* 25–650 mg/day OD or in two divided doses
- *Adverse drug reactions:* Cardiovascular adverse effects
- *Caution:* Best avoided in children.

Tolmetin

Brand names: Brexic, Minicam, Paricam, and Tolectin
- *Indications:* Juvenile idiopathic arthritis (JIA)
- *Available as:* Tablet 200 mg, 600 mg; Capsule 400 mg
- *Dose:* 5–10 mg/kg/dose 3–4 times a day.
- *Adverse drug reactions:* Gastrointestinal upset (including hematemesis and blood in stools), hives; difficulty breathing; edema of face, lips, tongue, or throat; worsening of preexisting heart illness.
- *Contraindications:* Bleeding disorder and renal failure
- *Caution:* Avoid in <2-year-old children.

Tramadol

It is a powerful analgesic acting on opiate receptors without respiratory depression.

Brand name: Trammgazac
- *Available as:* Tablet 50 mg, 100 mg; Injection 50 mg/mL.
- *Indications:* Severe pain.
- *Dose:* 50–100 mg q 8 hours (PO, IM, and IV).
- *Caution:* Avoid in <14-year-old children.

Chapter 6

Antacids

INTRODUCTION

Antacids are agents that neutralize or counter the acidity in the stomach. Ingredients like aluminum or magnesium act as bases (alkalis) to neutralize the stomach acid, thereby lowering the pH. Their action is quick though not sustained in relieving the symptoms of acid reflux as in gastroesophageal reflux disease (GERD), heartburn or indigestion (dyspepsia). Most proprietary brands contain both magnesium hydroxide and aluminum hydroxide that have laxative and constipating side effects, respectively. Antacid use should be only temporary. Prolonged use may cause kidney dysfunction.

Antisecretory drugs like proton pump inhibitors (PPIs), e.g., omeprazole, pantoprazole, etc., are good for achieving long-standing antacid effect, especially in subjects with GERD. Also effective in handling stomach acid are histamine-2 antagonists.

ANTACIDS

Aluminum Hydroxide

Brand names: Aludrox and Mucaine gel

- *Available as:* Tablet 840 mg; Gel 350 mg/5 mL. It is usually available in combination with magnesium hydroxide.
- *Indications:* Acute gastritis, stomach acidity, and GERD

- It is usually available in combination with magnesium hydroxide.
- *Dose:* 20–50 mg/kg/day in 4–5 divided doses, preferably 15 minutes before meal.
- *Adverse drug reactions:* Constipation, encephalopathy when administered to subjects with uremia because of aluminum deposits formed in the brain.
- *Caution:* Avoid in uremic patients. Prolonged treatment should be discouraged.

Magnesium Hydroxide

It is an antacid with a laxative property.
Brand names: Milk of Magnesia and Pedia-Lax
- *Available as:* Chewable tablet and liquid suspension
  - Usually available in combination with aluminum hydroxide
- *Indication:* Acute gastritis and constipation
- *Dose:* As in case of aluminum hydroxide
- *Drug interaction:* Antibiotics, lactulose, and phenytoin.

ALLIED DRUGS

Histamine-2 antagonist drugs and proton-pump inhibitors tackle acidity in stomach in a different way. For details, *see* **Chapter 18: Antireflux Drugs**.

Chapter 7

Anti-acne Drugs

INTRODUCTION

Acne is a common skin disorder, especially in adolescents. It is characterized by red pimples on the skin, more so on the face, due to inflamed or infected sebaceous glands. Main cause is thought to be a rise in androgen levels during puberty.

Left untreated, acne may cause cosmetic issues in the shape of pits and scar.

ADAPALENE

Brand names: Aclene, Adapen, and Adaple

- *Available as:* Gel 0.1%
- *Dose:* To be applied to face after it has been washed and dried up.
- *Caution:* Avoid sunlight exposure.

AZELAIC ACID

Brand name: Azderm

- *Available as:* Cream 10% and 20%.
- *Dose:* To be applied to the face after it has been washed and dried up. In the first week, a single application a day suffices. Later it should be twice daily.
- *Caution:* Avoid contact with lips and eyes and use beyond 6 months.

BENZOYL PEROXIDE

Brand names: Benzac AC, Pernox, and Persol

- *Available as:* Gel 2.5%
- *Dose:* To be applied to face after it has been washed and dried up once or twice daily.
- *Adverse drug reactions:* Erythema and peeling of skin.
- *Caution:* Start with small amount and less frequency to enable its tolerance by the affected skin.

TRETINOIN

Brand name: Retino-A

- *Available as:* Cream 0.025%, 0.05%, and 0.1% (for fair and dry skin); Gel 0.05% (for dark and oily skin).
- *Dose:* To be applied to face after it has been washed and dried up once or twice daily.
- *Caution:* Avoid sunlight exposure and contact with eyes, lips, and nostrils.

Chapter 8

Antiasthma Drugs/Bronchodilators

INTRODUCTION

Asthma is a hyper-reactivity of the airways to intrinsic or extrinsic factors, resulting in bronchoconstriction (bronchospasm), and shortness of breath and cough. Mucosal inflammation, causing edema and exudates in the airway invariably accompanies it. Asthma triggers include:

- Smoke, especially cigarette and tobacco smoke
- Dust, especially the mites, pollen, mild and detergents in house dust.
- Pollutants in air, airconditioner backlash
- *Pests*: Cockroaches and rats
- *Pets*: Dogs, cats, and mice
- Mold
- *Miscellaneous*: various allergies, exercise, respiratory infection, emotional outburst, changing weather, exposure to chill, throat irritants such as spicy and sore foodstuffs, preservatives in foodstuffs, dried fruits, and vegetables, onion, garlic, and carbonated drinks.

Antiasthmatic drugs, therefore, largely target bronchospasm and inflammation. Bronchodilators (salbutamol, levosalbutamol, and terbutaline) relax the muscles around the airway. Anti-inflammatory drugs (steroids) such as prednisolone, methylprednisolone, budesonide, fluticasone, beclomethasone, and mometasone reduce edema and mucous production in the airway. Additionally, biologic therapy may be indicated in cases with persistence of the manifestations in spite of use of bronchodilators and anti-inflammatory therapy, including inhaler. Inhalation therapy using nebulizer or inhaler is far superior.

ORAL/INJECTABLE DRUGS
Adrenaline (Epinephrine)

It is a sympathomimetic agent.
- *Available as:* 1 in 1,000 aqueous solution, 1 mg/mL.
- *Indications:* Bronchial asthma. Also, cardiac arrest, cardiac asthma, severe bradycardia, anaphylaxis, croup, and laryngeal edema.
- *Dose*: For relief of bronchospasm, 0.01 mL/kg/dose [intramuscular (IM), subcutaneous (SC)] with a maximum of 0.5 mL/dose. Repeat every 10–20 minutes for three or four times, if needed.
- *Adverse drug reactions (ADRs):* Nausea, vomiting, anxiety, restlessness, tachycardia, angina, hypertension, tremors, cold extremities, and gangrene.
- *Precaution:* Avoid its use in nervous or anxious patients, or those having hypertension, hyperthyroidism, ischemic heart disease, or in conjunction with trichloroethylene, halothane, cyclopropane, or monoamine oxidase inhibitors.

Aminophylline

Indications: Bronchodilator and neonatal apnea
- *Available as:* Tablets 100 mg, 200 mg; Injection 25 mg/mL

- *Dose:* 4–6 mg/kg/dose (IM and IV); 12 mg/kg/day (IM and IV) in three or four divided doses; 10 mg/kg/dose (PO) to be repeated every 6–8 hours.
  - An alternative and better method for controlling the acute attack of bronchial asthma consists in giving 4–6 mg/kg of aminophylline in over 15 minutes as an intravenous infusion. Then, continue giving 0.6–1 mL/kg every hour as a constant infusion.
  - For apneic attacks in newborn, the dose is 4–6 mg/kg/day (PO) in four divided doses.
- *Adverse drug reactions (ADRs):* Restlessness, palpitation, dizziness, nausea, hypotension, shock, cardiac arrest, sudden death (usually secondary to very rapid injection).
- *Caution:* Electrocardiography (ECG) monitoring desirable.

Bambuterol Hydrochloride

It is a terbutaline prodrug; long-acting β agonist.
Brand names: Asthafree, Bambudil, and Betaday

- *Available as:* Tablet 10 mg, 20 mg; Syrup 5 mg/mL, 10 mg/mL.
- *Indications:* Long-term treatment of persistent asthma
- *Dose:* 2–5 years; 5 mg at night; 6–12 years; 10 mg at night; >12 years 10–20 mg at night.
- *Adverse drug reactions:* Headache, fatigue, nausea, and tremors.
- *Contraindications:* Pregnancy and liver disease.
- *Caution:* Avoid <2 years and as a rescue therapy in acute asthma. Dose adjustment needed renal impairment.

Doxofylline

It is a new generation long-acting methylxanthine derivative.
Brand names: Asmadox, Doxiflo, and Freefil

- *Available as:* Tablet 400 mg; Syrup 100 mg/5 mL
- *Indication:* Asthma
- *Dose:* 6 mg/kg/dose twice a day
- *Adverse drug reactions:* Nausea, vomiting, epigastric pain, palpitations, headache, and insomnia
- *Caution:* Avoid <6 years.

Levosalbutamol

This levo version of salbutamol is twice more potent than salbutamol.

Brand name: Levolin

- *Available as:* Tablet 1 mg, 2 mg; Syrup 0.5 mg/5 mL, 1 mg/5 mL
- *Dose:* 0.5–2 mg/kg/dose q8–12 hours
- *Adverse drug reactions:* Fine tremors (most remarkable in hands) tachycardia, headache, tenseness, and arrhythmias.

Mometasone Sodium

Brand names: Furomet, Metasafe, and Metatop

- *Available as:* 50 mg/dose
- *Indications:* Asthma, allergic rhinitis, and nasal polyp.
- *Dose:*
  - *Less than 6 years:* One spray in each nostril once a day.
  - *More than 6 years:* Two sprays in each nostril once a day.
- *Adverse drug reactions:* Quite safe. Infrequently, hypersensitivity reactions. Rarely, cataract and glaucoma. Montelukast.

A singular leukotriene receptor blocker, employed as an "add-on" therapy in moderate asthma (chronic/recurrent); allergic rhinitis.

Montelukast

Brand names: Montair, Romilast, Telekast, and Ventair

- *Indications:* For prevention and treatment of chronic/recurrent/persistent bronchial asthma; also in nasobronchial allergy.
- *Available as:* Tablets 4, 5, 10 mg; Syrup 4 mg/5 mL
  - Montelukast 5 mg + bambuterol 5 mg (Romilast B5)
  - Montelukast 10 mg + bambuterol 10 mg (Romilast B10, Telekast plus)
- *Dose:*
  - *2–5 years:* 4 mg (PO) OD in the evening (preferably bedtime).
  - *6–14 years:* 5 mg (PO) OD in the evening (preferably bedtime).
  - *15 years and above:* 10 mg (PO) OD in the evening (preferably bedtime).
- *Drug interactions:* Phenobarbital, phenytoin, rifampicin, drugs metabolized by CYP2C8 such as rosiglitazone.
- *Adverse drug reactions:* Headache, dizziness, dyspepsia, fatigue, and raised liver enzymes.
- *Contraindication:* Pregnancy
- *Caution:* For the best outcome, it should be administered in the evening. Do not employ as a substitute for oral or inhaled steroid therapy.

Magnesium Sulfate

- *Available as:* Injection 1%, 10%, 25%, 50%, 1 mL ampule.
- *Indications:* Acute severe asthma; also, acute severe malnutrition.
- *Dose:* 25 mg/kg IV infusion in about 30 minutes
- *Adverse drug reactions:* Hypermagnesemia, hypotension, respiratory depression, and diarrhea.

- *Contraindications:* Severe renal impairment, heart block, and myocardial disease.
- *Cautions:* Renal insufficiency, concurrent therapy with digoxin.
- *Antidote:* Intravenous calcium gluconate.

Orciprenaline Sulfate

Brand name: Alupent

- *Available as:* Injection 1 mL containing 0.5 mg, 1 mg; Syrup 2 mg/mL; Tablet 10 mg and 20 mg.
- *Indication:* Bronchial asthma
- *Dose:* 0.02 mg/kg/dose (IM), 2–3 mg/kg/day (PO) in four divided doses.
- *Adverse drug reactions:* Palpitations, restlessness, finger tremors, nausea, sleep disturbances, headache, flushing, allergic reactions, and extra systoles.
- *Caution:* Avoid concurrent use of sympathomimetics or monoamine oxidase (MAO) inhibitors.
- *Contraindication:* Thyrotoxicosis.
- *Antidote:* A β-blocker agent.

Salbutamol

Brand names: Asthalin, Bronkotab, Bronkosyrup, Brethmol, and Salbetol

- *Indications:* Bronchial asthma; other lung conditions accompanied by significant bronchospasm.
- *Available as:* Tablet 2 mg, 4 mg; Syrup 2 mg/5 mL.
- *Dose:* 0.1–0.4 mg/kg/dose q 8 hours
- *Adverse drug reactions:* Fine tremors (most remarkable in hands), tachycardia, headache, muscle cramps, tenseness, and arrhythmias.

Terbutaline Sulfate

Brand names: Bricanyl and Bronkine
- *Available as:* Tablet 2.5 mg, 5 mg; Suspension 1.5 mg/5 mL; and Injection (SC) 0.5 mg/mL
- *Indications:* Bronchospasm as in bronchial asthma
- *Dose:* 0.2 mg/kg/day (PO), 0.005 mg/kg/dose (SC). Intravenous infusion may be given in difficult cases.
- *Adverse drug reactions:* Nervousness, muscle tremors, headache, muscle cramps, tachycardia, palpitation, drowsiness, nausea, vomiting, and sweating. These side effects are usually mild, their frequency reducing with continued therapy. No or little cardiac side effects since it has selective action on β-2 receptors in bronchial muscles and relatively slight effect on β-1 receptors in the heart.
- *Contraindications:* Thyrotoxicosis, known hypersensitivity to sympathomimetic amines, arrhythmias.
- *Caution:* As with all sympathomimetic stimulants, it should be used with special caution in patients with hypertension, coronary artery disease, congestive cardiac failure (CCF), hyperthyroidism or diabetes mellitus.

Theophylline

Brand names: Etophylate, Broncordil, and Deriphyllin
- *Available as:* Tablet 100 mg, 200 mg; elixir 30 mg, 125 mg/5 mL; Injection 110 mg/mL
- *Indications:* Bronchospasm and apnea of prematurity
- *Dose:* 10–20 mg/kg/day (PO) in two to three divided doses; 5 mg/kg/dose (IM, IV, and SC)
- *Adverse drug reactions:* Gastrointestinal tract upset, hypotension, cardiovascular collapse, increased gastric and urine excretion, irritability, tremors, and convulsions.

- *Caution:* Reduce dose by 50% in viral illness, high fever (>102°F), cor pulmonale, concurrent administration of drugs such as macrolides, quinolones, cimetidine, verapamil, and ibuprofen.

Zafirlukast

Brand name: Zuvair
- *Available as:* Tablet 10 mg, 20 mg.
- *Indications:* Add-on therapy in persistent asthma showing poor response to conventional therapy; asthma prophylaxis.
- *Dose:* 10–20 mg BD.
- *Adverse drug reactions:* Headache, dizziness, gastrointestinal upset, dyspepsia, fatigue; raised liver enzymes.
- *Drug interactions:* Warfarin, theophylline, aspirin, erythromycin, and smoking.
- *Contraindication:* Pregnancy, lactation, hepatic/renal impairment.
- *Caution:* Administer on empty stomach. Avoid in <12 years children.

INHALATION THERAPY

Beclomethasone Dipropionate

Brand names: Beclate Inhaler and Beclate Nasal Spray
- *Indications:* Persistent asthma; also, allergic and vasomotor rhinitis, and nasal polyposis (sheer symptomatic).
- *Dose:* Metered-dose inhaler.
  - *Mild asthma:* 200–400 mg/day in 2–4 divided doses.
  - *Moderate asthma:* 400–800 mg/day in 2–4 divided doses.
  - *Severe asthma:* 800–1,000 mg/day in 2–4 divided doses.

- Inhalation therapy needs to be continued for 10–12 weeks.
- *Nasal spray:* 50 mg dose of spray once daily or twice daily.
- *Adverse drug reactions:* Hoarseness, superadded fungus infection (candidiasis) involving mouth, and throat.
- *Caution:* Mouth and throat wash after every inhalation/spray.

Budesonide

Brand name: Pulmicort inhaler
- *Available as:* Inhaler
- *Indications:* Persistent asthma, also croup.
- *Dose:*
  - *Mild asthma:* 100–400 mg/day in two divided doses.
  - *Moderate asthma:* 400–600 mg/day in two divided doses.
  - *Severe asthma:* 600–800 mg/day in two divided doses.

Cromoglycate Disodium

Brand names: Cremolyn, Ifiral, and Intal.
- *Available as:* Rotacap 20 mg
- *Indication:* Prophylaxis of acute asthmatic attack. It reduces airway hyperactivity and inhibits mast cell degranulation (blocking mediator release).
- *Dose:* Inhalation of 1 rotacap thrice daily for 4–6 weeks. Repeat course after 3–6 months.
- *Adverse drug reactions:* Transient bronchospasm
- *Caution:* Avoid in children below 5 years.

Keep a specific bronchodilator injection handy for use in the event of bronchospasm developing as a side effect of cromoglycate.

Ipratropium Bromide

Brand name: Duolin metered-dose inhaler.
- *Available as:* Ipravent respirator solution for nebulization.
- *Dose:* 1–2 puffs thrice daily.
  - *For nebulization:* 250 mg, diluted in 2 mL saline, administered over 10 minutes every 20 minutes × 3 doses. This should be followed by 250 mg nebulization over 2–4 hours.

Fluticasone Propionate

Brand names: Flohale MDI and Flohale rotacaps.
- *Indication:* Persistent asthma.
- *Available as:* Inhaler 25 mg, 50 mg, 125 mg/dose (Flohale MDI)
  100 mg, and 250 mg/dose
  Also, available in combination with salmeterol.
- *Dose:*
  - *Mild persistent asthma*: 50–100 mg/dose in two divided doses.
  - *Moderate persistent asthma*: 100–200 mg/day in two divided doses.
  - *Severe persistent asthma*: 200–500 mg/dose (flohale rotacaps).
- *Adverse drug reactions:* Stuffy nose, sneezing, sore throat; low fever, cough, wheezing, chest tightness; hoarseness or deepened voice; white patches or sores inside mouth or on lips; headache; or nausea, vomiting, and gastrointestinal upset.
- *Caution:* Inhaler hygiene and maintenance.

Formoterol

It is a long-acting β-2 agonist.
Brand names: Foracort inhaler and Foracort rotacap.
- *Available as:* 6 mg/dose (along with budesonide 100 mg, 200 mg or 400 mg/dose)
- *Indications:* When one long-term therapy (say, inhaled corticosteroids) does not control breathing problems or when more than one long-term medication is clearly needed to control breathing problems.
- *Dose:* 12 mg/dose
- *Adverse drug reactions:* Stuffy nose, sneezing, sore throat; low fever, cough, wheezing, chest tightness; hoarseness or deepened voice; white patches or sores inside mouth or on lips; headache; or nausea, vomiting, and gastrointestinal upset.
- *Caution:* Inhaler hygiene.

Salmeterol

It is a β-2 agonist, long-acting bronchodilator meant for use in children >4 years of age.
Brand names: Salmeter, Serobid MDI, and Ventolin.
- *Indications:* Exercise-induced asthma and nocturnal asthma.
- *Dose:* 50–100 mg/day
- *Adverse drug reactions:* Palpitations/tachycardia, headache, and tremors.
- *Caution:* Avoid in children <4 years of age.

Terbutaline

Brand names: Bricanyl MDI, Bricanyl nebulizing solution.

Chapter 8: Antiasthma Drugs/Bronchodilators

- *Available as:* MDI 250 mg/metered dose, and nebulizing solution 10 mg/mL.
- *Dose:* Inhalation: 1–2 puffs three to four times daily.
  - *Nebulization:*
    - Less than 20 kg weight 2.5 mg.
    - More than 20 kg weight 5 mg.

Chapter 9

Anticancer (Antineoplastic) Drugs

INTRODUCTION

Cytotoxic drugs for pediatric cancer have been available since 1950s. Over and above these, we now have a diverse antineoplastic drugs, e.g., small-molecule kinase inhibitors, monoclonal antibodies, and other antibody-based therapies and genetically engineered cell therapy that have emerged as a part of the growing pediatric oncology armamentarium.

Today, quite a few anticancer or antineoplastic drugs are available. Chemotherapy may frequently be in combination with other treatments such as surgery and/or radiation therapy.

BUSULFAN

Brand name: Myleran

- *Available as:* Tablet 2 mg
- *Indications:* Chronic myeloid leukemia (CML), polycythemia vera, myelofibrosis, and essential thrombocythemia.
- *Dose:* 0.06 mg/kg/day (PO) until total leukocyte count (TLC) falls to 20,000/mm.^{3}
- *Adverse drug reactions (ADRs):* Bone marrow depression (especially the myeloid series, sometimes platelets), skin pigmentation, weakness, nausea, hypotension, heart block (third degree), and hyperuricemia.
- *Caution:* Hospitalize the patient during induction therapy.

Chapter 9: Anticancer (Antineoplastic) Drugs

CHLORAMBUCIL

It is a alkylating agent for myeloid elements (granulocyte precursors, platelets, and RBCs).

Brand name: Leukeran

- *Available as:* Tablet 2 mg, 5 mg
- *Indications:* Chronic lymphoblastic leukemia, Hodgkin's disease, and non-Hodgkin's lymphomas.
- *Dose:* 0.1–0.2 mg/kg (PO) as single dose or in divided doses.
- *Adverse drug reactions:* Nausea, vomiting, bone marrow depression, rarely skin rash, hyperpigmentation, fever, cystitis, hepatotoxicity, peripheral neuropathy, seizures; anemia, leukopenia, neutropenia, pancytopenia, thrombocytopenia, hyperuricemia, and pulmonary fibrosis.
- *Drug interactions:* Drugs lowering seizure threshold, myelosuppressives, and phenylbutazone.
- *Contraindications:* Neutropenia, thrombocytopenia, within 4 weeks of radiation or chemotherapy.
- *Caution:* Hematologic monitoring.

CYCLOPHOSPHAMIDE

Brand names: Endoxan-N and Cycloxan

- *Available as:* Tablet 50 mg; Injection 100 mg, 200 mg, and 500 mg.
- *Indications:* Malignancy, nephrotic syndrome not responsive to steroids.
- *Dose:* 2–3 mg/kg/day (PO and IV) or a total of 7 days dose (IV) once in a week. For resistant neoplasm, use 4–8 mg/kg/day. For maintenance, 2–5 mg/kg (PO) twice a week.

- *Adverse drug reactions:* Bone marrow depression, alopecia, gastrointestinal upset, fluid retention, cardiac toxicity, menstrual irregularity, hepatic damage, cystitis, colitis, pigmentation, and thrombocytopenia.
- *Drug interaction:* Barbiturates, digoxin, oral coagulants, myelosuppressive therapy, chloramphenicol, allopurinol, and radiotherapy.
- *Contraindications:* Leukopenia, thrombocytopenia, and bladder hemorrhage.
- *Caution:* Renal and hepatic failure.

DAUNORUBICIN

Brand name: Daunobin

- *Available as:* Vial containing 20 mg lympholized daunorubicin.
- *Indications:* Acute myeloblastic leukemia, alone or in association with other cytotoxic drugs; acute lymphoblastic leukemia (mainly in those subjects refractory to other antileukemic agents); AIDS-related Kaposi's sarcoma.
- *Dose:* A single injection in a dose of 0.5–3 mg/kg (IV). This dose is to be dissolved in 10–20 mL of normal saline and then injected into the tubing of a fast-running intravenous drip infusion of normal saline solution.

Repeat injections are given at 1–2 weeks intervals.

- *Adverse drug reactions:* Flushing, fever, chills, rash, alopecia, skin pigmentation, gastrointestinal upset, abdominal pain, chest tightness, backache, hyperuricemia, immunosuppression, myelosuppression.
- *Drug interaction:* Myelosuppressants (e.g., cyclophosphamide, methotrexate, and doxorubicin); live viral vaccines; heparin; and dexamethasone.

Chapter 9: Anticancer (Antineoplastic) Drugs

- *Contraindications:* Marked myelosuppression (as a result of earlier radiotherapy or cytotoxic therapy; cardiac impairment).
- *Caution:* Hematologic, cardiac, and renal monitoring of the subject on this drug is a must.

DOXORUBICIN

Brand name: Adriamycin
- *Available as:* Injection 10 mg/vial.
- *Indication:* Leukemia.
- *Dose:* 1.2–2.4 mg/kg/dose (IV) every 3 weeks.
- *Adverse drug reactions:* Cardiotoxicity, alopecia, and bone marrow depression.
- *Caution:* Avoid in hepatic or cardiac dysfunction.

L-ASPARAGINASE

Brand name: Leunase
- *Available as:* Injection 10,000 units/vial.
- *Indications:* Acute leukemia and malignant lymphoma.
- *Dose:* 50–200 units/kg/day by IV infusion.
- *Adverse drug reactions:* Hepatic dysfunction, pancreatitis, hyperglycemia, CNS depression (somnolence, confusion, disorientation), renal insufficiency, defect in clotting mechanism, thrombocytopenia, hypersensitivity, fever, chills, respiratory distress, and arthralgia.
- *Drug interaction:* Antitumor agents, vincristine, prednisolone, methotrexate, and thyroid function tests.
- *Contraindication:* Pancreatitis.
- *Caution:* Hypersensitivity.

MELPHALAN

Brand name: Alkeran
- *Available as:* Tablet 2 mg, 5 mg. Injection 100 mg/vial
- *Indications:* Malignancy including multiple myeloma.
- *Dose:* 2–4 mg/day.
- *Adverse drug reactions:* Nausea, vomiting, and bone marrow depression.
- *Contraindications:* Neutropenia, thrombocytopenia, and concurrent radiotherapy.

MERCAPTOPURINE

Brand names: 6-MP, Purinethol
- *Available as:* Tablet 50 mg
- *Indications:* Acute leukemias and chronic granulocytic leukemia.
- *Dose:* 2.5 mg/kg/day.
- *Adverse drug reactions:* Bone marrow depression, nausea, vomiting, diarrhea, jaundice, anorexia, oral and gastrointestinal ulcers, muscular wasting, and lupus (disseminated).
- *Caution:* The dose should be halved when used along with allopurinol.

METHOTREXATE

Brand names: Biotrexate and Neotrexate
- *Available as:* Tablet 2.5 mg; Injection 5 mg, 15 mg, and 50 mg/vial.
- *Indications:* Acute leukemias (lymphoblastic) including CNS prophylaxis, osteogenic sarcoma, choriocarcinoma, and bronchogenic carcinoma.

Chapter 9: Anticancer (Antineoplastic) Drugs

- *Additional indications:* Nephrotic syndrome, severe psoriasis, acute active rheumatoid arthritis refractory to other drugs.
- *Dose:* 0.12 mg/kg/dose (PO), 0.25–0.5 mg/kg/day (IT), 3–5 mg/kg/(IV) as single dose every other week.
- *Adverse drug reactions:* Anorexia, stomatitis, diarrhea, pain abdomen, bone marrow depression, rash (even Stevens–Johnson syndrome), superimposed infections, alopecia, testicular/ovarian dysfunction, menstrual disturbances, alveolitis, interstitial pneumonia, osteoporosis, renal toxicity, and hepatic toxicity.
- *Contraindications:* Preexisting bone marrow depression, leukopenia, thrombocytopenia, severe renal or hepatic dysfunction, immunodeficiency, and lactation.
- *Drug interactions:* Protein-bound drugs, hepatitis A and B vaccines, folic acid, folate antagonists, anticonvulsants, cotrimoxazole, probenecid, lipid-lowering agents, and penicillins.
- *Caution:* Monitor blood, hepatic, renal and pulmonary status before, during and after therapy. Ensure alkaline urine.

MITOMYCIN C

Brand name: Mutamycin

- *Available as:* 2 mg
- *Indications:* Malignancy, especially lymphosarcoma, adenocarcinoma, and seminoma.
- *Dose:* 0.05 mg/kg/day (IV) for 5 days.
- *Adverse drug reactions:* Bone marrow depression, leukopenia, thrombocytopenia, and ulceration of mouth.
- *Contraindications:* Bleeding tendencies and bone marrow depression.
- *Caution:* Local necrosis may occur from leakage.

MUSTINE HYDROCHLORIDE

(A nitrogen mustard)

Brand name: Mustargen

- *Available as:* Injection 10 mg/vial.
- *Indications:* Hodgkin's lymphoma; certain types of chronic leukemias; bronchogenic carcinoma.
- *Dose:* 0.1–0.4 mg/kg/dose (IV) with a maximum of 8 mg for 3–4 days.
- *Adverse drug reactions:* Nausea, vomiting, diarrhea, fever, anorexia, skin rash, alopecia, local thrombosis and thrombophlebitis, and bone marrow depression.
- *Contraindications:* Anemia, severe leukopenia, thrombocytopenia, and infectious granuloma (both coexisting and suspected).
- *Caution:* Never give IM.

VINBLASTINE

Brand name: Cytoblastin

- *Available as:* Dry powder providing 1 mg/mL after reconstruction.
- *Indications:* Leukemias, Hodgkin's disease, other responsive cancers as such or in combination with other agent(s).
- *Dose:* 0.1–0.2 mg/kg/week (IV).
- *Adverse drug reactions:* Transitory bone marrow depression, usually occurring within a week of the dose, alopecia, neurologic disturbances, hypertension, bone pain, malaise, bronchospasm, and dyspnea.
- *Contraindications:* Leukopenia, bacterial infection, and intrathecal (IT) administration.
- *Drug interaction:* Mitomycin C and phenytoin.

- *Caution:* Hematologic monitoring. If the WBC count falls below 4,000/mm^3, then omit the subsequent dose.

VINCRISTINE

Brand name: Cytocristine
- *Available as:* Injection 1 mg/mL.
- *Indications:* Acute leukemias.
- *Dose:*
  - 0.05–0.15 mg/kg/week until remission or toxicity occurs.
  - 1.5–2 mg/m^2/week.
- *Adverse drug reactions:* Muscle weakness, particularly of dorsiflexors of feet, hand and larynx, loss of reflexes and paresthesia, constipation, intestinal obstruction, alopecia, bone marrow depression, hypertension/hypotension, and bronchospasm.
- *Drug interaction:* Phenytoin and live vaccines.
- *Caution:* If the TLC falls below 4,000/mm^3, then omit the subsequent dose.

Chapter 10

Anticoagulants

INTRODUCTION

Also termed "blood thinners", these are chemical substances that prevent or reduce coagulation of blood, thereby prolonging the clotting time and safeguarding against thromboembolism. Closely related to these are the antiplatelet drugs that inhibit platelet aggregation (clumping together). Anticoagulants inhibit the coagulation cascade by clotting factors that happens after the initial platelet aggregation.

Therapeutic effect of anticoagulants is derived:
- Indirectly by inhibition, or
- Directly by biding to antithrombin or by preventing their synthesis from vitamin K-dependent factors in the liver.

Anticoagulants are available in many different forms, including oral and injectable drugs. Their use aims at by entreating and preventing life-threatening conditions secondary to blood clots, e.g., strokes, heart attacks, pulmonary embolisms, etc.

ACENOCOUMAROL

Acting via inhibition of coagulation by reducing synthesis of vitamin K dependent coagulation factors, it behaves such as a vitamin K antagonist—just like warfarin. It is a derivative of coumarol.

Brand names: Acitrom and Sintrom
- *Indications:* Prophylaxis and treatment of venous thrombosis and pulmonary embolism.
- *Available as:* Tablets 1 mg, 2 mg, 3 mg, and 4 mg.
- *Dose:* 1–8 mg/day (PO) OD
- *Adverse drug reactions:* Bleeding headache, anorexia, skin necrosis, alopecia (reversible); bleeding; allergy; hepatotoxicity.
- *Contraindications:* Hemorrhagic conditions, impaired hepatic/renal function, infective endocarditis, pericarditis, pericardial effusion, and pregnancy.

HEPARIN

Brand names: Beparine, Heparne, and V-parin
- *Indications:* Situations warranting anticoagulant therapy, e.g., venous thrombosis, thromboembolism, pulmonary embolism; prophylactically to cut-down risk of post-operative vascular complications; disseminated intravascular coagulopathy, and purpura fulminans.
- *Available as:* Injection 1 and 5 thousand units/mL (1 mg is equivalent to 120 units).
- *Dose:* Therapeutic-loading (bolus) dose 50 units/kg (IV) slowly over 10–12 min followed by 50–100 units/kg to be added to IV infusion every 4 hours. Alternatively, maintenance can be 10–30 units/kg/h as IV infusion.
- *DVT prophylaxis:* 5,000 units/dose (SC) every 8–12 hours as long as the patient remains ambulatory.
- *Peripheral IV-line flushing:* 10 units/mL every 4 hours, each flush needing 1–2 mL.
- *Central IV-line flushing:* 100 units/mL, each flush needing 2–3 mL, once in 24 hours.

- *Arterial lines/TPN:* 0.5–1 unit/mL solution.
- *Adverse drug reactions:* Anaphylaxis, rash, fever, flushing, bronchospasm, nasal congestion, alopecia, osteoporosis, severe itching, burning of feet, and bleeding.
- *Contraindications:* Gastric ulcer, bleeding diathesis, shock, infective endocarditis; thrombocytopenia.
- *Drug interaction:* Agents that have antithrombotic or antiplatelet effect (e.g., streptokinase, urokinase, aspirin, dipyridamole, NSAIDs such as ibuprofen and ketorolac).
- *Caution:* APTT monitoring recommended.
- *Antidote:* Protamine sulfate.

LOW-MOLECULAR-WEIGHT HEPARIN (ENOXAPARIN)

Unlike natural heparin, low-molecular-weight heparin (LMWH) can be given subcutaneously and does not need APTT monitoring.

Brand names: Clexane, LMWX, and Lupenox

- *Available as:* Injection 10 mg/0.1 mL
- *Indications:* Thromboembolism (both prophylaxis and treatment), disseminated intravascular coagulation (DIC), and purpura fulminans.
- *Dose:* 1–1.5 mg/kg (SC) BD or TDS (therapeutic): Half of this dose is for prophylaxis.
- *Adverse drug reactions:* Gastrointestinal upset, bleeding, and thrombocytopenia.
- *Contraindications:* Gastric ulcer, bleeding diathesis, shock, infective endocarditis; thrombocytopenia.
- *Drug interaction:* Agents that have antithrombotic or antiplatelet effect (e.g., streptokinase, urokinase, aspirin, dipyridamole, NSAIDs such as ibuprofen and ketorolac).

Chapter 10: Anticoagulants

- *Caution:* Monitor platelet count. A fall <100,000/mm^3 is an indication for withdrawal of the agent.
- *Antidote:* Protamine sulfate in case of an accidental overdose.

PHENINDIONE

Brand name: Dindevan
- *Available as:* Tablet 50 mg
- *Indication:* Thromboembolism
- *Dose:* 0.5–4 mg/kg/day q 12 hours
- *Adverse drug reactions:* Hemorrhage, agranulocytosis, eosinophilia, hepatitis, and renal damage
- *Contraindications:* Hemorrhagic states, renal or hepatic dysfunction, and lactation
- *Caution:* Renal impairment, hypertension, and vitamin K deficiency.

WARFARIN

An anticoagulant that antagonizes hepatic vitamin K synthesis, depleting vitamin K-dependent clotting factors II, VI, VII, IX, and X.

Brand names: Coumadin, Sofarin, Uniwarfin, and Warf
- *Available as:* Tablets 1 mg, 2 mg, 5 mg; Injection 50 mg.
- *Dose:* 0.2 mg/kg (PO) followed by 0.1 mg/kg/24 hours. Younger infants need higher dose (0.3 mg/kg/24 hours). Dose is dependent on patient.
- *Adverse drug reactions:* Bleeding, hemoptysis, and skin necrosis.
- *Drug interactions:* Aspirin, barbiturates, carbamazepine, cimetidine, omeprazole, phenytoin, rifampicin, vitamin K, ritonavir, and delavirdine.

- *Caution:* Avoid foods with high vitamin K content, e.g., green leafy vegetables.

XANTINOL NICOTINATE

Brand name: Complamina

- *Indications:* Disordered cerebral function, circulatory cerebral disturbances, intermittent claudication, endangiitis obliterans, and diabetic angiopathy.
- *Available as:* Tablet 150 mg; Injection 300 mg/ampule.
- *Dose:* 150–600 mg twice daily after meals; Injection 300–900 mg (IM and IV infusion).
- *Adverse drug reactions:* Flushing and hypotension.
- *Contraindications:* Recent myocardial infarction, decompensated cardiac insufficiency, acute hemorrhage and after compensation with cardiac glycosides.

Chapter 11

Anticonvulsants

INTRODUCTION

A seizure or convulsion is a sudden change in movement or awareness (sensorium) due to a sudden burst of electrical energy from the neurons. As a result, over and above the movements, the sensation and consciousness may be affected. Fundamentally, seizures are alterations in the brain's electrical activity as a result of such factors as biochemical changes (excess sodium), injury, tumor or infection/inflammation. The manifestations may be dramatically noticeable, subtle, or all together absent. A focal onset seizure (partial seizure) starts in just one area of the brain. Generalized seizures involve all areas of the brain from the time they start. These may be tonic, clonic, tonic-clonic or absent (petit mal) seizures. When seizures are unprovoked and recurrent, the term "epilepsy" is applied.

Also termed "antiepileptic drugs" (AEDs) or "antiseizure drugs", these are a diverse group of drugs that are used to prevent and control seizure activity. *Anticonvulsants suppress the excessive rapid firing of neurons during seizures. They also prevent the spread of the seizure activity within the brain. Since they are supposed to be mood elevators, anticonvulsants are also increasingly being used in the treatment of bipolar disorder and borderline personality disorder, as also in treatment of neuropathic pain.*

STANDARD ANTICONVULSANT DRUGS

Carbamazepine

Brand names: Carbatol, Tegrital, and Mazetol

- *Indications:* Seizure disorder and trigeminal neuralgia.
- *Available as:* Tablets 100 mg, 200 mg, 400 mg; Suspension 100 mg/5 mL.
- *Dose:* 10–20 mg/kg/day (PO) in two to three divided doses.
- *Adverse drug reactions:* Nausea, anorexia, drowsiness, cardiomegaly, hypertension, rash, bone marrow depression, and difficulty in accommodation.
- *Contraindications:* Known hypersensitivity to drug or tricyclic compounds, atrioventricular block, with or within 2 weeks of MAI therapy, glaucoma, alcoholism, and psychosis.
- *Caution:* Liver or renal disease and blood dyscrasias.

Clobazam

Brand names: Clozam, Cloba, Lobazam, and Frisium

- *Available as:* Tablet 5 mg, 10 mg, and 20 mg.
- *Indications:* Febrile seizure prophylaxis; add-on anticonvulsant in generalized tonic-clonic, complex partial, generalized tonic, absence, myoclonic and atonic seizures, and Lennox-Gastaut syndrome.
- *Dose:* Febrile seizures prophylaxis: 1 mg/kg/day (PO) q 12 hours for 2 or 3 days.
- *Other situations:* Initial 0.1 mg/kg/day. Maintenance 0.3–1 mg/kg/day OD (preferably bedtime) or q 12 hours.
- *Adverse drug reactions:* Dryness of mouth, constipation, anxiety, impaired consciousness asthenia/poor weight gain, tiredness, insomnia, and tremors.
- *Contraindications:* Hypersensitivity to benzodiazepines and myasthenia gravis.

Clonazepam

Brand names: Clotrin and Rivotril

- *Indications:* Anticonvulsant (focal, resistant petit mal, and myoclonus).
- *Available as:* Tablet 0.5 mg, 1 mg, and 2 mg.
- *Dose:* 0.01–0.03 mg/kg/day (PO) q 8–12 hours. The dose should be increased by increments of 0.25–0.5 mg until a maximum of 0.2 mg/kg/day is attained.
- *Adverse drug reactions:* Syndrome of drowsiness, somnolence, fatigue, and lethargy occurs in one-half of the users. Muscular incoordination, ataxia, hypotonia, dysarthria, dizziness, behavior disturbances in the form of irritability, aggression, and hyperactivity, both anorexia and hyperphagia. Increased salivary and bronchial secretion and exacerbation of seizures are the other undesirable reactions that have been encountered.
- *Contraindications:* Advanced liver disease, sleep apnea, respiratory depression, acute pulmonary insufficiency, and acute narrow-angle glaucoma.
- *Caution:* Do not use together with valproate to safeguard against petit mal status.
- *Drug interaction:* Alcohol, central nervous system (CNS) stimulants and depressants, anticonvulsants, cimetidine, disulfiram, and anticholinergics.

Diazepam

Brand names: Calmpose, Valium, Tenavil, and Direc-2

- *Indications:* Symptomatic relief of anxiety; muscle relaxation; acute convulsive episode; chronic prophylaxis for febrile convulsions.
- *Available as:* Tablet 2 mg, 5 mg; Syrup 2 mg/5 mL; Injection 5 mg/mL; Rectal 2 mg/mL.

- *Dose:*
  - 0.1–0.3 mg/kg/dose (IM and IV) or 1 mg/year of age to a maximum dose of 10 mg.
  - 0.1–0.8 mg/kg/day (PO) in three to 4 divided doses.
  - 0.5 mg/kg/dose (R) **(Figs. 1A to K)**.
- *Adverse drug reactions:* Rise in ocular tension, hypersensitivity, drowsiness, ataxia, nervousness, hiccup, fall in blood pressure (BP), respiratory depression, thrombophlebitis; local mechanical irritation in case of rectal diazepam.
- *Caution:* Do not mix diazepam with other drugs. Also do not dilute it.

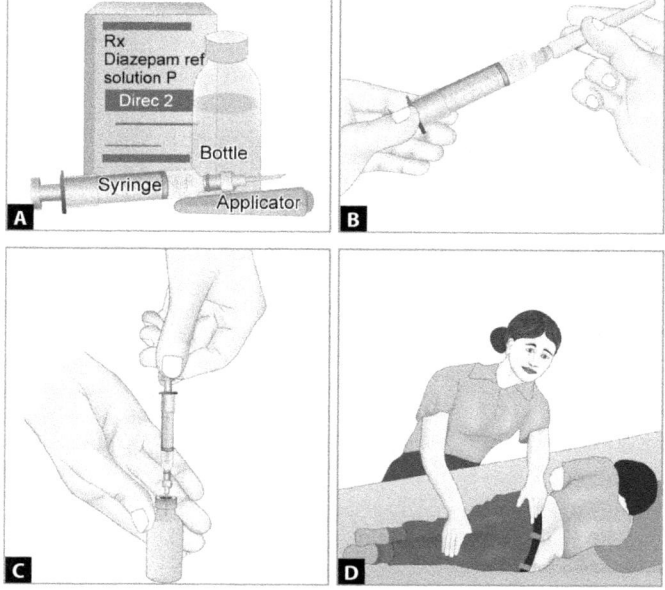

Figs. 1A to D

Chapter 11: Anticonvulsants

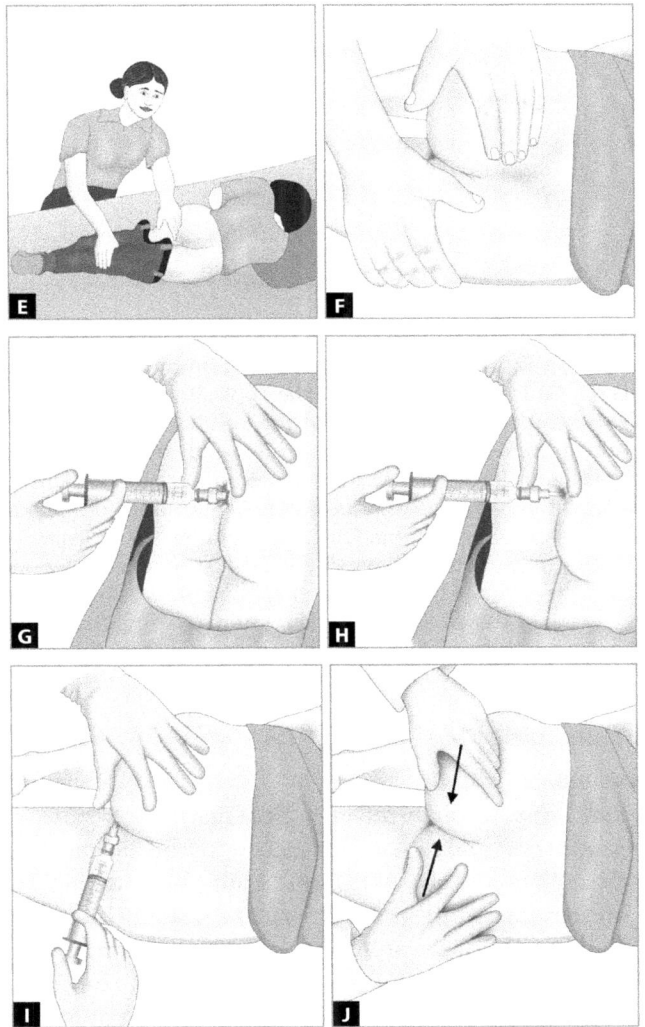

Figs. 1E to J

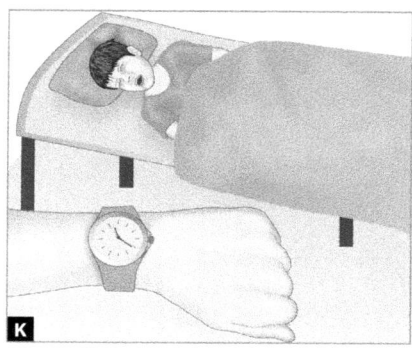

Figs. 1A to K: Directions for administration of rectal diazepam (Direc-2): (A) The medicine; (B) Fix the applicator on to the syringe; (C) Draw out required amount of the solution from the bottle; (D) Turn the patient on side, facing you; (E) Bend upper leg forward to expose rectum; (F) Separate buttocks to expose rectum; (G) Lubricate the applicator using a suitable lubricator. Gently insert the applicator completely into the rectum. For children under 15 kg insert only half way; (H) Empty the solution in the syringe completely by slowly pressing the piston of the syringe until it stops; (I) Remove the syringe and the applicator slowly from the rectum; (J) Press the patient's buttocks together for a few minutes to prevent leakage; (K) Keep person on side facing you, note time and continue to observe.

Ethosuximide

Brand name: Zarontin

- *Indication:* Absence seizures (petit mal).
- *Available as:* Tablet/capsule 250 mg; Syrup 250 mg/5 mL.
- *Dose:* 15 mg/kg/day 9 (PO) q 12 hours. Increase in weekly increments until absence attacks seize. This usually happens at a dose varying between 20 and 40 mg/kg/day. This dose should be continued. Usually, the dose of 250 mg/day for <6 years and 500 mg/day for >6 years with a maximum of 1,500 g/day suffices.

- *Adverse drug reactions:* Rash, gastritis, vomiting, mental dullness, suicidal ideation, eosinophilia, hematuria, nephrotic syndrome, and blood dyscrasias.
- *Drug interaction:* Isoniazid (INH) and other anticonvulsants.
- *Contraindications:* Porphyria and pregnancy.
- *Caution:* Hepatic and renal dysfunction, and lactation.

Fosphenytoin

It is a water-soluble prodrug of phenytoin (1 mg phenytoin = 1.5 mg fosphenytoin).

Brand names: Fosolin and Fosphen

- *Indications:* Acute seizures (tonic-clonic and partial), status epilepticus.
- *Available as:* Injection (IV and IM), 50 mg/mL.
- *Dose:*
  - Emergency 15–20 mg/kg (IV); nonemergency 10–15 mg/kg (IV and IM).
  - Maintenance dose 4–6 mg/kg/day (IV and IM).
  - IV infusion rate should not exceed 3 mg/kg/min.
- *Adverse drug reactions:* Cardiovascular collapse, hypotension; hyperplasia of gums, rash, blood dyscrasia, bone marrow depression, liver damage, neurologic manifestations (nystagmus, choreoathetosis, and hyperactivity), lymphadenopathy, arthropathy, and nephrosis.
- *Contraindication:* Porphyria.
- *Caution:* Make sure IV infusion rate remains <3 mg/kg/min.

Gabapentin

It is used as an add-on therapy.

Brand names: Gabapin and Neurontin
- *Indications:* Partial seizures and diabetic neuropathy.
- *Dose:* 15 mg/kg/day q 8 hours followed by increase in increments to 30–60 mg/kg/day q 8 hours.
- *Adverse drug reactions:* Nausea, vomiting, rhinitis, dizziness, somnolence, tiredness, ataxia, headache, diplopia, nystagmus, and tremors.
- *Caution:* Avoid <12 years of age.

Lacosamide

It is used as an adjunctive therapy.

Brand names: Lacasa, Lacosam, and Lacoset
- *Available as:* Tablet 50 mg, 100 mg, 150 mg, and 200 mg.
- *Indications:* Adjunctive therapy in refractory partial onset seizures; also, diabetic neuropathy.
- *Dose:* 1 mg/kg/day BD. Depending on the response, it may be increased to 2–12 mg/kg/day in increments and subsequent days.
- *Adverse drug reactions:* Nausea, vomiting, dizziness, headache, fatigue, somnolence, tremors, and ataxia.

Lamotrigine

It is used as an add-on therapy with valproate.

Brand names: Lametec and Lamitor
- *Indications:* Partial seizures, generalized seizures, absence seizures (atypical), tonic-clonic seizures, atonic generalized seizures; Rett syndrome.
- *Available as:* Tablet 2.5 mg, 5 mg, 25 mg, 50 mg, and 100 mg.
- *Adverse drug reactions:* Hypersensitivity skin rash/reaction which may turn out to be life-threatening.
- *Contraindications:* Advanced liver dysfunction.

Levetiracetam

Brand names: Kepra, Levilex, Levroxa, and Torleva

- *Indications:* Refractory partial seizures, tonic-clonic seizures, absence seizures, and myoclonic seizures.
- *Available as:* Tablet 250 mg, 500 mg, 750 mg, 1,000 mg; Syrup 100 mg/mL.
- *Dose:* 10 mg/kg/day q 12 hours followed by an increase by 10 mg/kg every week until 40 mg/kg/day is reached.
- *Adverse drug reactions:* Nervousness, somnolence children <6 months.
- *Contraindication:* Infants <6 months of age.

Lorazepam

It is a benzodiazepine possessing sedative and antianxiety property; and effective in status epilepticus.

Brand name: Lorpose

- *Indications:* Poorly or uncontrolled status epilepticus.
- *Available as:* Tablet 1 mg and 2 mg.
- *Dose:*
  - *Sedation:* 0.05 mg/kg/dose.
  - *Status epilepticus:* 0.05 mg/kg/dose (IV and IM), to be repeated after 15–20 minutes and again after another 15–20 minutes, if indicated.
- *Adverse drug reactions:* CNS depression, impaired alertness, amnesia, and dependence.
- *Contraindication:* Hypersensitivity to benzodiazepines, sleep disorder (apnea), respiratory depression, and narrow angle glaucoma.
- *Drug interaction:* Alcohol and other CNS depressants.

Midazolam

Brand names: Mezolam and Fulsed

- *Indications:* Poorly or uncontrolled status epilepticus.
- *Available as:* Injection 1 and 5 mg/mL.
- *Dose:*
  - Intranasal (pending establishment of IV access) 0.2 mg/kg.
  - Buccal (pending establishment of IV access) 0.3 mg/kg.
  - *After IV access is established:* A bolus of 0.2 mg/kg (IV and IM) followed by 0.1–0.2 mg/kg/h.
- *Adverse drug reactions:* Respiratory depression and narrow angle glaucoma.

Nitrazepam

Brand names: Nitravan and Nitravet

- *Indications:* Partial epilepsy, infantile spasms (salaam seizures), partial epilepsy; also, as hypnotic in insomnia.
- *Available as:* Tablet 2.5 mg, 5 mg, and 10 mg.
- *Dose:* 0.25–1 mg/kg/day (PO) OD or q 12 hours.
- *Adverse drug reactions:* Paradoxical stimulation, behavior problems, irritability, excessive sweating, blurring of vision, dryness of mouth, and urinary incontinence.
- *Contraindications:* Porphyria, myasthenia gravis, acute narrow angle glaucoma, and benzodiazepine hypersensitivity.

Oxcarbazepine

It is a ketoderivative of carbamazepine.

Brand names: Oxycarb and Selzic

- *Indications:* Partial, seizures, and generalized tonic-clonic seizures.

- *Available as:*
  - Tablet 150, 300, 600 mg.
  - Syrup 300 mg/5 mL.
- *Dose:* 8–10 mg/kg/day which should be increased in increments of 10 mg/kg every week to a maximum of 40 mg/kg/day.
- *Adverse drug reactions:* Rash, headache, easy fatigability, dizziness, ataxia, and hyponatremia.
- *Caution:*
  - Reduce dose to one-half in renal insufficiency/failure.
  - Avoid in children <6 years of age.

Paraldehyde

Brand name: Available under generic name only

- *Indications:* Status epilepticus for sedation.
- *Available as:* Injection 2, 5, and 10 mL, each mL providing 1 g.
- *Dose:*
  - 0.1–0.2 mL/kg/dose or 1 mL/year/dose (PO, IM, and IV), 0.3–0.6 mL/kg/dose (PR).
  - Higher limit of dose is for hypnotic or anticonvulsant effect and the lower for simple sedation.
- *Adverse drug reactions:* Very bad smell from breath, gastric irritation, pulmonary hemorrhage, respiratory depression, cardiac depression, cardiac failure, and hepatotoxicity.
- *Caution:* Never use plastic syringe in view of risk of reaction with plastic.

Phenobarbital Sodium

Brand names: Gardenal and Luminal

- *Indications:* Seizures (neonatal, tonic-clonic, prophylaxis of febrile seizures, and epilepsy); for sedation; and for sleep.

- *Available as:* Tablet 15 mg, 30 mg, 60 mg, 100 mg; Syrup 20 mg/5 mL injection 100 and 200 mg/mL.
- *Dose:*
  - 15–20 mg/kg/dose (IV bolus) over 15–30 minutes for an acute attack of convulsions. Subsequently, 5 mg/kg every 15–30 minutes. Total dose must not exceed 30 mg/kg/day.
  - 3–5 mg/kg/day (PO and IV) in divided doses as maintenance therapy or for sedation.
- *Adverse drug reactions:* Rash, vertigo, idiosyncrasy, respiratory depression, drowsiness, rickets during prolonged therapy, behavior problems, and paradoxical hyperactivity.
- *Drug interaction:* Valproic acid, chloramphenicol, felbamate, steroids, and griseofulvin.
- *Contraindications:* Porphyria, asthma (severe), hepatic insufficiency, and renal insufficiency.

Phenytoin Sodium (Diphenylhydantoin Sodium)

Brand names: Dilantin, Epileptin, Epsolin, and Eptoin

- *Indications:* Epilepsy; IV infusion in status epilepticus; ventricular tachyarrhythmia.
- *Available as:* Capsule 100 mg; suspension 100 mg/5 mL; injection (IV and IM) 100 mg/mL.
- *Dose:* 3–8 mg/kg/day (PO) as single dose or in two divided doses; 10–15 mg/kg (IV and IM).
- *Adverse drug reactions:* Hyperplasia of gums, rash, blood dyscrasia, bone marrow depression, liver damage, neurologic manifestations (nystagmus, choreoathetosis, and hyperactivity), lymphadenopathy, arthropathy, and nephrosis.

Chapter 11: Anticonvulsants

Primidone

Brand name: Mysoline
- *Indications:* Epilepsy; partial seizures and tonic-clonic seizures.
- *Available as:* Tablet 250 mg; suspension 250 mg/5 mL.
- *Dose:* 40–50 mg/kg/day in divided doses.
- *Adverse drug reactions:* Nausea, drowsiness, giddiness, rash, megaloblastic anemia, ataxia, polyuria, and oculomotor paresis.

Topiramate

Brand names: Topamac, Topamax, and Topex
- *Indications:* Refractory partial seizures, primary generalized tonic-clonic seizures, absence seizures, infantile myoclonic seizures (Salaam seizures and West syndrome), Lennox–Gastaut syndrome. This is best employed as an "add-on" therapy.
- *Available as:* Tablets 25 and 100 mg.
- *Dose:*
  - *Seizures:* 1 mg/kg/day. Increase in increments to 3–9 mg/kg/day OD or q 12 hours.
  - *Migraine prophylaxis:* 0.5 mg/kg/day.
- *Adverse drug reactions:* Nausea, anorexia, weight loss, dizziness, headache, and ataxia.
- *Drug interaction:* Phenytoin, carbamazepine, valproic acid, CNS depressants, carbonic anhydrase inhibitors, and anticholinergics.
- *Contraindication:* Lactation.
- *Caution:* Avoid administering with other carbonic anhydrase inhibitors since coadministration may cause additive effect leading to renal calculi; avoid in renal and hepatic insufficiency.

Valproate Sodium

Brand name: Valparin
- *Indications:* Epilepsy.
- *Available as:* Tablet 200 mg; Syrup 200 mg/5 mL.
- *Dose:* Start with 15 mg/kg/day in two to three divided doses. May increase dose by weekly increments of 5–10 mg/kg/day up to a maximum recommended dose of 30 mg/kg/day.
- *Adverse drug reactions:* Anorexia, nausea, vomiting, sedation, ataxia, incoordination, and hepatotoxicity.
- *Caution:* Concomitant use with clonazepam may lead to petit mal (absence) status.

Vigabatrin

It is used as an add-on therapy in epilepsy.
Brand name: Sabril
- *Indications:* Refractory partial seizures, infantile spasms (infantile myoclonic seizures, salaam seizures, and West syndrome), Lennox–Gastaut syndrome.
- *Available as:* Tablet 500 mg.
- *Dose:* 20–40 mg/kg/day (PO). This should be increased in increments to 80–100 mg/kg/day q 8–12 hours.
- *Adverse drug reactions:* Gastrointestinal (GI) upset, behavioral problems, defects of field of vision. CNS depression.
- *Precautions:* It is important to conduct baseline ophthalmic examination at the outset and then half yearly.

Zonisamide

It is an anticonvulsant with unclear mechanism of action.
Brand names: Zonisamide and Zonigran.
- *Indication:* Absence seizures (atypical), partial seizures, and tonic-clonic seizures.

- *Dose:* 4–8 mg/kg/day q 12 hours.
- *Adverse drug reactions:* Susceptibility to hypohidrosis and hyperthermia while on this agent, skin rash, and renal calculi.
- *Caution:* Avoid <16 years.

OTHER AGENTS EMPLOYED FOR SEIZURE CONTROL

Adrenocorticotropic Hormone

Brand name: Acthar
- *Indication:* Infantile spasms (infantile myoclonic seizures, salaam seizures, and West syndrome).
- *Available as:* Injection 40 and 80 IU/mL.
- *Dose:* 20–40 IU/day (IM and SC) for 6 weeks. During next 4–12 weeks, it may be tapered.
- *Adverse drug reactions:* Cushing disease, euphoria, psychosis, superadded fungal infections, tuberculosis, immunosuppression, cataract, acne, skin and muscle atrophy, and adrenal suppression.
- *Contraindications:* Acute psychosis, hypertension, congestive cardiac failure (CCF), and peptic ulcer.

Prednisolone

Brand names: Omnacortil, Predone, and Wysolone
- *Indication:* Infantile spasms (infantile myoclonic seizures, salaam seizures, and West syndrome); several other indications include asthma, nephritic syndrome, idiopathic thrombocytopenic purpura, and rheumatic carditis with CCF.
- *Available as:* Tablet 5 mg, 10 mg, 20 mg, 40 mg; Syrup 5, 10, and 15 mg/5 mL.
- *Dose:* 2 mg/kg/day q 12 hours × 2–6 weeks. During the next 4–12 weeks, it may be tapered.

- *Adverse drug reactions:* Edema, Cushing disease, peptic ulcer, euphoria, psychosis, superadded fungal infections, tuberculosis, immunosuppression, cataract, acne, skin and muscle atrophy, and adrenal suppression.
- *Contraindications:* Acute psychosis, hypertension, CCF, and peptic ulcer.

Pyridoxine (Vitamin B_6)

- *Indication:* Pyridoxine dependent seizures, drug-induced (INH and hydralazine) pyridoxine deficiency causing neuritis.
- *Dose:* 50–100 mg/dose (IM and IV). Thereafter, same maintenance dose but orally.
- *Adverse drug reactions:* Nausea, folic acid deficiency, and liver dysfunction.
- *Caution:* Large IV doses may precipitate seizures; serum phenobarbital and phenytoin concentration may be reduced.

Thiopental

It is a barbiturate induction agent, widely employed as anesthetic that may be used in refractory status epilepticus.
Brand names: Anesthal and Pentothal.
- *Available as:* 250 mg, 500 mg, and 1 g.
- *Dose:* Loading dose 5–10 mg/kg (IV) slowly over 2–5 minutes. Thereafter, 2–10 mg/kg/h as IV infusion if seizures remain uncontrolled.
- *Adverse drug reactions:* Severe drowsiness and dizziness
- *Contraindications: Porphyria,* liver or kidney disease, severe anemia, myasthenia gravis, asthma, a thyroid disorder, or Addison's disease.

Chapter 12

Antidiarrheals

INTRODUCTION
Antidiarrheal drugs are the agents that reduce the frequency, volume, and fluidity of the stools, thereby providing symptomatic relief.

FURAZOLIDONE
Brand name: Furoxone
- *Available as:* Tablet 100 mg; Syrup 33.5 mg/5 mL
- *Indications:* Nonspecific diarrhea, bacterial diarrhea, diarrhea associated with giardiasis, and cholera. Occasionally, enteric fever.
- *Dose:* 6–8 mg/kg/day (PO) in three to four divided doses for 5–10 days.
- *Adverse drug reactions:* Gastrointestinal tract upset, hemolytic anemia, rash, hypotension, headache, nausea, vomiting, fever, and arthralgia.

COLISTIN SULFATE
Brand name: Walamycin
- *Available as:* Suspension 12.5 mg/5 mL
- *Indications:* Acute bacterial diarrhea due to gram-negative organisms, especially neomycin-resistant *E. coli*.
- *Dose:* 5–8 mg/kg/day (PO) in divided doses.

- *Adverse drug reactions:* Pruritus, dizziness, vertigo, slurred speech, tingling sensations, circumoral paresthesia or numbness, renal damage, and hypersensitivity.

DIPHENOXYLATE HYDROCHLORIDE

An antimotility drug.

Brand name: Lomotil
- *Available as:*
  - Tablet 2.5 mg
  - Liquid 2.5 mg/5 mL
  - Drops 0.5 mg/mL (15 drops). Subtherapeutic dose of atropine is also added to the proprietary preparation.
- *Indications:* Symptomatic control of diarrhea through the antimotility and antisecretory action on gut.
- *Dose:* 0.2–0.3 mg/kg/day in divided doses.
- *Adverse drug reactions:* Drowsiness, constipation, flushing, nausea, vomiting, rash, restlessness, insomnia, narcosis, respiratory depression, and paralytic ileus.
- *Contraindications:* Atropine or diphenoxylate intolerance/allergy, pseudomembranous enterocolitis, and jaundice.
- *Caution:* Avoid in infants and children under 6 years of age.

LOPERAMIDE HCL

It is an antimotility drug.

Brand names: Diamod, Diatlop, Imodium, Imogen, Imotil, and Loparet
- *Available as:*
  - Tablet/capsule 2 mg
  - Liquid 0.2 mg/mL
- *Indications:* Symptomatic relief of diarrhea through the antimotility and antisecretory action on gut.

- *Dose:* 0.3 mg/kg/day; 0.1 mg/kg/dose.
- *Adverse drug reactions:* Dryness of mouth, abdominal cramps, drowsiness, constipation, vomiting, dizziness, headache, gastric distention, rash, and increased micturition.
- *Caution:* Avoid in infants and children under 6 years of age.

RACECADOTRIL

It is an inhibitor of enkephalinase, and it prevents water and electrolyte losses in diarrhea.

Brand names: Enuff, Lomorest, and Racotil

- *Available as:*
  - Sachets 10 mg and 30 mg
  - Capsule 100 mg
- *Indication:* Secretory diarrhea.
- *Dose:* 1.5 mg/kg (PO) TDS.
- *Adverse drug reactions:* Vomiting, constipation, increased thirst, headache, vertigo, abdominal pain, hypokalemia, bacterial overgrowth, and toxic megacolon.
- *Contraindications:* Pregnancy, lactation, and renal insufficiency.

PROBIOTICS

These are friendly live bacterial products that promote growth of normal flora of the gut and displace pathogenic bacteria. The examples of the commonly used probiotics in the products are *Saccharomyces boulardii, Lactobacillus acidophilus,* and *Lactobacillus sporogenes*.

Brand names: Econorm, Ecoflora, and Darolac

- *Available as:* Sachets/tablet 5–10 billion organisms.

- *Indications:* As adjuncts to antidiarrheal therapy, broad-spectrum antibiotic therapy; ever increasing spectrum of other indications including inflammatory bowel disease (IBD), necrotizing enterocolitis, *Helicobacter pylori* gastritis, irritable bowel syndrome, and infantile colic, etc.
- *Dose:* 5–10 billion organisms/day twice daily.
- *Adverse drug reactions:* Infrequent. Nausea, vomiting, constipation, abdominal distention, hyperactivity, and aggression. Rarely, sepsis.
- *Contraindication:* Septicemia.

ORAL REHYDRATION SALTS

Brand names: Electrobion, Punarjal, and Walyte

- *Available as:* Sachets 6 g (for 200 mL water), 30 g (for 1 L water). **Table 1** gives contents of different types of oral rehydration salts (ORS). Additionally, **Table 2** gives the contents as well as composition of new formula (low osmolarity) ORS.
- *Indications:* Prophylaxis of diarrheal dehydration and treatment of mild-to-moderate dehydration; continuation therapy following rehydration with IV fluids in severe dehydration. Nondiarrheal uses of ORS include situations such as postsurgery fluid administration where maintenance fluids are required after the IV administration is over.

Administration/Dose

- *Adverse drug reactions:* Hypernatremic edema in neonates and infants with the standard ORS.
- *Caution:* In case of vomiting, do not push ORS. Giving it in "sips" is not only safe but also helpful in tiding over the difficult period.

TABLE 1: Contents of standard oral rehydration salts (ORS) and low osmolarity ORS.

Component	Standard ORS	Low osmolarity ORS
Contents		
Sodium chloride	3.5 g	2.6 g
Sodium bicarbonate (citrate)	2.5 g (2.9 g)	2.9 g
Potassium chloride	1.5 g	1.5 g
Glucose	20.0 g	13.5 g
Osmolarity		
Sodium	90 mmol	75 mmol
Chloride	80 mmol	65 mmol
Citrate	10 mmol	10 mmol
Potassium	80 mmol	20 mmol
Glucose	111 mmol	75 mmol
Total osmolarity	311	245

Source: Adapted from Gupte S, Anderson RA. In: Gupte S (Ed). The Short Textbook of Pediatrics, 13th edition. New Delhi: Jaypee Brothers Medical Publishers (P) Ltd.; 2020. pp. 441-80.

TABLE 2: Content and concentration of new formula (low osmolarity) World Health Organization-oral rehydration salts (WHO-ORS).

New formula WHO-ORS			
Content		Concentrations	
NaCl	2.6 g	Na^+	75 mM
KC1	1.5 g	K^+	20 mM
Trisodium citrate	2.9 g	Cl^-	65 mM
Glucose	13.5 g	Citrate	10 mM
Water	1 L	Glucose	75 mM

Total osmolarity 245 mOsm/L

(*Note:* Available as Oretral-A, Electrobion, Electral 21 g sachet for 1,000 mL; Walyte, Relyte 4.2 g sachet for 200 mL).

SUPER ORS

The term "super ORS" refers to an ORS that, in addition to rehydrating, decreases purging rates (reduction in volume and frequency of motions), improves diarrhea by enhancing absorption, and provides nutrition.

- Addition of certain actively transported amino acids (alanine and glycine)
- Boiled rice powder 40–50 g/L is an efficient substitute for glucose.
- Wheat, maize, and potato based ORS.
- Zinc, dextrose, and lactobacillus based super ORS. Zinc is useful in so many ways, including enhanced absorption of fluids from the gut and prevention of future attacks of severe diarrhea.

Chapter 13

Antiemetics

INTRODUCTION

These are the drugs that are effective against vomiting and nausea. Typically, these are used to tackle (both prevent and treat) nausea/vomiting associated with gastritis, gastroenteritis, motion sickness and the side effects of opioid analgesics, general anesthetics, antipsychotic medication, and cancer chemotherapy.

CHLORPROMAZINE

Brand names: Largactil and Megatil
- *Available as:* Tablet 10 mg, 25 mg, 50 mg, and 100 mg. Injection 25 mg/mL (2 mL ampule)
- *Dose:* 0.5 mg/kg/dose
- *Caution:* Avoid in infants.

DIMENHYDRINATE

Brand names: Dramamine, Draminate, and Gravol
- *Available as:* Syrup 15.6 mg/5 mL; Injection 50 mg/mL
- *Dose:* 5 mg/kg/day (PO, IM, and IV)

DOMPERIDONE

Brand names: Domperon, Domstal, and Gastractiv
- *Indications:* Nausea and vomiting and gastric motility disorders (reflux esophagitis, duodenogastric reflux, and dyspeptic symptoms)

- *Available as:* Tablet 10 mg; Suspension 1 mg/mL
- *Dose:* 0.2–0.4 mg/kg at 4–8 hours intervals
- *Adverse drug reactions:* Mild abdominal cramps, rarely extrapyramidal manifestations, rise in serum prolactin
- *Caution:* Avoid concomitant administration of anticholinergic agents.

GRANISETRON

It is usually reserved for cancer chemotherapy. Several times (15–20 times), it is more potent than ondansetron.

Brand name: Cadigran, Grandem, and Granicap

- *Available as:* Tablet 1 mg, 2 mg; Syrup 1 mg/5 mL; Injection 1 mg/mL
- *Dose:* 10–20 µg/kg/dose (IV) over 15–60 minutes before chemotherapy; two to three times postchemotherapy, if needed
- *Caution:* Avoid in children <2 years of age.

METOCLOPRAMIDE HYDROCHLORIDE

Brand names: Perinorm, Reglan, and Maxeron

- *Indications:* As an antiemetic; as a galactagogue; as an appetizer and weight-gaining agent; gastritis, reflux esophagitis; hyperacidity; heartburn; dyspepsia; chalasia; and hiccup
- *Available as:* Tablet 10 mg; Syrup 5 mg/5 mL; Injection 5 mg/mL
- *Dose:* 0.5 mg/kg/day in three divided doses. After first year, may give up to 1 mg/kg/day
- *Adverse drug reactions:* Extrapyramidal manifestations (spasticity, nuchal rigidity, oculogyric crisis, nystagmus, protrusion of tongue, and opisthotonos), somnolence,

nervousness, asthenia, gynecomastia, lactorrhea, diarrhea, and motor restlessness
- *Antidote:* Diazepam
- *Contraindication:* Epilepsy
- *Precaution:* Avoid its concurrent use with a phenothiazine or atropine and other anticholinergic agents.

ONDANSETRON HCL

It is a serotonin 5-HT3 receptor antagonist.

Brand names: Emeset and Vomiof
- *Indications:* Best indicated in chemotherapy and radiotherapy-induced vomiting; may be employed for controlling vomiting in other conditions
- *Available as:* Tablet 4 mg, 8 mg. Syrup 2 mg/5 mL. Injection 2 mg/mL
- *Dose:*
  - Less than 4 years 2 mg (PO) q 4 hours
  - 4–12 years 4 mg (PO) q 4 hours
  - More than 12 years 8 mg (PO) q 4 hours
  - Injectable 0.15 mg/kg IM and IV
- *Adverse drug reactions:* Constipation, headache, flushing, liver dysfunction, seizures, and arthralgia
- *Contraindications:* Hypersensitivity, liver dysfunction, nausea, and vomiting during postoperative period.

PALONOSETRON

It is popular in case of cancer chemotherapy.

Brand name: Palnox
- *Available as:* Injection 0.25 mg (250 µg)/mL
- *Dose:* Prophylaxis for postoperative vomiting 75 µg single dose

- Vomiting associated with cancer chemotherapy 250 µg
- *Caution:* Avoid rapid injection as it is also used in intestinal obstruction.

PROMETHAZINE HYDROCHLORIDE

Brand name: Phenergan
- *Indications:* Vomiting, motion sickness; for obtaining tranquilizing effect and sedation
- *Available as:* Tablet 10 mg. Elixir 5 mg/5 mL. Injection 25 mg/mL
- *Dose:* 0.5 mg/kg/dose (PO and IM)
- *Adverse drug reactions:* Allergic reactions, confusion, dizziness, disorientation, somnolence, headache, tremors, twitching, ataxia, solar dermatitis, and dystonia
- *Antidote:* For dystonic reaction, it is chlorpromazine.

PROCHLORPERAZINE

Brand name: Stemetil
- *Available as:* Tablet 5 mg, 25 mg; Injection 12.5 mg/mL
- *Dose:*
  - More than 2 years or >10 kg. 0.4 mg/kg/day (PO) q 6–8 hours
  - 0.2 mg/kg/day (IM) q 6–8 hours
- *Adverse drug reactions:* Orthostatic hypotension. Extrapyramidal symptoms
- *Caution:* Avoid in children <2 years of age.

TRIFLUOPERAZINE

Brand names: Manocalm, Neocalm, Trazine, and Siquil
- *Indications:* Vomiting, motion sickness, for sleep
- *Available as:* Tablet 10 mg; Injection 10 mg, 20 mg/mL

- *Dose:* 0.5–0.2 mg/kg/day (PO), 0.25 mg/kg/day (IM)
- *Adverse drug reactions:* Faintness, palpitations, nasal stuffiness, dry mouth, constipation, orthostatic hypotension, hyper- or hypothermia, agranulocytosis, pigmentary degeneration of retina, extrapyramidal syndromes, especially, dystonic reactions
- *Contraindications:* Hepatic dysfunction, coma, and bone marrow depression.

Chapter 14

Antifibrillatory Drugs

INTRODUCTION

By definition, arrhythmia is an abnormality in the rate and rhythm of heartbeat (rapid, irregular, and unsynchronized) as a result of abnormal contractions of the heart muscle fibers of the heart very high, very low, or erratic electrical impulses. Diagnosis is confirmed by ECG or a small portable ECG recording device worn by the patient for 24 hours or more.

Fibrillations may be atrial or ventricular. In atrial fibrillation, electrical pulses coming from the sinoatrial node are overwhelmed by disorganized electrical impulses usually originating in the roots of the pulmonary veins, leading to irregular conduction of impulses to the ventricles which generate the heartbeat. Ventricular fibrillation is a common cause of cardiac arrest and is usually fatal if not reversed by defibrillation.

Over and above pharmacotherapy, treatment revolves around cardioversion and surgical intervention.

ADENOSINE

It is a powerful short-acting vasodilator (not used as vasodilator), employed for correcting the irregular rhythm of ventricles (not atriums).

Brand names: Adenocar, Adenoject, Adenox, Cadsine, and Carnosine

- *Available as:* Injection 3 mg/mL (2 mL ampule)

- *Indication:* Paroxysmal supraventricular tachycardia (PSVT)
- *Dose:* 0.3 mg/kg (IV) direct into the vein or as a rapid bolus. The injection site needs to be closest to heart
- *Adverse drug reactions:* Facial flushing, nausea, bronchospasm, light-headedness, headache, and seizures
- *Contraindication:* Second and third degree AV block, sick sinus syndrome (SSS)
- *Caution:* Asthma child on digoxin or verapamil. Each IV bolus should be followed by a rapid 5–10 mL saline flush.

AMIODARONE HYDROCHLORIDE

It is an antiarrhythmic agent.

Brand names: Cordarone X and Eurythmic

- *Available as:* Tablet 200 mg; Injection 50 mg/mL
- *Indications:* Life-threatening ventricular arrhythmia; also refractory congestive cardiac failure (CCF)
- *Dose:* Oral dose: <1 year 10–20 mg/kg/24 hours in two divided doses for 10 days. Follow with 5–10 mg/kg/24 hours. After 1–4 weeks or control of arrhythmia, cut doses in half
- *Intravenous (IV) dose:* 5 mg/kg over 1 hour. Follow with continuous infusion of 5–15 µg/kg/min
- *Adverse drug reactions:* Proarrhythmias (bradyarrhythmias, tachyarrhythmias, or heart block), fatigue, malaise, nightmares, behavioral changes, hypothyroidism, hyperglycemia, slate blue color of skin, photosensitivity, rash, hepatotoxicity, pulmonary toxicity, photophobia, and thrombocytopenia
- *Monitoring:* Keep an eye on clinical signs and symptoms of toxicity; liver, lung, and thyroid function tests; chest X-ray, electrocardiograph ECG; and eye examination.

ATROPINE SULFATE

A muscarinic receptor antagonist that inhibits the effects of excessive vagal activation on the heart manifested as sinus bradycardia.

Brand name: Isopto
- *Available as:* 0.5 mg/mL
- *Indications:* Heart block (sinus bradycardia). Also, premedication (before surgery) to inhibit secretions and salivation, and organophosphate poisoning
- *Dose:* Sinus bradycardia 0.02 mg/kg IV
  - Premedication <5 kg 0.2 mg/kg 30 minutes preoperatively followed by q 4–6 hours
  - 5 kg 0.1–0.2 mg/kg/dose with a maximum of 0.4 mg/dose
  - Poisoning 0.02–0.05 mg/kg q 10–20 minutes until atropine effect manifested by tachycardia, mydriasis, and fever. Follow with q 1–4 hours for at least 24 hours
- *Adverse drug reactions:* Tachycardia, palpitations, delirium, ataxia, dry, hot skin, tremors, and impaired vision
- *Caution:* Avoid in narrow angle glaucoma, intestinal obstruction, tachycardia, and thyrotoxicosis.

DISOPYRAMIDE PHOSPHATE

A sodium-channel blocker, employed as an *antiarrhythmic medication* in the treatment of *ventricular tachycardia*. It has anticholinergic effect, contributing to adverse effects.

Brand names: Norpace, Regubeat, and Rhythmodan
- *Available as:* Capsule 100 mg, 150 mg; Injection 10 mg/mL

- *Indications:* Ventricular arrhythmias, and atrial tachyarrhythmias
- *Dose:*
  - *Oral:* 10–20 mg/kg/day in two divided doses
  - *Intravenous:* 5 mg/kg (loading). Follow with oral dose for maintenance
- *Adverse drug reactions:* Constipation, dizziness, malaise, blurring of vision, and cholestatic jaundice
- *Contraindications:* Second and third degree AV block and shock (cardiogenic)
- *Caution:* Avoid concurrent use of erythromycin and clarithromycin.

LIGNOCAINE HYDROCHLORIDE (LIDOCAINE HYDROCHLORIDE)

It is a class 1 antiarrhythmic drug.

Brand name: Xylocard

- *Available as:* Injection 21.33 mg/mL (2% 50 mL vial); Topical gel/ointment/aerosol spray
- *Indications:* Short-term control of ventricular arrhythmias, e.g., tachycardia, premature beats, fibrillation; also, for local anesthesia; and also, as local anesthesia
- *Dose:* 1 mg/kg/dose, IV bolus q 5 minutes up to a maximum of 5 mg/kg (total dose). This should be followed by IV infusion of 10–50 µg/kg/min, not exceeding maximum dose of 5 mg/kg/day
- *Adverse drug reactions:* Nausea, vomiting, arrhythmias, heart block, lethargy, coma, seizures, blurring of vision, paresthesia, diplopia, and rash
- *Caution:* Avoid concurrent use of epinephrine preparation.

PHENYTOIN SODIUM (DIPHENYLHYDANTOIN SODIUM)

It is a sodium-channel protein inhibitor.

- *Indications:* Ventricular tachyarrhythmia (digoxin-induced in particular). Also, epilepsy and IV infusion in status epilepticus.
- *Dose for ventricular tachyarrhythmia (usually from digoxin):* 1.25 mg/kg (IV) every 5 minutes up to a total of 15 mg/kg or until arrhythmia is controlled or development of hypotension. Follow with a maintenance dosed of 5–10 mg/kg/day in two divided doses. Total loading dose must not exceed 1.5 g.
- For remaining details, *see* Chapter 11 (Anticonvulsants).

PROCAINAMIDE

Brand names: Pronestyl and Procan

- *Available as:* Tablet 250 mg; Injection 100 mg/mL (0 mL vial)
- *Indications:* Ventricular tachycardia, premature ventricular contractions, paroxysmal atrial tachycardia, and atrial fibrillation
- *Dose:* Loading dose 3–6 mg/kg/dose (IV) over 5 minutes with a maximum of 100 mg/dose. Repeat q 5–1 minutes if needed with a max of 15 mg/kg total dose. Follow with a maintenance dose of 15–50 mg/kg/24 hours (PO) q 3–6 hours; 20–30 mg/kg/24 hours with a maximum of 4 g/24 hours; continuous IV infusion of 20–80 µg/min with a maximum of 2 g/24 hours
- *Adverse drug reactions:* Hypotension, arrhythmias, AV block, confusion, agranulocytosis, Coombs-positive hemolytic anemia, systemic lupus erythematosus (SLE)-like syndrome, fever, and rash

- *Contraindications:* Heart block, myasthenia gravis
- *Drug interactions:* Cimetidine, β-agonists, and anticholinergic agents
- *Monitoring:* Maintain procainamide concentration 4–10 μg/mL (therapeutic) and 10–30 mg/mL
- *Caution:* Watch for positive antinuclear antibody reaction and general cardiodepression.

PROPRANOLOL HYDROCHLORIDE

It is a sodium-channel blocker.

Brand names: Ciplar and Inderal

- *Indications:* Tachyarrhythmias. Also, hypertension, hypercyanotic spells of Fallot tetralogy (both preventive and therapeutic); infantile tremor syndrome; coronary heart disease; migraine; and hyperthyroidism
- *Available as:* Tablet 10 mg, 40 mg, 80 mg; Injection 1 mg/mL
- *Dose:*
  - 0.15–0.25 mg/kg/dose (IV) for hypercyanotic spells
  - 0.5–1 mg/kg/day (PO) in divided doses for arrhythmia and prevention of hypercyanotic spells
  - 2 mg/kg/day (PO) q 6 hours in hyperthyroidism
- *Adverse drug reactions:* Vomiting, diarrhea, fever, hypotension, bradycardia, cardiac failure, rash, and laryngospasm
- *Caution:* Poor cardiac reserve, CCF, general anesthesia, clonidine therapy. In ischemic heart disease (IHD), it should not be withdrawn abruptly
- *Contraindications:* Second or third degree heart block, bronchospasm, acidosis, prolonged fasting, and verapamil therapy.

QUINIDINE SULFATE

It is a myocardial depressant.

Brand name: Quinidine
- *Available as:* Tablet 200 mg; Injection 80 mg/mL
- *Indications:* Arrhythmias (supraventricular tachycardia, paroxysmal ventricular tachycardia, and premature atrial/ventricular contractions)
- *Dose:* Test dose 2 mg/kg. Then 30 mg/kg/day (PO) q 6 hours
- *Adverse drug reactions:* Syncope, hypotension, heart block, fever, abdominal discomfort, bone marrow depression, thrombocytopenia, widened QRS complexes, and long Q-T interval
- *Drug interactions:* Verapamil, cimetidine, phenytoin, phenobarbital, digoxin, and rifampicin
- *Contraindications:* Hypotension, CCF, and heart block.

VERAPAMIL

It is a calcium-channel blocker, and it is more effective than digoxin in controlling ventricular rate.

Brand names: Isoptin, Veramil, Voratril, and Voraprim
- *Available as:* Tablet 40 mg, 80 mg; Injection 2.5 mg/mL (2 mL ampule)
- *Indication:* PSVT, atrial fibrillation, and atrial flutter. Also hypertension, including hypertensive crisis
- *Doses:*
  - Infants 4–8 mg/kg/day (PO) in three divided doses
  - 0.1–0.2 mg/kg (IV) over 2 minutes
  - Children 0.1–0.3 mg/kg (IV) over 2 minutes
  - A continuous ECG monitoring and BP monitoring are mandatory

- *Adverse drug reactions:* Allergic reactions (urticaria, bronchospasm, swelling face, lips and tongue, etc.)
- *Contraindications:* <2 years of age, cardiogenic shock, CCF (uncomplicated), and AV block
- *Caution:* Avoid in liver damage and with β-blockers. If the child is on disopyramide, it should not be given 48 hours before and 24 hours after verapamil.

15
Chapter

Antihistaminic Drugs

INTRODUCTION

Too much excretion of the chemical, histamine by the body's immune system causes allergic reactions that may manifest in varied ways such as urticaria, allergic rhinitis, etc.

Antihistaminic agents, antihistamines, or histamine antagonists are the medications that counter the effect of the histamine released during an allergic reaction by blocking the action of the histamine on the tissue. They do not stop the allergic reaction but protect tissues from some of its effects. The old or first generation antihistamines frequently cause some sedation (drowsiness) and dryness of mouth; infrequently, urinary retention and cardiac abnormalities may complicate. The so-called newer, second generation, or nonsedating antihistamines are considered relatively safer though somewhat less effective. Drowsiness, if at all, is mild. Adverse effects like dryness of mouth, drowsiness, urine retention (in males), and palpitations are infrequent.

ASTEMIZOLE

It is a second generation H1-receptor antagonist; long-acting and least-sedating.

Brand names: Acemiz, Astelong, and Stemiz
- *Available as:* Tablet 10 mg and suspension 10 mg/5 mL

- *Dose:* 0.2 mg/kg/day as a single dose on empty stomach as first thing in the morning.
- *Adverse drug reactions:* Very safe; drowsiness, if at all, is only slight.
- *Caution:* Avoid in children under 6 years of age.

AZATADINE MALEATE

Brand name: Zadine
- *Available as:* Tablet 1 mg and syrup 0.5 mg/5 mL
- *Dose:* 1–6 years: 0.25 mg BD
- *More than 6 years:* 0.5–1 mg BD
- *Caution:* Avoid in infants.

CETIRIZINE DIHYDROCHLORIDE

Brand names: Alerid, Allerzine, Cetriwal, Cetzine, Zyncet, and Zyrtec
- *Indications:* As an antiallergic; symptomatic treatment of perennial and seasonal rhinitis, urticaria
- *Available as:* Tablet 10 mg; syrup 5 mg/5 mL
- *Dose:* 2.5–5 mg for age group 2–6 years
- 5–10 mg for age group 6–12 years
- *Adverse drug reactions:* Drowsiness, dryness of mouth, headache, dizziness, agitation, gastrointestinal disturbance. Infrequently, aggressive reactions, seizures, somnolence, fatigue, arthralgia, diarrhea, bronchospasm, epistaxis, irritability, and insomnia
- *Contraindication:* Hypersensitivity to hydroxyzine, lactation
- *Caution:* Avoid in children <6 months (preferably <2 years), and renal and hepatic impairment.
- *Drug interaction:* Central nervous system (CNS) depressants.

CHLORPHENIRAMINE MALEATE

Brand name: Piriton
- *Available as:* Tablet 4 mg; syrup 2.5 mg/5 mL; injection 10 mg, 100 mg/mL
- *Dose:* 0.35 mg/kg/day (PO and SC) in four divided doses. Also, it may be given as a single stat dose and for prolonged action 0.2 mg/kg (PO).
- *Adverse drug reactions:* Drowsiness.

CLEMASTINE FUMARATE

Brand names: Clamist, Tavegyl, and Tavist
- *Indications:* Allergy, especially pertaining to conjunctiva and skin; allergic rhinitis
- *Available as:* Tablets 1 mg, 1.34 mg; syrup 0.67, 0.5 mg/5 mL
- *Dose:*
   - 2–6 years 0.05 mg/kg/day q BD or TDS
   - 6–12 years 0.5 mg/dose q BD
   - >12 years 1 mg/dose q BD
- *Adverse drug reactions:* Dryness of mouth, constipation, drowsiness, headache, and dizziness
- *Contraindications:* Narrow angle glaucoma and bladder-neck obstruction
- *Caution:* Avoid in infants and children <2 years.

CYPROHEPTADINE HCL

Brand names: Ciplactin, Ciproval, Periactin, Peritol, and Practin
- *Indications:* Antiallergic (urticaria and hay fever); also, appetite stimulant; migraine prophylaxis
- *Available as:* Tablet 4 mg; syrup 2 mg/5 mL
- *Dose:* 0.25 mg/kg/day in three or four divided doses
   - *More than 6 years:* 0.5–1 mg BD

Chapter 15: Antihistaminic Drugs

- *Adverse drug reactions:* Drowsiness, nausea, dry mouth, paradoxical excitement, gastritis, hypotension, dizziness, anticholinergic effects, and blood dyscrasias.
- *Contraindications:* Glaucoma, asthma, urinary retention, lactation; neonatal period; concurrent with monoamine oxidase (MAO) inhibitors
- *Caution:* Avoid in asthma, hypertension, high intraocular tension, hyperthyroidism, hypertension, cardiovascular disease.

DESLORATADINE

A tricyclic H1-antihistamine, a major active metabolite of loratadine; long-acting, and nonsedating.

Brand names: Claridin, Cozy, Deslor, D-Loratidine and Lorfast

- *Available as:* Tablet 5 mg
- *Indications:* Allergic rhinitis; an emerging indication is acne.
- *Dose:*
    - 1–5 years 1 g OD
    - 6–11 years 2.5 mg OD
    - >12 years 5 mg OD
- *Adverse drug reactions:* Dry mouth, fatigue, headache, gastrointestinal upset (especially vomiting); infrequently, slight drowsiness.

DIMETHINDENE MALEATE

Brand name: Foristal

- *Indications:* Allergic states such as allergic dermatoses, pruritic and ocular allergies
- *Available as:* Tablet 1 and 2.5 mg (sustained action)
- *Dose:* 1 mg TDS. 2.5 mg BD

- *Adverse drug reactions:* Drowsiness and dryness of mouth.
- *Contraindications:* Epilepsy, vulnerability to urinary retention, and lactation.
- *Caution:* Avoid in children <6 years.

DIPHENHYDRAMINE HCL

Brand name: Benadryl

- *Indications:* Antiallergic, sedative; antidote in phenothiazine toxicity/idiosyncrasy
- *Available as:* Capsule 25 mg, 50 mg; elixir 12.5 mg/5 mL
- *Dose:* 5 (4–6) mg/kg/day in three to four divided doses
- *Adverse drug reactions:* Drowsiness, dryness of mouth, nausea, and nervousness; very infrequently thrombocytopenia
- *Drug interaction:* CNS depressants (including alcohol)
- *Contraindications:* Asthma, narrow-angle glaucoma, obstructive urinary tract, and gastrointestinal conditions.
- *Caution:* Lactation, myasthenia gravis; avoid driving/handling machinery.

FEXOFENADINE

Brand name: Allegra

- *Indications:* Allergic rhinitis and dermatological conditions
- *Available as:* Tablets 120 and 180 mg; Suspension 30 mg/5 mL
- *Dose:* Less than 12 years 30 mg BD. More than 12 years 60 mg BD.
- *Adverse drug reactions:* Drowsiness, dryness of mouth, throat and nose, headache, dizziness, nausea, tachycardia, palpitations, fatigue, diarrhea, backache, dyspnea, taste disturbance, menstrual problems, and anaphylactoid reactions.

- *Drug interaction:* Antacids containing aluminum or magnesium, erythromycin, ketoconazole, and fruit juices.
- *Contraindication:* Lactation.

HYDROXYZINE HCL

Brand name: Atarax
- *Indications:* Pruritus, urticaria, dermatoses; premedication in surgery
- *Available as:* Tablet 10 and 25 mg; Syrup 10 mg/5 mL; Drops 6 mg/mL. Injection 25 mg/mL.
- *Dose:* 2 mg/day (PO) q 6 hours. <1 year 0.5–1 mg/kg/dose (IM) q 4–6 hours.
- *Adverse drug reactions:* Drowsiness, anticholinergic effect, involuntary motor activity at high doses.
- *Drug interaction:* CNS depressants (including alcohol) and coumarin anticoagulants.
- *Contraindication:* Lactation
- *Caution:* Avoid under the age of 1 year when it may be precipitative acute porphyria and cause electrocardiogram abnormalities.

KETOTIFEN

Brand name: Ketasma
- *Available as:* Tablet 1 mg
- *Indications:* Allergic rhinitis, allergic conjunctivitis, and allergic bronchial asthma for prophylaxis
- *Dose:* 0.5 mg BD. Gradually, the dose should be built up to 1–2 mg BD.
- *Adverse drug reactions:* Drowsiness, dizziness, dryness of mouth, impaired reactions; very infrequently cystitis, hepatitis, and seizures.

- *Drug interaction:* CNS depressants (including alcohol)
- *Contraindication:* Lactation
- *Caution:* The drug should be taken after food. Avoid in epileptic subjects.

LEVOCETIRIZINE

Levo form of cetirizine, more potent and longer-acting with minimal sedation.

Brand names: L-cetrizet, Levocet, Teczine, and Xyzal
- *Indications:* Seasonal and perennial allergic rhinitis; chronic urticaria
- *Available as:* Tablet 5 mg
- *Dose:*
  - <6 years 0.125 mg/kg/day OD
  - >6 years 2.5 OD
- *Adverse drug reactions:* Somnolence, dryness of mouth, fatigue, rhinitis, arthralgia, and migraine
- *Caution:* Avoid in children <6 years.

LORATADINE

Brand names: Lorfast, Loridin, and Lorin
- *Available as:* Tablet 10 mg; syrup 5 mg/5 mL
- *Indications:* H1-receptor antagonist antihistamine, indicated in treatment of allergic symptoms
- *Dose:* Weight <30 kg—5 mg/day. Weight >30 kg—10 mg/day
- *Adverse drug reactions:* Somnolence, headache, depression, anxiety, and easy fatigability
- *Contraindications:* <3 years
- *Caution:* Avoid combining with agents inhibiting hepatic enzymes. Else, prolonged QT interval may develop.

METHDILAZINE HCL

Brand name: Dilosyn
- *Available as:* Tablet 8 mg; syrup 4 mg/5 mL; injection 22.5 mg/mL
- *Indications:* Allergy, pruritus, and neurodermatitis.
- *Adverse drug reactions:* Drowsiness, CNS stimulation, impaired alertness, seizures, hypotension, arrhythmias, and gastrointestinal and genitourinary upset.
- *Drug interaction:* Levodopa, CNS depressants, MAO inhibitors, phenothiazines, adrenaline, and thiazide diuretics.
- *Contraindications:* Dehydration, coma, concomitant high-dose antidepressants, levodopa; jaundice; avoid in children <3 years.
- *Caution:* Narrow angle glaucoma, obstructive gastrointestinal and genitourinary conditions, and lactation.

PHENIRAMINE MALEATE

Brand names: Avil and Avil retard
- *Available as:* Tablet 25, 50, and 75 mg; injection 22.75 mg/mL
- *Indications:* Allergy, allergic dermatitis, common cold, insect bite; emergency allergic disorders, anaphylactic shock, severe angioneurotic edema
- *Dose:* 1–5 mg/kg/day (PO and IM)
- *Adverse drug reactions:* Sedation, anticholinergic effects, blurred vision, agranulocytosis, increased ICP, muscle weakness, rarely, hemolytic anemia.
- *Drug interactions:* Anticholinergics (atropine), alcohol, MAO inhibitors, and CNS depressants.

PROMETHAZINE HCL

Brand name: Phenergan
- *Available as:* Tablet 10 and 25 mg; syrup 5 mg/5 mL; injection 25 mg/mL
- *Indications:* Vomiting, motion sickness, and mild sedation for a procedure.
- *Dose:* Vomiting 0.5 mg/kg/dose (PO, IM, IV, and PR) q 4–6 hours.
- Motion sickness 0.5 mg/kg/dose (PO) 30 minutes prior to beginning of travel.
- *Adverse drug reactions:* Drowsiness, dizziness, disorientation, dryness of mouth, photosensitivity, excitation, seizures, gastrointestinal upset, blurred vision, blood dyscrasia, jaundice, agranulocytosis, hypo-/hypertension, and severe tissue injury from intravenous (IV) injection.
- *Drug interaction:* CNS depressants, anticholinergics, MAO inhibitors, and alcohol.
- *Caution:* Bronchitis, hypertensive crisis, epilepsy, glaucoma, impaired respiratory, renal or hepatic function, obstructive gastrointestinal or urinary tract conditions, and bone marrow depression.

PSEUDOEPHEDRINE

Brand name: Sudafed
- *Available as:* Tablet 60 mg; syrup 30 mg/5 mL
- *Indications:* As decongestant in URI
- *Dose:* Less than 12 years, 4 mg/kg/day q 6–8 hours. More than 12 years 30–60 mg/dose q 6–8 hours.
- *Adverse drug reactions:* CNS stimulation, insomnia, nervousness, excitability, palpitations, and fixed drug eruption.

- *Drug interaction:* MAO inhibitors, antacids, and kaolin.
- *Contraindications:* Diabetes, cardiovascular disease, uncontrolled hypertension, and pregnancy.
- *Precaution:* Avoid concomitant use of MAO inhibitors to cut down risk of hypertensive reactions including hypertensive crisis.
- *Special remarks:* The use of pseudoephedrine in the pharmacological industry is now discouraged on account of its abuse as a CNS stimulant (like amphetamine and dexedrine).

TERFENADINE

Brand name: Terfed

- *Available as:* Tablets 60 and 120 mg; Suspension 30 mg/5 mL
- *Indications:* An antihistaminic employed for symptomatic treatment of perianal and seasonal allergies, especially, allergic rhinitis; less sedation than with earlier antihistamines.
- *Dose:*
  - 3–6 years—30 mg/day in two divided doses
  - 6–12 years—60 mg/day in two divided doses
  - Adolescents—120 mg/day in two divided doses
- *Adverse drug reactions:* Dry mouth, muscle cramps, syncope, tremors, sweating, abdominal pain, dyspepsia, headache, dizziness, gastrointestinal upset, rash, alopecia, anaphylaxis, angioedema, palpitations, visual disturbances, bronchospasm, paresthesia, ventricular arrhythmias in high doses in cases with hepatic dysfunction, dyselectrolytemia, or QT prolongation.
- *Contraindications:* Liver and heart disease, concomitant use of such drugs as macrolides, ketoconazole, or itraconazole.
- *Caution:* Ventricular arrhythmias, electrolyte disturbances, and hepatic impairment.

TRIPROLIDINE HYDROCHLORIDE

An anticholinergic antihistamine. Quick-acting decongestant.

Brand name: Actifed

- *Available as:* Combination with paracetamol and phenylpropanolamine. Tablet 2.5 mg; syrup 0.265 mg/5 mL
- *Indications:* Nasal congestion and flu-like symptoms
  - *Dose:* 6 months–4 years, 0.3 mg/dose QID; 4–6 years 0.9 mg dose QID 6–12 years, 1.25 mg/dose, QD (maximum 10 mg/daily)
- *Adverse drug reactions:* Drowsiness, agitation
- *Caution:* Avoid driving and swimming.
- *Contraindications:* Glaucoma, hyperthyroidism, hypertension, and chronic constipation.

16 Antihypertensive Drugs

INTRODUCTION

Hypertension is defined as a hike in blood pressure. In other words, the force of blood circulation pushing against the walls of the blood vessels is consistently very high. High blood pressure causes harm by increasing the workload of the heart and blood vessels with reduced efficiency. With passage of time, the delicate tissues inside the arteries get damaged. In the damaged vasculature, low-density lipoprotein (LDL) *cholesterol* forms plaque along tiny tears in the artery walls, (*atherosclerosis*). Eventually, hypertension causes varied insults to heart and other systems, the most glaring being fibrillations, myocardial infarction, and stroke.

The most important and most widely used antihypertensive drugs are thiazide diuretics, calcium-channel blockers, angiotensin-converting enzyme (ACE) inhibitors, angiotensin-II receptor blockers (ARBs) and β-blockers. They achieve the blood pressure-lowering effect through varying mechanisms.

AMILORIDE

A potassium-sparing and sodium-channel blocker, amiloride works by directly blocking the epithelial sodium channel (ENaC), thereby inhibiting sodium reabsorption in the late distal convoluted tubules, connecting tubules, and collecting ducts in the nephron.

Brand names: Amitru, Biduret, Furosemide, Lasride, and Midamor

- *Available as:* Typically, in combination with a loop diuretic or thiazide diuretic
  Tablets: Amiloride 5 mg + Furosemide 40 mg (Lasride)
  Tablets: Amiloride 2.5 mg + Hydrochlorothiazide 25 mg (Biduret)
- *Indications:* Adjunctive therapy with thiazides in hypertension, congestive cardiac failure (CCF)
- *Dose:* 0.5–0.6 mg/kg/day as a single dose or in two divided doses.
- *Adverse drug reactions:* Nausea, vomiting, abdominal discomfort, flatulence, anorexia, hyperkalemia, and hyponatremia.
- *Contraindications*: Hyperkalemia, hyponatremia, poor renal function, and Addison's disease
- *Caution*: Avoid simultaneous use of aspirin and aceclofenac.

AMLODIPINE

A calcium-channel blocker.

Brand names: Amlopres and Amlosun

- *Available as*: Tablet 2.5 mg, 5 mg, and 10 mg
- *Indications:* First-line treatment either as monotherapy or in combination with thiazide-type diuretics, ACE inhibitors, or angiotensin-II receptor antagonists for all patients regardless of age.
- *Dose:* 0.05–0.5 mg/kg/day as a single dose or in two divided doses daily.

Chapter 16: Antihypertensive Drugs

- *Adverse drug reactions:* Dizziness, fatigue, abdominal pain, nausea, flushing; rarely jaundice from hepatotoxicity.
- *Caution*: Avoiding to get up too fast from a sitting or lying position. Else the patient may feel dizzy.

ATENOLOL

An adrenergic receptor antagonist (β-blocker)

Brand names: Altol, Aten, Tenolol, and Ziblok
- *Available as:* Tablet 25 mg, 5 mg, and 100 mg
- *Dose:* 0.5–2 mg/kg/day (PO) OD
- *Adverse drug reactions:* Hypotension, bradycardia, headache, wheezing, CCF, angina, Raynaud's phenomenon, arthralgia, peripheral neuropathy, and diabetes.
- *Contraindications:* Asthma, CCF, bradycardia, heart block, and peripheral arterial disease.

CAPTOPRIL

It is an ACE inhibitor.

Brand names: Aceten, Agiepril, and Acetein
- *Indications:* Hypertension (especially renovascular), CCF, angina
- *Available as:* Tablet 25 mg
- *Dose:* 0.1–0.4 mg/kg/day 1 to 4 times daily. Increase by increments to 2.0 mg/kg/day (maximum).
- *Adverse drug reactions:* Bradycardia, hypotension, neutropenia, due to hemopoietic depression, proteinuria, nephrotic syndrome, hyperkalemia, dysgeusia causing feeding difficulties, rash, abdominal pain, nausea, and vomiting.
- *Caution:* Avoid concomitant use of indomethacin, ibuprofen, potassium, and diuretics.

CLONIDINE HYDROCHLORIDE

It is a centrally acting α-agonist hypotensive agent.

Brand names: Arkamin, Catapres, Cloneon, and Clonid
- *Indications:* Essential and secondary hypertension; also attention-deficit/hyperactivity disorder (ADHD).
- *Available as:* Tablet 100 µg
- *Dose:* 5–10 µg/kg/day
- *Adverse drug reactions:* Dry mouth, drowsiness, constipation, sleep disturbances, impotence, allergic manifestations, and rebound hypertension with sudden stoppage of therapy.
- *Caution:* (i) Avoid concomitant use of tranquilizers, sedatives, and alcohol-containing preparation, (ii) Restrict activity involving risk of accidents, and (iii) Initiation and termination of therapy should be gradual as sudden withdrawal can cause rebound hypertension.
- *Contraindication:* Sick sinus syndrome (SSS).

DIAZOXIDE

A benzothiadiazine derivative and a peripheral vasodilator used for hypertensive emergencies and refractory hypoglycemia. By a potassium-channel activation, it causes local relaxation in smooth muscles of blood vessels.

Brand names: Eudemine and Hyperstat
- *Indications:* Hypertensive crisis and refractory hypoglycemia
- *Available as:* Tablet 15 mg. Injection 15 mg/mL (300 mg/20 mL ampule)
- *Dose:* 8–15 mg/kg/dose (PO) q 8–12 hours, 4–5 mg/kg/dose (IV). If no response, repeat after half an hour.
- *Adverse drug reactions:* Burning at injection site, transient tachycardia, hypotension, weight gain, and edema.

DILTIAZEM

It is a calcium-channel blocker.

Brand names: Angizem and Cardizem
- *Available as:* Tablet 30, 60, 90, and 120 mg
- *Indication:* Hypertension (especially low-renin type); angina, supraventricular tachycardia (SVT), atrial fibrillation/flutter; migraine.
- *Dose:* 1.5–2 mg/kg/day in two or three divided doses.
- *Adverse drug reactions:* Dizziness, weakness, headache, nausea, and rash.
- *Contraindications:* SSS and atrioventricular (AV) block.
- *Drug interaction:* β-blockers *and* quinidine.
- *Caution:* Avoid chewing or crushing the tablet.

ENALAPRIL MALEATE

It is an ACE inhibitor.

Brand names: Enalapril and Minipril
- *Available as:* Tablet 2.5, 5, 10, and 20 mg
- *Dose:* 0.1–0.5 mg/kg/day (PO) q 12–24 hours with a maximum of 40 mg/day.
- *Contraindications:* Outflow obstruction, aortic stenosis, and renal artery stenosis (bilateral).

EPLERENONE

It is an aldosterone-receptor blocker.

Brand names: Eplecard, Eperenone, and Eptus
- *Available as*: Tablet 25 and 50 mg
- *Dose*: 0.5 mg/kg/day (PO) as a single dose. Depending on response, dose may be gradually increased to 1 mg/kg.

- *Adverse drug reactions*: Postural hypertension, gynecomastia, hyperkalemia, hyperglyceridemia, and atrial fibrillation.
- *Caution*: Avoid in children, except adolescents.

GUANETHIDINE SULFATE

Brand name: Ismelin
- *Indication:* Hypertension including renal hypertension
- *Available as:* Tablet 10 and 25 mg
- *Dose:* 0.2 mg/kg/day in one or two doses
- *Adverse drug reactions:* Hypotension (postural), syncope after excretion, rising blood urea nitrogen (BUN), diarrhea, and retrograde ejaculation.
- *Contraindications:* Pheochromocytoma and recent attack of myocardial infarction.

HYDRALAZINE HYDROCHLORIDE

Brand names: Apresoline, Nepresol, and Zinepress
- *Indications:* Hypertension including renal and essential types
- *Available as:* Tablet 10, 25, and 100 mg; Injection 20 mg/1 mL ampule.
- *Dose:* 0.75 mg/kg/day (PO) in four to six divided doses; 0.15 mg/kg/dose (IM and IV)
- *Adverse drug reactions:* Tachycardia, anorexia, sweating, palpitations, headache, nausea, vomiting, dizziness, and rheumatoid and lupus-like syndromes. Nasal congestion, flushing, lacrimation, conjunctivitis, paresthesia, edema, tremors, muscle cramps, rash, fever, polyneuritis, angina, anemia, and gastrointestinal tract (GI) bleeding occur less frequently.

- *Contraindications:* Systemic lupus erythematosus (SLE), porphyria, and mitral valve stenosis/regurgitation (rheumatic).

LABETALOL

Brand names: Normadate, Lobet, and Trandate
- *Available as:* Tablet/capsule 50, 100, 200, and 400 mg; injection 5 mg/mL.
- *Indications:* Hypertension including hypertensive crisis.
- *Dose:*
  - *Hypertension:* 5–10 mg/kg/day (PO) q 12 hours
  - *Hypertensive crisis:* 0.25–1 mg/kg/dose (IV). After 5 minutes, the same dose needs to be repeated.
  - 0.4–3 mg/kg/h as continuous IV infusion
- *Adverse drug reactions:* Urinary retention, hypotension, congestive heart failure (CHF), and AV conduction defects.
- *Caution:* Avoid in coexisting asthma, hypoglycemia state, and CCF.

METHYLDOPA

Brand names: Aldomet and Emdopa
- *Available as:* Tablet 125, 250, and 500 mg; injection 50 mg/mL.
- *Indications:* Hypertension
- *Dose:* 10 mg/kg/day (PO) in divided doses, increasing to the maximum of 65 mg/kg/day, if need be, at 2 days or more intervals.
  20–40 mg/kg/day (IV) for hypertensive crisis
- *Adverse drug reactions:* Hepatotoxicity, dizziness, headache, drowsiness, irritability, emotional lability, orthostatic hypotension, dark urine (due to Coombs' positive hemolytic anemia), nasal stuffiness, fever, and GIT upset.

- *Contraindications:* Mental depression, when monoamine oxidase (MAO) inhibitors are being administered, liver dysfunction, and pheochromocytoma.

METOPROLOL

Brand names: Betaloc, Cardibeta, Metapro, and Meteor
- *Available as*: Tablet 12.5, 25, and 50 mg
- *Indications*: Hypertension. Also, hypercyanotic spells in tetralogy of Fallot.
- *Dose*:
  - *Hypertension:* 1–4 mg/kg/day (PO) with maximum of 6 mg/kg/day in two divided doses.
  - *Hypercyanotic spells:* 0.1 mg/kg over 1–2 minutes. Repeat after 5–10 minutes, if required.
- *Adverse drug reactions:* Dizziness, fatigue, confusion, depression, bronchospasm, and bradycardia.

MINOXIDIL

It is a direct-action peripheral vasodilator.

Brand names: Gromane, Loniten, and Minitop
- *Available as:* Tablet 2.5, 5, and 10 mg. Topical solution (2% and 5%).
- *Indications:* Severe hypertension that fails to respond to maximum therapeutic doses of a diuretic and two other antihypertensive drugs; baldness.
- *Dose:* 0.2 mg/kg/day as a single dose (PO). Followed by stepwise increase to 0.25–1 mg/kg/day.
  - Topical sol is required to be applied generously to the affected scalp area at bedtime daily for 3–6 months for effective outcome.
- *Adverse drug reactions:* Hypertrichosis and pericardial effusion.

NIFEDIPINE

Brand names: Calcigard, Calcigard retard, Depin, and Depin retard

- *Available as:*
  - Capsule 5 and 10 mg
  - Retard (sustained-release) Tablet 20 mg
- *Indication:* Hypertensive crisis
- *Dose:* 0.2–0.5 mg/dose (PO) every 4–6 hours; 3–5 mg/kg/dose (sublingual) for severe hypertension.
- *Adverse drug reactions:* Headache, dizziness, flushes, tachycardia, edema, rash, fatigue, increased micturition, fatigue, tremors, paresthesia, cramps, gingival hyperplasia, visual disturbances, GI upset (nausea and vomiting), hepatic dysfunction; rarely ischemic pain.
- *Drug interaction:* Antihypertensives, β-blockers, diltiazem, digoxin, cimetidine, quinidine, rifampicin, anticonvulsants (phenobarbital, phenytoin, and carbamazepine), antibiotics (erythromycin and clarithromycin), antiasthmatics (theophylline, terbutaline, salbutamol), and anticoagulants.
- *Contraindications:* Cardiogenic shock, severe aortic stenosis, lactation, and porphyria.
- *Caution:* Avoid its concomitant use with large dose of β-blockers and in diabetes mellitus, and CCF.
- *Special remarks:* Though widely employed, in the wake of possibility of a sudden and high reduction in blood pressure, it is no longer favored in hypertensive emergencies.

NITROPRUSSIDE

Brand names: Nipress, Pruside, and Sonide
Available as: Injection 50 mg/mL

- *Indication*: Hypertensive crisis. Also, acute heart failure, induction, and maintenance of controlled hypotension during anesthesia in surgery, cerebral vasospasm following subarachnoid hemorrhage.
- *Dose:* 0.3–0.5 µg/kg/min (IV) with a maximum of 0.8 µg/kg/min
- *Adverse drug reactions*: Hypotension and cyanide toxicity.
- *Contraindications*: Coarctation of aorta, hypotension, and arteriovenous shunt.
- *Caution*: Evaluate blood pressure (BP) for at least 5 minutes before titrating to a higher or lower dose to achieve the desired BP; monitor BP during IV infusion.

PHENOXYBENZAMINE

Brand name: Dibenzyline
- A reversible nonselective α-adrenergic blocker
- *Available as*: Capsule 10 mg
- *Indication*: Hypertension associated with pheochromocytoma
- *Dose:* 0.2 mg/kg/dose (PO) BD
- *ADR*: Orthostatic hypotension.

PHENTOLAMINE

A reversible nonselective α-adrenergic blocker.

Brand names: Fentanar and Regitine
- *Available as:* Injection 10 mg/mL
- *Indications*: Hypertensive crisis, most notably during pheochromocytoma surgery
- *Dose*: 0.05–0.1 mg/kg/dose
- *Adverse drug reactions*: Orthostatic hypotension.

Chapter 16: Antihypertensive Drugs

PRAZOSIN HYDROCHLORIDE

It is an α-1 blocker.

Brand names: Minipress, Prazocip XI, and Prazopress
- *Available as*: Tablet 2.5 and 5 mg
- *Indications:* Hypertension and acute severe heart failure. Also, in autonomic crisis in scorpion sting.
- *Dose:* 0.1 mg/kg/dose every 6 hours.
- *Adverse drug reactions:* Remarkable hypotension, fatigue, unconsciousness, syncope, and priapism
- *Contraindication*: Known allergy to the drug.
- *Caution*: Avoid concomitant use of other drugs likely to cause hypotension to safeguard against cumulative effect.

PROPRANOLOL

It is a β-blocker.

Brand names: Betabloc, Ciplar, and Inderal
- *Indications:* Hypertension, cyanotic spells of Fallot tetralogy; infantile tremor syndrome; coronary heart disease; migraine; hyperthyroidism
- *Available as:* Tablet 10 mg, 40 mg, 80 mg; Injection 1 mg/1 mile
- *Dose:*
  - 0.5–1 mg/kg/day in two to four divided doses for hypertension
  - 0.15–0.25 mg/kg/dose (IV) for cyanotic spells
  - 0.5–1 mg/kg/day (PO) in divided doses for arrhythmia
  - 2 mg/kg/day (PO) q 6 hours in hyperthyroidism
- *Adverse drug reactions:* Vomiting, diarrhea, fever, hypotension, bradycardia, cardiac failure, rash, and laryngospasm

- *Caution:* Poor cardiac reserve, CCF, general anesthesia, and clonidine therapy. In ischemic heart disease (IHD), it should not be withdrawn abruptly.
- *Contraindications:* Second or third degree heart block, bronchospasm, acidosis, prolonged fasting, and verapamil therapy.

RAMIPRIL

It is an ACE-inhibitor.

Brand names: Cardace, Cardiopril, Ramihart, and Ramipres
- *Available as:* Tablet 1.25, 2.5, 5, and 10 mg
- *Indications:* Hypertension; also, CCF.
- *Dose:* 0.05 mg/kg OD.
- *Adverse drug reactions:* Nausea, fatigue, light-headedness, chest pain, bradycardia, and hyperkalemia.
- *Contraindications:* ACE-inhibitor allergy, and pregnancy.
- *Caution:* Avoid in children; may use in adolescents.

RESERPINE

It is an indole alkaloid, used as antihypertensive and antipsychotic.

Brand name: Serpasil
- *Dose:* 0.07 mg/kg/dose (IM) for acute hypertension as in acute nephritis; 0.02 mg/kg/day (PO) in three to four divided doses for chronic hypertension.
- *Adverse drug reactions:* Nasal stuffiness, flushing, drowsiness, bradycardia, depression, and diarrhea.

SODIUM NITROPRUSSIDE

It is a vasodilator.

Chapter 16: Antihypertensive Drugs

Brand names: Nipride and Sonide
- *Available as:* Injection 50 mg/mL in 2 mL vial. Dry powder needs to be dissolved in 5% dextrose.
- *Indication:* Hypertensive crisis
- *Dose:* 0.5–8.0 µg/kg/min. If we dissolve 50 mg in an L of 5% dextrose solution, a concentration of 5 µg/mL is obtained.
- *Adverse drug reactions:* Hypothyroidism, thiocyanate production.

VERAPAMIL

Brand names: Isoptin, Veramil, Voratril, and Voraprin
- *Available as:* Injection 2 mL vial
- *Indication:* Hypertensive crisis
- *Dose:*
  - *Hypertension:* 2–4 mg/kg/day (PO) q 8 hours
  - *Hypertensive crisis:* 0.15 mg/kg (IV) as loading (bolus) dose followed by 0.005 mg (5 µg)/kg/min as infusion. If we dissolve 5 mg in 100 mL of 5% dextrose, a concentration of 5 µg/mL is obtained. A continuous electrocardiogram (ECG) monitoring and BP monitoring are mandatory.
- *Contraindications:* <2 years of age, cardiogenic shock, CCF (uncomplicated), and AV block.
- *Caution:* Avoid in liver damage and with β-blockers.

Chapter 17

Antimyasthenic Drugs

INTRODUCTION

Myasthenia gravis is a chronic neuromuscular disease that has an autoimmune origin. It is characterized by weakness of the skeletal muscles. The subject's immune system produces antibodies that destroy or block many of the muscle receptor sites for neurotransmitter, acetylcholine. The left out few normal receptor sites are able to receive only limited signals, resulting in muscle weakness. Manifestations include difficulty in chewing, swallowing, speaking (slurring), making facial expression, and weakness of arms, legs, and neck muscles.

Antimyasthenics are the drugs used to treat myasthenia gravis, a rare disease characterized by weakness and early fatigue of muscles which are under voluntary control. The disease is caused by a breakdown in the normal communication between nerves and muscles at the neuromuscular junction.

EDROPHONIUM

Brand name: Tensilon

Available as: Injection 10 mg (ampule)

- *Indications:* Confirmation of diagnosis, differentiation of disease from cholinergic crisis, and treatment of disease

- *Dose:*
  - <12 months 0.1 mg (IV and IM) followed by 0.4 mg in case of poor response
  - >12 months 0.04 mg/kg/dose (IV and IM) followed by 0.16 mg/kg/dose in case of poor response after 1 minute with a maximum total dose of 5 mg for <30 kg and 10 mg for >30 kg weight
- *Adverse drug reactions:* Drowsiness, diaphresis, hypotension, arrhythmias, fasciculations, seizures, bronchospasm, laryngospasm, and cholinergic crisis
- *Contraindications:* Arrhythmias and gastrointestinal obstruction
- *Caution:* It is advisable to give a test dose for hypersensitivity. Atropine and resuscitation equipment needs to be kept ready to combat cholinergic crisis if it develops.

NEOSTIGMINE

Brand names: Myostigmin, Prostigmin, and Tilstigmin
- *Available as:* Tablet 15 mg; Injection 0.5 mg
- *Indications:* Treatment, reversal of nonpolarizing neuromuscular blocking agents
- *Dose:*
  - For diagnosis, 0.025–0.04 mg/kg (IM) as a single dose
  - For treatment, in neonates 0.05–0.1 mg, 15 minutes before giving feed. To start with parenteral route is recommended and then oral
  - For treatment in infants and children 2 mg/kg/24 hours q 3-4 hours (PO), 0.01–0.04 mg/kg/dose q 2-3 hours (IM, SC, and IV)
- *Adverse drug reactions:* Excessive salivation, mucous production and sweating, increased mucus, muscle

twitching, abdominal cramps, nausea, vomiting, diarrhea, dizziness/headache, rash, and increased micturition
- *Contraindications:* Urinary tract and intestinal obstruction
- *Caution:* Adjustment of dose in renal disease.

PYRIDOSTIGMINE

Brand names: Distinon, Mestinon, and Mustone
- *Available as:* Tablet 60 mg
- *Indications:* Treatment of myasthenia and reversal of nonpolarizing neuromuscular blocking agents
- *Dose:*
  - Infants born to mothers with myasthenia 0.05–0.15 mg/kg/dose
  - Children suffering from myasthenia 7 mg/kg/24 hours in five to six divided doses
- *Adverse drug reactions:* Headache, excessive salivation, bradycardia, meiosis, frequency of micturition, and seizures
- *Caution:* Keep atropine ready to counter muscarine adverse reactions.

18
Chapter
Antireflux Drugs

INTRODUCTION

The term, *gastroesophageal reflux (GER),* denotes retrograde movement of the acidic gastric contents into the esophagus as a result of laxity of the lower esophageal sphincter. This is a common physiological problem in neonates and infants in the first 6 months of life, usually responding to postural modification during and after feeding. When it persists with such symptoms as vomiting, abdominal discomfort, and failure to thrive, often causing such complications as recurrent respiratory infections and even asthma-like manifestations, it is called *gastroesophageal reflux disease (GERD).*

Though antacids may provide a temporary relief, dependable pharmacotherapy is through prokinetics, H_2-receptor antagonists, or proton-pump inhibitors.

PROKINETICS

For GERD subjects, especially with abdominal distention, heaviness, etc., prokinetics are of value. They facilitate relaxation of the lower esophageal sphincter and emptying of the gastric contents. They are best used in conjunction with H_2-receptor antagonists or proton pump inhibitors.

Domperidone

It is effective in GERD but not as much as metoclopramide. For details, *see* Chapter 13 (Antiemetic Drugs).

Metoclopramide

Among prokinetics, it is the best for GERD. For details, *see* Chapter 13 (Antiemetic Drugs).

H$_2$-ANTAGONISTS

H$_2$-antagonists, also called H$_2$-blockers, are a sort of antihistamines that block the action of histamine at the histamine H$_2$-receptors of the parietal cells in the stomach. As a result, the production of histamine and, therefore, acid in stomach is cut down. H$_2$-antagonists are employed in the treatment of GERD, reflux esophagitis and peptic ulcer, and for prevention of stress ulcers in systemic illnesses including sepsis. Earlier, they surpassed the antacids. In recent years, they are being surpassed by proton pump inhibitors (PPIs) that are found to be more effective at both healing and alleviating symptoms of ulcers and reflux esophagitis than the H$_2$-blockers.

Cimetidine

Brand name: Tagamet
- *Available as:* Tablet 200 mg
- *Indications:* For inhibiting gastric acid secretions; stress ulcers
- *Dose:* 20–40 mg/kg/day in divided doses, preferably with every meal
- *Adverse drug reactions (ADRs):* With limited experience in pediatric practice, none recorded so far. However, the likely side effects include constipation, diarrhea, headache, vertigo, drug rash, gynecomastia, confusion, arthralgia, muscle pain, and granulocytopenia
- *Drug interactions:* Antacids (containing Mg, Ca, and Al), sucralfate, theophylline, probenecid, warfarin, and cyclosporine

- *Contraindications:* Hypersensitivity to quinolones
- *Caution:* Avoid the drug 1-2 hours before and 4 hours after the antacids
  - Avoid with theophylline and nonsteroidal anti-inflammatory drugs (NSAIDs)
  - Avoid in epileptics
- *Caution:* In subjects with renal failure, the dose must be reduced.

Famotidine

It is a histamine-2 (H-2) receptor blocker that inhibits the gastric secretions; nine times more potent than cimetidine and 32 times more potent than ranitidine.

Brand names: Facid, Famocid, Famont, Famowal, Famtac, Fudone, and Topcid
- *Available as:* Tablet 20 mg, 40 mg. Suspension 40 mg/5 mL. Injection 10 mg/mL (2 mL ampule)
- *Indications:* Gastroesophageal reflux disease and gastric ulcers. Also, an adjunct in standard drug-resistant schizophrenia
- *Dose:* 0.4 mg/kg/day
- *ADRs:* Dizziness/headache and constipation/diarrhea
- *Caution:* Reduce dose in poor renal and hepatic function.

Ranitidine

Brand names: Ranitin, Ranitiget, and Ranial.
- *Available as:* Tablet 150 mg, 300 mg. Injection 25 mg/mL
- *Indications:* Gastric/duodenal ulcer, stress ulcer, reflux esophagitis
- *Dose:* 1-4 mg/kg/day (O, IM, and IV) in two to three divided doses

- *ADRs:* Impaired renal function
- *Contraindication:* Malignancy
- *Caution:* Reduce dose in poor renal and hepatic function. Avoid in patients with acute porphyria in whom it may precipitate attack.

PROTON PUMP INHIBITORS

Proton pump inhibitors are a class of drugs that target the terminal step (proton pump) in gastric acid production, causing irreversible inhibition of gastric acid secretions. A significant advance over H_2-antagonists, these agents need to be taken on empty stomach. Over and above therapy of gastric ulcers, these are effective in *H. pylori* infection.

Esomeprazole

Brand names: Esomac, Esotrax, and Nexpro
- *Available as:* Tablet 20 and 40 mg
- *Indications:* Treatment of GERD, esophagitis, and duodenal ulcer. Prevention of stress ulcers and NSAID-associated ulcers
- *Dose:* 0.5–0.8 mg/kg/day, single daily dose
- *ADRs:* Esomac, Esotrax, and Nexpro
- *Caution:* Avoid <1 year age.

Lansoprazole

Brand names: Esomac, Esotrax, and Nexpro
- *Available as:* Capsule 15 and 30 mg
- *Indications:* Treatment of GERD, esophagitis, and duodenal ulcer. Prevention of stress ulcers and NSAID-associated ulcers
- *Dose:* 0.5 mg/kg/day, single daily dose

- *ADRs:* Abdominal discomfort, constipation, dizziness, headache, and leukopenia
- *Caution:* Avoid <1 year of age.

Omeprazole

Brand names: Lomac, Lomicid, and Ocid
- *Available as:* Capsule 10 and 20 mg
- *Indications:* Treatment of GERD, esophagitis, and duodenal ulcer. Prevention of stress ulcers and NSAID-associated ulcers
- *Dose:* 0.5–0.7 mg/kg/day single daily dose
- *ADRs:* Abdominal discomfort, constipation, dizziness, headache, and leukopenia
- *Caution:* Avoid <2 years of age.

Pantaprazole

Brand names: Lippan, Pantocid, and Pantop
- *Available as:* Tablet/capsule 20 and 40 mg
- *Indications:* Treatment of GERD, esophagitis, and duodenal ulcer. Prevention of stress ulcers and NSAID-associated ulcers
- *Dose:* 0.5–0.8 mg/kg/day, single daily dose on empty stomach (preferably 1 hour before breakfast)
- *ADRs*: Abdominal discomfort, constipation, dizziness, headache, and leukopenia
- *Caution:* Avoid in children <6 years of age.

Sucralfate

An antiulcer medication, containing an aluminum salt, works by forming a protective barrier over the ulcer. This protects the ulcer from the acid of the stomach, allowing it to heal.

Brand names: Pepsigard, Sucrace, Sucral Kid, and Ulcekon
- *Available as:* Tablet 1 g. Syrup 0.5 g and 1 g/5 mL
- *Indications*: Duodenal, gastric, and NSAID-associated ulcers. Topically chemotherapy-associated stomatitis; burns
- *Dose:* 1 tablet BID 1 hour before food in grown-up children
- *ADR:* Constipation
- *Drug interaction:* Antacids, cimetidine, ranitidine, digoxin, thyroxine, ketoconazole, and tetracyclines
- *Caution:* Avoid in severe renal dysfunction.

Chapter 19

Antipsychotic Drugs

INTRODUCTION

Strictly speaking, antipsychotics or neuroleptics are a class of medication primarily used to manage psychosis (including delusions, hallucinations, paranoia, or disordered thought). In paranoia, the patients carry an erroneous suspicion of being under some sort of a threat though, in actuality, there is hardly any such evidence.

This chapter, however, mostly deals with neuropsychiatric drugs frequently employed in children.

AMITRIPTYLINE HYDROCHLORIDE

Brand names: Tryptanol, Sarotena, Amiline, and Amitryn

- *Available as:* Tablet 10 and 25 mg
- *Indications:* Nocturnal enuresis and depression
- *Dose:* 1.5 mg/kg/day in depression, 10–25 mg at bedtime in enuresis
- *Adverse drug reactions:* Signs of atropinism such as dilated pupils, malar flushing, dry mouth, hyperpyrexia, urinary retention, drowsiness agitation, hallucination, convulsions, coma, tachycardia, bundle branch block, CCF, allergic skin rash, black tongue, parotid swelling, gynecomastia, and alopecia
- *Contraindications:* Narrow-angle glaucoma, severe heart disease, cardiovascular insufficiency, and retention of urine.

ATOMOXETIN

A selective norepinephrine reuptake inhibitor with slow but sustained action.

Brand names: Attentrol, Axepta, and Tomoxetin
- *Indication:* Attention-deficit hyperactivity disorder (ADHD)
- *Available as:* Tablet 10 mg, 18 mg, 25 mg, 40 mg, and 60 mg
- *Dose:* 0.5–1.2 mg/kg/day in a single dose or in two divided doses. Start with 5 mg/kg and gradually build up to the upper limit of the dose
- *Caution*: Avoid in children <6 years of age.

CHLORAL HYDRATE

Brand names: Acquachloral, Noctec, and Somnos
- *Available as:* 250 and 500 mg/5 mL
- *Indications*: Sedative and hypnotic
- *Dose:* 10–20 mg/kg/dose (O, R), 25 mg/kg/day (O, R) as sedative, 50 mg/kg/day (O, R) as hypnotic in divided doses with a maximum of 2 g/dose
- *Adverse drug reactions:* GIT upset, excitement, delirium, hypersensitivity, hepatic, and renal dysfunction.

CHLORPROMAZINE HYDROCHLORIDE

Brand names: Largactil
- *Indications:* Tranquillizer, often used for sedative effect
- *Available as:* Tablets 10, 25, and 100 mg
  - *Syrup:* 5 and 25 mg/5 mL
  - *Injections:* 25 mg/mL ampule
- *Dose:* 0.5–1 mg/kg/dose O, IM, 2 mg/kg/day (PO) in four to six divided doses

- *Adverse drug reactions:* Extrapyramidal symptoms, sweating, salivation, pallor, jaundice, constipation, photosensitivity, retention of urine, and blood dyscrasia.

CHLORDIAZEPOXIDE

Brand names: Librium and Equibrom
- *Available as:* Tablets 5 and 10 mg
- *Indications:* Tranquilizing effect
- *Dose:* 0.5 mg/kg/day (PO) in divided doses
- *Adverse drug reactions:* Agitation, drowsiness, confusion, rash, GIT upset, ataxia, hepatic dysfunction, and blood dyscrasia.

IMIPRAMINE

Brand names: Depsonil and Tofranil
- *Available as:* Tablet 25 mg
- *Indications:* Nocturnal enuresis and depression
- *Dose:* 1.5 mg/kg/day (PO) in two to four divided doses. In enuresis, 25 mg/day at bedtime for 2 months
- *Adverse drug reactions:* Rash, sweating, hypotension, heart block, jaundice, leukopenia, fine tremors, and reactions resembling atropine toxicity.

HALOPERIDOL

Brand names: Serenace and Depidol
- *Available as:* Tablet 0.25 mg, 1.5 mg, 5 mg, and 10 mg. Drops 0.1 mg/drop (2 mg/mL). Suspension 10 mg/5 mL
- *Indications:* Anxiety, tension, reactive anxiety-depression, as such or in association with neurosis or other psychosomatic disorders, and rheumatic chorea

- *Dose:* 0.05 mg/kg/day; usually the daily dose varies between 1 and 5 mg
- *Adverse drug reactions:* Slight drowsiness and extrapyramidal manifestations (dystonia)
- *Caution:* Avoid using this agent in a patient who is already on a central nervous system (CNS) depressant; also in patients with basal ganglia lesions and below 12 years of age.

NITROXAZEPINE HCL

Brand name: Sintamil
- *Available as:* Tablet 25 and 75 mg
- *Indications:* Nocturnal enuresis and depression
- *Dose:* 25–50 mg bedtime
- *Adverse drug reactions:* Constipation, dryness of mouth, giddiness, headache, burning sensation, restlessness, skin rash, excessive perspiration, tremors, and palpitations
- *Caution:* Avoid its use in epilepsy, liver or kidney damage, cardiovascular disorders, glaucoma, urinary retention, and suicidal tendency
- *Contraindication:* Concurrent use of monoamine oxidase inhibitors.

PYRITINOL (PYRITHIOXINE)

Brand name: Encephabol
- *Available as:* Tablet 100 mg, 200 mg; Suspension 80.5 mg/5 mL
- *Indications:* ADHD, MBD, postencephalitic sequelae, and perinatal distress

- *Dose:* Infants—2.5 mL, one to three times a day. Children— 2.5-5 mL (or tablet) thrice daily. Give for at least 3-4 weeks
- *Adverse drug reactions:* Pruritus, rash, gastrointestinal tract (GIT) upset, disturbed taste, rise in body temperature, leukopenia, thrombocytopenia, hepatotoxicity, albuminuria, and myasthenia-like symptoms.

20
Chapter

Antispasmodics/Antiflatulence Drugs

INTRODUCTION

Abdominal complaints such as colic, flatulence and distention are common in infants whereas recurrent/chronic abdominal pain is a frequent complaint by the children and adolescents.

Antispasmodics are medications that are used to treat various medical conditions that involve contraction and relaxation of the smooth muscles of the gut.

An *antiflatulent* is a drug used for the alleviation or prevention of disturbing abdominal distention from excessive intestinal gas (flatulence).

ATROPINE SULFATE

It is an anticholinergic drug.
- *Indications:* Antispasmodic, antiarrhythmic, and premedication in anesthesia.
- *Available as:* Tablet 0.3, 0.4, and 0.6 mg; Injection 0.6 mg/mL.
- *Dose:* 0.01 mg/kg/dose (SC) with a maximum of 0.4 mg/dose. Repeat every 4–6 hours prn.
- *Adverse drug reactions:* Dryness of mouth, flushing, fever, tachycardia, blurring of vision, photophobia, dilated pupils, rash, constipation, retention of urine, and central nervous system (CNS) manifestations such as restlessness and delirium.

DICYCLOMINE

An anticholinergic agent employed for relief of abdominal discomfort from intermittent spasm of the smooth muscles of the gut and allied conditions; often available in combination with an analgesic (paracetamol and mefenamic acid) and/or simethicone.

Brand name: Colimex, Cyclopan, and Meftal-Spas

- *Available as:* Tablet 20 mg; Suspension 10 mg/5 mL. Drops [usually in combination with paracetamol, or a nonsteroidal anti-inflammatory drug (NSAID)]
- *Indications:* An anticholinergic agent effective as an antispasmodic in colic and irritable bowel syndrome
- *Dose:* 5 mg/dose in infants above 6 months. 10 mg/dose in children. 40 mg/dose in adolescents.
  The dose may be repeated every 6–8 hourly.
- *Adverse drug reactions:* Blurring of vision, dryness of mouth, drowsiness, and retention of urine.
- *Contraindications:* Obstructive uropathy, obstructive gastrointestinal disease, paralytic ileus, intestinal atony, severe ulcerative colitis, myasthenia gravis, and infants under 6 months.
- *Precaution:* Gastroesophageal reflux with reflux esophagitis.

DIMETHYLPOLYSILOXANE

Brand name: Dimol

- *Available as:* Tablet 40 mg; Drops 40 mg/mL.
- *Indications:* Flatulence, colic, before infant feeding for facilitating burping; before X-ray of abdomen; to dispel gas.
- *Dose:* ¼ to ½ tablet or liquid added to infant's formula or administered directly for "burping".

- *<6 months:* 5–10 drops 15 minutes before feed.
- *>6 months:* 10–20 drops 15 minutes before feed.

DROTAVERINE HCL

Brand names: Drotin and Drovin
- *Indication:* Antispasmodic
- *Available as:* Tablets 40 and 80 mg; Injection 20 mg/mL.
- *Dose:* 0–6 years 20 mg TDS, >6 years 40 mg TDS.
- *Drug interaction:* Reduces therapeutic effect of levodopa.
- *Contraindications:* Severe renal, hepatic, and cardiac insufficiency.
- *Adverse drug reactions:* Anticholinergic effects.
- *Caution:* Monitor renal and hepatic status.

HYOSCINE BUTYLBROMIDE

Brand name: Buscopan
- *Indications:* Antispasmodic (gastrointestinal and biliary tract), esophagospasm and cardiospasm, colonic motility disorders; hiccup.
- *Available as:* Tablet 10 mg; Suppositories 7.5 and 10 mg; Injection 20 mg/mL.
- *Dose:* Oral 6–12 years 10 mg TDS. Later 10–20 mg TDS.
- *Injection:* 10–20 mg (IM and IV).
- *Adverse drug reactions:* Anticholinergic effects, vision disturbances, tachycardia, and palpitations.
- *Contraindications:* Glaucoma and myasthenia gravis.
- *Precaution:* Pregnancy.

OXYPHENONIUM BROMIDE

Brand name: Antrenyl
- *Available as:* Tablets 5 and 10 mg; Drops 10 mg/mL.

- *Indications:* Antispasmodic, useful in peptic ulcer, gastritis, hyperacidity, and hypermotility.
- *Dose:*
  - 1–2 tablets 4 times daily.
  - *2–6 years:* 5–8 drops 1–3 times daily.
  - *6–12 years:* 8–15 drops 1–3 times daily.
- *Adverse drug reactions:* Mild blurring of vision, dry mouth, dizziness, tremors, and urinary retention.

PIPENZOLATE METHYLBROMIDE

Brand name: Pipcal

- *Available as:* Drops 4 mg/mL (in combination with same amount of dimethylpolysiloxane)
- *Dose:*
  - On an average 2.5–5 mg (O) TDS
  - <6 months 4 drops before a feed
  - 6 months to 1 year, 8–10 drops before a feed
  - 1–3 years, 16 drops before a feed
- *Adverse drug reactions:* Practically none.

PROPANTHELINE BROMIDE

Brand name: Probanthine

- *Available as:* Tablet 15 mg.
- *Dose:* 15 mg TDS, preferably an hour before main meals.
- *Caution:* Do not exceed total dose of 120 mg/day.
- *Adverse drug reactions:* Drowsiness, gastrointestinal upset, palpitations, urinary hesitancy and retention, anhidrosis, constipation, and dryness of skin.

SIMETHICONE

It is an antiflatulent drug and is helpful in preventing vomiting.

Brand names: Colimex DF, Coliwin, and Espumisan
- *Available as:* Drops 80 mg/mL; Capsule 80 mg.
- *Dose:*
  - Infants and up to 2 years: 20 mg 6 hourly.
  - >2 years: 40 mg 6 hourly.

VALETHAMATE BROMIDE

It is primarily used in obstetric practice for dilatation of the cervix, and is a useful antispasmodic in children.

Brand names: Epidosin, Dilaton, Osdil, Valamate, and Valosin.
- *Indications:* Abdominal pain as such or associated with surgical conditions.
- *Available as:* Tablet 10 mg
- *Dose:* 0.2 mg/kg (PO). TDS. 0.1 mg/kg two to three times a day (IM and IV).
- *Adverse drug reactions:* Dryness of mouth, visual disturbances (blurring of vision), and palpitations.
- *Contraindications:* Intestinal obstruction and glaucoma.
- *Caution:* Avoid in liver and kidney disorders.

21 Chapter

Antitoxins

INTRODUCTION

Antitoxins are antibodies that are capable of neutralizing specific biological toxins such as cause snakebite envenomation, diphtheria, gas gangrene, or tetanus. Antitoxins are used prophylactically as well as therapeutically.

ANTISNAKE VENOM (ASV)

Four antivenom sera derived from common krait, cobra, Russel viper, and saw-scaled viper make up the currently available VSV.

- *Available as:* 10 mL vials. This is for intravenous (IV) infusion administration, in 250 mL of one-fifth saline at a rate of 20 mL/kg/h
- *Indications:* Poisonous snakebite, clinically presenting with hematologic or neurologic manifestations, inflammation around the bite
- *Dose:* It is calculated on the basis of severity of manifestations rather than age, body weight or surface area. Children need to be given 50% (1.5 times) higher dose in order to neutralize the injected venom which is relatively large enough in terms of the bodyweight and size
  - *Mild envenomation:* 50 mL (5 vials)
  - *Moderate envenomation:* 50–150 mL (5–15 vials)
  - *Severe envenomation:* 150–200 mL (15–20 vials)
  - Dose is, however, variable from center to center

- *Caution:* (1) Before administering antisnake venom (ASV), it is safe to test for the horse-serum allergy by injecting 0.02 mL of 1:10 diluted AVS and, in case of presence of hypersensitivity, desensitize the child. (2) Most effective when administered early enough to neutralize venom in the circulation before it reaches the target site
- *Adverse drug reactions:* Hypersensitivity.

TETANUS ANTITOXIN (TAT)

Brand names: Anti-TET, Tetanus antitoxin
- *Available as:* 750 IU, 1,000 IU, 1,500 IU, 5,000 IU, 10,000 IU
- *Indications:* Prophylaxis and treatment of tetanus
- *Dose:* Prophylaxis: 3,000–5,000 IU (SC and IM)
- *Therapeutic:* 10,000 IU (IM and IV); 250 IU/day for 3 days (IT)
- *Adverse drug reactions:* Hypersensitivity and serum sickness
- *Cautions:* Important to do test for hypersensitivity before administering it. In some instances, desensitization may be needed.

DIPHTHERIA ANTITOXIN

This is the mainstay of treatment of diphtheria. It neutralizes only free toxin and, therefore, should be administered as early as possible. Its efficacy decreases once the mucocutaneous symptoms of diphtheria appear.
- *Available as:* Ampules (10 mL) providing 10,000, and 20,000 IU. It is diluted in 1:20 isotonic NaCl solution. Administration should be slow (up to 1 mL/min)
- *Indications:* Treatment of diphtheria; Schick test-positive contacts
- *Dose:* Pharyngeal/laryngeal diphtheria of <48 hours duration—20,000–40,000 units (IV) as a single administration

Chapter 21: Antitoxins

- Nasopharyngeal diphtheria—40,000–60,000 units (IV) as a single administration
- Extensive diphtheria with diffuse neck swelling—80,000–120,000 units (IV) as a single administration
- Schick test-positive contacts—500–2,000 units IM. Simultaneously, a dose of diphtheria toxoid is given IM in the other arm. After a gap of 6 weeks, three doses of diphtheria toxoid (each at 4 weeks interval) for active immunization

- *Adverse drug reactions:* Hypersensitivity reactions
- *Precaution:* Dose is based not on child's age but on duration and extent of illness. Test for hypersensitivity before administering the antitoxin a "must"
- *Special remarks:*
  - In mild cases, IM rather than IV administration suffices
  - In order to achieve eradication of infection, it is necessary to also give erythromycin, benzyl penicillin (penicillin G), or procaine penicillin.

GAS GANGRENE ANTITOXIN

Brand name: AGGSall scorpion stings caused by red scorpion.
- *Available as:* Injection 10,000 IU/vial
- *Dose:* 30–75,000 IU (IM, SC, and IV).

SCORPION ANTIVENOM (ANTISCORPION VENOM AND SCORPION VENOM ANTITOXIN)

Though available, it is only infrequently used. It is effective only when administered within 30 minutes of the scorpion sting. Indications are all stings by red scorpion (the deadly species prevalent in Indian subcontinent) in symptomatic subjects. Currently, injection prazosin is considered the gold standard for treatment of scorpion sting.

Chapter 22

Antitussives and Cough Expectorants

INTRODUCTION

By definition, antitussives are drugs that suppress cough by acting on the central nervous system (CNS) and peripheral nervous system, e.g., a large group of opioid and nonopioid drugs. Because the cough reflex is necessary for clearing the upper respiratory tract of obstructive secretions, antitussives should not be used in a productive cough.

Codeine phosphate and hydrocodone bitartrate are by and large the most potent opioid antitussives. However, their use is not recommended in children.

Dextromethorphan hydrobromide is an effective antitussive with no dependence liability.

Antitussives are administered orally, usually in a syrup with a mucolytic (say bromhexine and ambroxol) or expectorant and alcohol, or, sometimes in a capsule with an antihistaminic and a mild analgesic.

Expectorants are bronchomucotropic agents that help in the removal of secretions or exudate from the throat, trachea, and bronchi. They liquefy viscid mucus or mucopurulent exudates through the decongestant action. Hence, they are used in the treatment of productive coughs to help to expel the exudates and secretion.

ANTITUSSIVES

Pholcodine (Homocodine)

It acts primarily on the CNS, causing depression of the cough reflex, partly by a direct effect on the cough center in the medulla.

Brand names: CRM, Tixylix, and Tedykoff-LX

- *Available as:* 1.5 mg/5 mL
- *Indications:* Dry cough, especially when painful
- *Dose:* 2–3 mg/day in divided doses
- *Adverse drug reactions (ADRs):* Gastrointestinal upset (especially constipation), drowsiness, dizziness, excitation, respiratory distress, and ataxia.
- *Caution:* Avoid in constipated subjects.

Dextromethorphan Hydrochloride

A D-isomer of a codeine isomer, employed as an antitussive agent; believed to be free of addictive effect.

Brand names: Lastuss and Suppressa

- *Available as:* As such and as a principal ingredient in cough suppressant preparations such as actifed DM, Alex cough formula.
- *Dose:* 1–2 mg/kg/day (PO) in three to four divided doses.
- *ADRs:* CNS depression or excitement, sleep disturbances, and hallucinations.
- *Caution:* Do not exceed a maximum dose of 60 mg/day.

EXPECTORANTS

Guaifenesin

An expectorant available in combination with such ingredients as ambroxol, bronchodilator, etc.

Brand names: Axalin Expectorant Codicoff and Dilo-BM Expectorant

- *Available as:* Syrup 100 mg/5 mL
- *Indications:* Symptomatic relief of dry, nonproductive coughs, and the presence of mucus in the airway.
- *Dose:* 10–15 mg/kg/day in 4–6 divided doses with enough of water.

MUCOLYTICS

Ambroxol

It is a secrotolytic agent.

Brand name: Mucolite
- *Available as:* Tablets 30 mg, Elixir 30 mg/5 mL.
- *Indication:* Situations needing reduction in the viscosity of the airway mucus (phlegm, e.g., rhinopharyngitis, acute bronchitis, pneumonia, and asthma).
- *Dose*: 0.5–1 mg/kg/day in two or three divided doses.
- *ADRs:* Nausea, vomiting, diarrhea, and abdominal discomfort.
- *Caution:* Avoid prolonged use beyond 5–7 days.

Bromhexine

It is a mucolytic agent that liquefies the thick respiratory mucus (phlegm) in the nose, trachea, and lungs so that it is easily coughed out.

Brand Names: Bisolvon and Intima
- *Available as:* Tablets 8 mg, Elixir 4 mg/5 mL. It is also available in combination with other ingredients in cough mixtures.
- *Dose:* 0.5–0.7 mg/kg/day in three divided doses.
- *ADRs*: Dizziness, headache, nausea, upper abdominal pain, vomiting, diarrhea, rash, red spots or bumps, itching, sweating, and changes in serum aminotransferase levels.
- *Caution:* Gastric ulcer, renal, and hepatic disease.

Chapter 23

Cardiotonic Drugs

INTRODUCTION

Cardiotonic drugs (cardiotonics) are drugs that increase the efficiency and contractions of the heart, thereby causing more blood to be pumped throughout the circulatory system, supplying all tissues of the body. Cardiotonic drugs usually affect intracellular calcium levels in the heart muscle to achieve the desired increase in muscle contractility. Their role is in cardiac insufficiency, i.e., a failure of the heart to pump enough blood to supply oxygen and nutrients to various organs and tissue. The manifestations of cardiac insufficiency include shortness of breath, easy fatigability, and edema. It is usually caused by arterial hypertension and ischemic heart disease.

ADRENALINE (EPINEPHRINE)

Brand name: Adrine
- *Available as:* Injection (amp) 0.1 mg/mL of 1:10,000 solution.
- *Indications:* Cardiac arrest, anaphylactic shock, allergic reactions, also, bronchial asthma/bronchospasm, hypoglycemia, open-angle glaucoma.
- *Dose:*
  - *Neonates:* IV, intratracheal 0.01–0.03 mg/kg (0.1–0.3 mL/kg) of 1:10,000 solution q 3–5 minutes.

- *Infants and children:* SC—0.01 mg/kg (0.01 mL/kg/dose of 1:10,000 solution or 0.005 mL/kg/dose suspension).
- IV: 0.01 mg/kg (0.1 mL/kg of 1:10,000 solution (maximum 1 mg).
- IT: 0.1 mg/kg/dose (0.1 mL/kg of 1:10,000 solution) (maximum 0.2 mL/kg).
- *Continuous infusion:* 0.1–1 µg/kg/min per response.
- *Nebulization:* 0.25–0.5 mL of 2.25% racemic epinephrine diluted in 3 mL of normal saline.
- *Glaucoma:* Instill one to two drops in the eye OD or BD.
- *Adverse drug reactions (ADRs):* Tachycardia, hypertension, nervousness, restlessness, irritability, headache, tremors, weakness, nausea, vomiting, and acute urinary retention.

AMRINONE LACTATE

It is an inotrope and vasodilator; increases cellular levels of cyclic adenosine monophosphate.

Brand name: Amicor
- *Available as:* Injection 5 mg/mL (20 mL ampule).
- *Indications:* Low cardiac output states.
- *Dose:*
    - *Neonates:* 0.75 mg/kg IV bolus over 2–3 min. Follow with 3–5 µg/kg/min continuous infusion IV.
    - *Infants and children:* 0.75 mg/kg IV bolus over 2–3 min. Follow with 5–10 µg/kg/min continuous infusion IV.
- *Adverse drug reactions:* Hypertension, arrhythmias, and thrombocytopenia.
- *Caution:* Excess diuresis may result from increased cardiac output.

DIGOXIN

Digitalis glycoside with positive inotropic and negative chronotropic effect.

Brand name: Lanoxin

- *Available as:* Tablet 0.25 mg, injection 0.25 mg/mL, Elixir 0.05 mg/mL.
- *Indications:* Congestive cardiac failure (CCF) caused by poor myocardial contractility.
- *Dose:* It is outlined in **Table 1**.

Half of the total calculated dose in given stat. Divide the remaining one-half in two doses, each to be given at 8 hours intervals. Maintenance dose is about one-fourth to one-third of the total digitalizing dose. This is given as a single administration or in two divided doses daily.

The above description applies to oral administration. Parenteral dose should be about two-thirds of the oral dose.

- *Adverse drug reactions:* Bradycardia, pulsus bigeminus, extrasystole, sinus arrhythmia, heart block, visual disturbances, nausea, vomiting, diarrhea, feed intolerance, anorexia, delirium, and gynecomastia.
- *Caution:* Use of digoxin in CCF is now discouraged on the ground that it merely improves the contractility of the exhausted heart muscle temporarily.

TABLE 1: Total digitalizing dose of digoxin.

Age group	24 hours dose (mg/kg)
Newborn full-term	0.03–0.04
Premature	0.02–0.25
Infants and children	0.04–0.06
Adolescents	1.0–1.5 mg in divided doses

DOBUTAMINE HYDROCHLORIDE

It is a β-adrenergic stimulant, works like dopamine as an inotropic.

Brand names: Dobucin, Dobustat, Dobutam, and Dobutrex.
- *Available as:* Injection 50 and 250 mg/vial.
- *Indication:* To increase cardiac output in circulatory failure.
- *Dose:*
  - *Newborn:* 2–20 µg/kg/min (IV) as continuous infusion.
  - *Children:* 25–40 µg/kg/min (IV) as continuous infusion.
- *Adverse drug reactions:* Palpitations, tachycardia, ectopics, angina, tachyarrhythmias, tingling, paresthesia, and cramps.
- *Caution:* Never mix with soda bicarbonate.

DOPAMINE

It is a sympathomimetic amine vasopressor that is the naturally occurring immediate precursor of norepinephrine.

Brand name: Dopinga
- *Available as:* 200 mg/5 mL ampule.
- *Indications:* Shock syndrome accompanying acute CCF and imminent renal failure. Also, acute pancreatitis; activation and support of diuretic therapy; during artificial respiration with positive end-expiratory pressure (PEEP); to stabilize cardiorespiratory function during epidural anesthesia; acute intoxication with antiarrhythmic agents, say barbiturates, that are excreted by the kidneys.
- *Dose:* Start with 0.002–0.005 mg/kg/min. If needed, increase by increments of 0.005 mg/kg/min up to 0.050 mg/kg/min.

To prepare a solution containing 0.400 mg/mL, mix 100 mg dopamine in 250 mL 5% distilled water or an electrolyte solution with pH < 7.0. Do not use a bicarbonate solution.

- *Adverse drug reactions:* Mild nausea and vomiting occasionally.
- *Contraindications:* Pheochromocytoma, manifest left ventricular hypertrophy.
- *Cautions:*
  - Volume deficiencies must be corrected prior to its administration.
  - Marked increase in heart rate and repeated arrhythmia indicate that no further increase in dose needs to be made.
  - Abrupt cessation of the infusion must never be done.

MEPHENTERMINE SULFATE

Brand names: Ephentine and Mephentine

- *Available as:* Tablet 10 mg. Injection 15 and 30 mg/mL (10 mL vial).
- *Indication:* Hypotension (secondary to spinal anesthesia or surgery); as vasopressor in hypercyanotic spells (Fallot's tetralogy).
- *Dose:* 0.4 mg/kg/dose. This may be given as slow IV infusion or as a bolus.
- *Adverse drug reactions:* Nausea, vomiting, loss of appetite, hypersalivation, headache, generalized weakness, anxiety, confusion, irritability, restlessness, psychosis, dyspnea, urinary retention, cerebral hemorrhage, ventricular arrhythmias, and pulmonary edema.
- *Contraindications:* Hypovolemic shock and chlorpromazine-induced shock.

- *Caution:* Avoid concurrent use of tricyclic antidepressants and monoamine oxidase (MAO) inhibitors.

MILRINONE

It is an inotropic and vasodilator drug.

Brand names: Milicor and Primacor
- *Available as:* Injection 10 mg/L Adrons 0 mL ampule.
- *Indications:* CCF refractory to diuretics, digoxin, and vasodilators.
- *Dose:* Loading dose 50–75 µg/kg followed by 0.25–1 µg/kg/min continuous IV infusion.
- *Adverse drug reactions:* Vomiting, hypokalemia, hypotension, and dysrhythmia.
- *Precaution:* This is only a short-term therapy.

NOREPINEPHRINE (NORADRENALINE)

It is similar to adrenaline, and it works by constricting the blood vessels and increasing blood pressure and blood glucose levels.

Brand names: Adrenor, Adronis, and Norad
- *Available as:* Injection 2 mg/mL.
- *Indications:* Cardiac arrest (as adjunct), acute hypotension, and shock (both vasodilatory and septic).
- *Dose:* 0.05–0.1 µg/kg/min. Depending on the beneficial effect, dose may be treated to as high as 0.2 µg/kg/min.
- *Adverse drug reactions:* Cardiac disturbances and plasma volume depletion.
- *Contraindications:* Hypovolemia, mesenteric or peripheral vascular thrombosis, cyclopropane and halothane anesthesia, and profound hypoxia/hypercapnia.

Chapter 23: Cardiotonic Drugs

- *Caution:* Monitor BP.
- *Drug interactions:* Tricyclic antidepressants and MAO incompatibilities.

VASOPRESSIN

Brand names: E-pressin, Pitressin, and Vasopin

- *Available as:* Injection 20 IU/mL.
- *Indications:* Catecholamine refractory septic shock, diabetes insipidus, and acute gastrointestinal bleeding.
- *Dose:*
    - Catecholamine refractory vasodilatory septic shock 0.3–2 IU/kg/min.
    - Diabetes insipidus 2.5–10 units/dose BD, TDS, or QID.
    - Gastrointestinal bleeding 0.002–0.01 units/kg/min as continuous IV infusion.
- *Adverse drug reactions:* Nausea, vomiting, flatulence, abdominal pain, tremors, sweating, circumoral pallor, fever water intoxication, hyponatremia, hypertension, bradycardia, and arrhythmia.
- *Contraindications:* Asthma, heart failure, and epilepsy.

Chapter 24: Chelating Agents

INTRODUCTION

Chelating agents (chelants and chelators) are sequestering chemical compounds = usually organic—that react with metal ions to form a stable, water-soluble complex which is then excreted. These agents are used to reduce the blood and tissue levels of heavy metals such as iron, lead, mercury, and copper.

DEFERASIROX

It is an oral iron chelator which is used once daily.

Brand names: Defrijet, Desirox, and Exjade

- *Available as:* Tablet 250 and 500 mg.
- *Indications:* Iron overload, both acute (as in accidental too heavy intake) and chronic [(as in thalassemia major following multiple blood transfusions, sickle-cell disease (SCD), and the myelodysplastic syndromes (MDS)]
- *Dose:* 20–30 mg/kg (PO) once daily. Initial dose of 20 mg/dose should be built up by increments of 5 mg/kg every 3–6 months.
- *Adverse drug reactions:* Skin rash, gastrointestinal upset, raised liver enzymes, and acute kidney injury.
- *Contraindications:* Hypersensitivity, acute kidney injury, and severe acute hepatitis.
- *Caution:* Monitor ferritin levels which must be maintained >500 ng/mL. Avoid in <2 years.

Chapter 24: Chelating Agents

DEFERIPRONE

Thrice daily oral iron chelator

Brand name: Kelfer

- Thrice daily oral iron chelator.
- *Available as:* Tablet 250 mg and 500 mg.
- *Indications:* Acute and chronic iron overload.
- *Dose:* 25 mg/kg/dose (PO) thrice daily.
- *Adverse drug reactions:* Gastrointestinal upset, arthropathy, musculoskeletal pain, neutropenia, and urine discoloration.
- *Contraindications:* Pregnancy, Henoch-Schönlein purpura (HSP), and periorbital edema with skin rash.
- *Caution:* Parents need to be told about *red urine*—a normal finding on this therapy. Rough sports and sharp objects should be avoided.

DEFEROXAMINE [ALSO KNOWN AS DESFERRIOXAMINE]

It is an injectable iron chelator.

Brand name: Desferal

- *Available as:* Injection 500 mg vial.
- *Indications:* Iron overload, both acute and chronic.
- *Dose:* Acute overload—IM route: A stat dose of 1,000 mg needs to be followed by two doses of 500 mg every 4 hours. If needed, further doses of 500 mg may be given at 4–12 hours interval. Total 24 hours dose must not exceed 6 g.
- *IV route:* A maximum of 15 mg/kg/hour for the first 1 g. If need to, further 125 mg/hour. Total 24 hours dose must not exceed 6 g.
- Chronic overload—SC route: 20–40 mg/kg/day (SC, employing a battery-driven pump) over 8–12 hours.

- *IM route:* 500–1,000 mg/day.
- Furthermore, each unit of blood transfusion should be accompanied by 2 g IV (10–15 mg/kg) by a separate infusion line.
- *Adverse drug reactions:* Injection site reactions, allergic reactions, tachycardia, hypotension, abdominal discomfort, diarrhea, hearing loss, blurred vision, and urine discoloration.
- *Contraindication:* Acute kidney injury.
- *Caution:* In chronic therapy, it is advisable to have periodic eye and auditory checkups.

DIMERCAPROL (BRITISH ANTI-LEWISITE)

Brand name: British anti-Lewisite (BAL)
- *Available as:* Injection 100 mg vial.
- *Indications:* Chelation of mercury, gold, arsenic, and lead poisoning.
- *Dose:* 2.5–4 mg/kg/dose (deep IM) every 4–6 hours for 2 days. The 2.5 mg/kg/dose every 12 hours for 10 days.
- *Adverse drug reactions:* Painful injection site, vomiting, fever, and hypertension.

PENICILLAMINE (D-PENICILLAMINE)

Check in miscellaneous for overlap.
It is a copper chelator.

Brand names: Artamin, Cilamin, Cuprimine, Distamin, Penamine, and Pendramine.
- *Available as:* Tablet/capsule 50, 125, and 250 mg.
- *Indications:* Heavy metal (copper and lead) poisoning; Wilson disease, rheumatoid arthritis, and cystinuria.
- *Dose:* 20–40 mg/kg/day (PO) in 3–4 divided doses.

- *Adverse drug reactions:* Abdominal pain, nausea, vomiting, loss of appetite, diarrhea, abdominal discomfort/pain, decreased sense of taste, itching or rash, ringing in the ears, sores in the mouth, poor wound healing, and increased wrinkling of the skin.
- *Caution:* Advisable to provide supplements of vitamin B_6 and zinc concurrently with d-penicillamine therapy.

Chapter 25

Colony-stimulating Factors

INTRODUCTION

Colony-stimulating factors (CSFs) are secreted glycoproteins that bind to receptor proteins on the surfaces of hemopoietic stem cells, thereby activating intracellular signaling pathways and promote production of white blood cells (WBCs), mainly granulocytes such as neutrophils. This occurs in response to an infection. Exogenous CSFs stimulate the stem cells in the bone marrow, thereby producing more of the particular WBCs. CSFs include:
- Granulocyte colony-stimulating factor (G-CSF)
- Granulocyte-macrophage colony-stimulating factor (GM-CSF)
- Erythropoietin
- Promegapoietin

ERYTHROPOIETIN (RECOMBINANT HUMAN)

Erythropoietin (hematopoietin) is a glycoprotein cytokine secreted by the kidney in response to cellular hypoxia. It stimulates red blood cell production (erythropoiesis) in the bone marrow. Recombinant human erythropoietin (rhEPO), exogenous erythropoietin, are produced by recombinant DNA technology in cell culture.

Brand names: Epoetin, Epox, and Eprex
- *Available as:* 2,000 IU, 4,000 IU/2 mL vial.
- *Indications:* Anemia of prematurity, chronic renal failure (CRF)/end-stage renal disease (ESRD) secondary to HIV/AIDS, retroviral treatment or chemotherapy of neoplasia.
- *Dose:* Anemia of prematurity 150–500 IU/kg/dose (SC) two to three times a week for 8–12 weeks. For adequate response, it is important to provide supplements of iron, folic acid, and vitamin $B_{12,}$ simultaneously.
  - CRF/ESRD 50–100 IU/kg/dose two to three times a week.
- *Adverse drug reactions:* Headache, edema, arthralgia, seizure, and hypertension. Increased risk of death, myocardial infarction, stroke, venous thromboembolism, and tumor recurrence.
- *Caution:* Avoid shaking the vial as a safeguard against denaturing of the glycoprotein.

GRANULOCYTE COLONY-STIMULATING FACTOR

Granulocyte colony-stimulating factor (G-CSF) specifically promotes neutrophil proliferation and maturation.

Brand name: Neupogen
- *Available as:* Injection 300 µg/mL.
- *Indications:* Severe neutropenia which may be neonatal, congenital, idiopathic, or secondary to chemotherapy in malignancies.
- *Dose:* 5–10 µg/kg/day (SC and IV) OD for a maximum of 2 weeks.
- *Adverse drug reactions:* Injection site inflammation, constipation, diarrhea, anorexia, headache, liver dysfunction, and tiredness.
- *Caution:* Avoid it 24 hours before and within 24 hours of chemotherapy.

GRANULOCYTE MACROPHAGE COLONY-STIMULATING FACTOR

Granulocyte macrophage colony-stimulating factor (GM-CSF), a monomeric glycoprotein that functions as a cytokine, is a white blood cell growth factor, stimulating stem cells to produce various granulocytes (neutrophils, eosinophils, and basophils) and monocytes.

Brand name: Leukine

- *Available as*: Injection 500 μg/mL.
- *Indications*: Neutropenia following bone marrow transplantation, pushing myeloid recovery after chemotherapy/bone marrow insult, neutropenia from HIV or sepsis.
- *Dose*:
  - Neonates 10 μg/kg/day (SC) OD for 5 days.
  - Infants and children 250 μg/kg (IV infusion, SC) for 21 days.
- *Adverse drug reactions:* Injection site reactions, diarrhea, weakness, light headedness, and low blood pressure.

PROMEGAPOIETIN

A cytokine that is employed during the course of chemotherapy to promote blood cell regeneration, especially platelets stimulating production of megakaryocytes by the bone marrow. Enhances megakaryocyte production is via stimulation of ligands for interleukin-3 and c-mpl.

Indications: (1) Severe thrombocytopenia induced by high-dose cancer chemotherapy; (2) Immune thrombocytopenic purpura that is not responding to steroids, immunoglobulins, and splenectomy; and (3) Acute radiation syndrome involving hemopoietic system.

Adverse drug reactions (ADRs): Fever, vomiting, and thrombocytopenia.

Chapter 26

Diuretics

INTRODUCTION

Diuretics are agents that promote enhanced production of urine (diuresis) along with surplus sodium and other electrolytes through varying mechanisms. These are used in hypertension, congestive heart failure (CHF), liver disease, kidney disease, water intoxication, edema, etc. through different dynamics. Antidiuretics such as vasopressin reduce the excretion of water in urine.

Clinically employed diuretic classes are—loop diuretics (high ceiling), thiazides (low ceiling), carbonic anhydrase inhibitors, potassium-sparing diuretics, calcium-sparing diuretics, osmotic diuretics, diuretics in the form of hypotonic aqueous preparations such as pure water, coffee, and tea cause excretion of free water and are termed "*aquaretics*".

ACETAZOLAMIDE

Brand names: Acetamide, Diamox, Dorzox eye drops, and Zolamide

- *Available as:* Tablet/capsule: 250 mg. Syrup: 250 mg/5 mL. Injection: 500 mg/mL, ophthalmic drops.
- *Indications:* Congestive heart failure (CHF), hypertension, cerebral edema, hydrocephalus, glaucoma, epilepsy, etc.
- *Dose:* 5 mg/kg/day (PO and IM) once daily as a diuretic in CHF; 8–30 mg/kg/day (PO) in three or four divided

doses as antiepileptic, in cerebral edema, hydrocephalus or glaucoma. For glaucoma, ophthalmic drops (as such or in combination with other intraocular-lowering agents) too are available.

- *Adverse drug reactions:* Drowsiness, confusion, abnormal sensations, paralysis, convulsions, hepatic dysfunctions, urticarial rash, fever, crystalluria, glycosuria, melena, hematuria, renal stone, polyuria, acidosis, blood dyscrasias, and transient myopia.
- *Caution:* Potassium supplements may be warranted during therapy with this agent.
- *Contraindications:* Significant renal or hepatic damage, hyperchloremic acidosis, sodium and potassium depletion, adrenal failure, sulfonamide sensitivity.

BUMETANIDE

Brand names: Bumet and Bumex

It is a loop diuretic and antihypertensive agent, 40-fold more potent than furosemide.

- *Available as:* Tablet: 0.5, 1, and 2 mg. Injection: 0.25 mg/mL.
- *Indications:* Edematous states, fluid overload, especially when refractory to furosemide.
- *Doses:*
  - 0.015–0.02 mg/kg/dose (PO) q 12–24 hours with a maximum of 10 mg/24 hours.
  - 8–30 mg/kg/day q 8 hours with a maximum of 1 g/day in epilepsy.
- *Adverse drug reactions:* Dehydration with electrolyte (sodium and potassium) depletion, muscle cramps, gynecomastia; thrombocytopenia and leukopenia.
- *Contraindications:* Anuria and hepatic encephalopathy.
- *Caution:* Avoid in preexisting hypokalemia.

CHLORTHALIDONE

Brand names: Hydrazide, Hythalton, and Thalizide
- *Available as:* Tablet: 12.5, 25, and 100 mg.
- *Dose:* 1–2 mg/kg/dose as a single dose daily or on alternate days.
- *Contraindication:* Anuria.
- *Caution:* Renal dysfunction.

CHLOROTHIAZIDE

Brand names: Chlotride and Diuril
- *Available as:* Tablet: 250 and 500 mg.
- *Indication:* Diuretic.
- *Dose:* 20 (7–40) mg/kg/day (PO) in two divided doses.
- *Adverse drug reactions:* Weakness, dizziness, hepatic dysfunction, blood dyscrasias, hyperglycemia, glycosuria, paresthesia, glomerulonephritis, pancreatitis, hypokalemia, and thrombocytopenia in newborn.
- *Contraindication:* Anuria.

ETHACRYNIC ACID

Brand name: Edecrin
- *Available as:* Tablet: 25 and 50 mg. Injection: 50 mg.
- *Indication:* Urinary tract infection.
- *Dose:*
  - 25 mg (PO), to be given as a single dose. Then, increase by increments of 25 mg.
  - 0.5–1 mg/kg/dose (IV) OD or BD.
- *Adverse drug reactions:* Gastrointestinal tract upset, rash, jaundice, hypoglycemia, hypokalemia, hyponatremia, peripheral circulatory failure, muscle cramps, weakness, and bone marrow depression.

FUROSEMIDE (FRUSEMIDE)

It is a sulfonamide loop diuretic and antihypertensive drug, acting through inhibition of reabsorption of electrolytes in ascending limb of loop of Henle and inhibiting reabsorption of sodium and chloride and increasing potassium excretion in distal tubule and a direct effect on electrolyte transport at proximal tubule and renal vasodilatory effect.

Brand names: Furoped and Lasix

- *Available as:* Tablet 40 mg. Oral solution: 10 mg/mL. Injection: 10 mg/mL.
- *Indications:* As diuretic in edema of CCF, nephrotic syndrome, cirrhosis; hypertension particular accompanied by CCF or renal disease; hypocalcemia, etc.
- *Dose:* 1–3 mg/kg/dose (PO), 0.5–1.5 mg/kg/dose (IM and IV). (Parenteral dose being half of the oral dose). This dose may be doubled if required but the maximum of 6 mg/kg/day must not be exceeded.
- *Adverse drug reactions:* Fluid and electrolyte imbalance, nausea, weakness, cramps, anesthesia, dizziness, urinary frequency, sweating, thirst, rash, bone marrow depression, thrombocytopenia, hyperuricemia; orthostatic hypotension.
- *Contraindications:* Hypokalemia, hyponatremia, Addison's disease, and lactation.
- *Caution:* Avoid in neonates who may develop ototoxicity secondary to renal maturity and in premature neonates in first week because of the increased risk of patent ductus arteriosus (PDA) through prostaglandin E-mediated process.

HYDROCHLOROTHIAZIDE

Brand name: Esidrix
- *Available as:* Tablet 25 and 50 mg.
- *Indications:* Edema of CCF, hepatic cirrhosis, and renal disease.
- *Dose:* 2 mg/kg/day (P) in two divided doses.
- *Adverse drug reactions:* Hyperglycemia, glycosuria, jaundice, blood dyscrasia, paresthesia, weakness, dizziness, neonatal thrombocytopenia, acute glomerulonephritis, pancreatitis, azotemia, and electrolyte imbalance.

MANNITOL

- *Indications:* Cerebral edema, oliguria, water intoxication, and hyponatremia.
- *Available as:* 200 mg/mL (350 and 500 mL bottles, providing 70 and 100 g mannitol).
- *Dose:* 7–10 mL/kg/day by drip.
- *Adverse drug reactions:* Hypersensitivity, thrombosis, or pain from extravasation, hyperglycemia, glycosuria, headache, nausea and vomiting, circulatory overload, hyponatremia, and convulsions.

METOLAZONE

Brand names: Diurem, Memtiz, Metiz, and Zytanix
- *Available as:* Tablet 2.5, 5, and 10 mg.
- *Dose:* 0.2–0.4 mg/kg/day once a day.
- *Caution:* Renal dysfunction, deteriorating level of consciousness.
- *Contraindications:* Coma and anuria.

SPIRONOLACTONE

Brand names: Aldactone and Lactone
- *Available as:* Tablet 25 mg.
- *Indications:* For obtaining diuresis.
- *Dose:* 1.5–3 mg/kg/day (PO) in one to three divided doses. The agent is usually given along with a thiazide.
- *Adverse drug reactions:* Hyperkalemia, drowsiness, hirsutism, gynecomastia, minor gastrointestinal tract (GIT) upset, and skin rash.
- *Contraindications:* Anuria, hyperkalemia, and renal insufficiency and sensitivity to spironolactone.
- *Caution:* Do not give potassium and do periodic serum electrolytes.

TRIAMTERENE

Brand name: Ditide

A diuretic and antihypertensive agent, competing with aldosterone for receptor sites in distal renal tubules.
- *Available as:* Tablets 50 mg (in combination with 25 mg of benzthiazide).
- *Indication:* For obtaining diuresis, hypertension.
- *Dose:* 2–4 mg/kg/day (PO) in one or two doses.
- *Adverse drug reactions:* Nausea, vomiting, headache, constipation, fatigue, hyperkalemia, hyponatremia, and hyperchloremic metabolic acidosis.
- *Contraindications:* Hyperkalemia and renal failure.
- *Caution:* Avoid concurrent administration of potassium.

Chapter 27

Drugs for Attention-deficit Hyperactivity Disorder

INTRODUCTION

The one of the most common neurodevelopmental disorders, *attention-deficit hyperactivity disorder (ADHD),* is characterized by a range of symptoms such as problems in attention and concentrating, hyperactivity, impulsiveness, forgetfulness, and inability to finish task (say homework). Drug treatment revolves around central nervous system (CNS) stimulants and CNS nonstimulants. Pharmacotherapy needs to be complemented with behavioral therapy, support at home and school, exercise, and balanced nutrition, and education.

AMPHETAMINE

Brand name: Dexedrine
- *Available as:* Tablet/capsule 5 and 10 mg.
- *Indication:* Attention-deficit hyperactivity disorder (ADHD)
- *Dose:* 0.15–0.5 mg/kg/day with enhancement of the initial dose in increment of 2.5 mg/day at weekly intervals.
- *Adverse drug reactions:* Agitation, insomnia, dizziness, and headache.

- *Caution:* Avoid, if the child has used an monoamine oxidase (MAO) inhibitor, such as isocarboxazid, linezolid, methylene blue injection, phenelzine, rasagiline, selegiline, or tranylcypromine in the past 14 days.

METHYLPHENIDATE

Brand names: Addwize and Ritalin
- *Available as:* Tablet 10 and 20 mg.
- *Indications:* ADHD and narcolepsy.
- *Dose:* 0.3–1 mg/kg/day (PO) before breakfast and lunch. In weekly increment of 5–10 mg, dose may be increased to a maximum of 2 mg/kg.
- *Adverse drug reactions:* Appetite loss, dry mouth, anxiety/nervousness, nausea, and insomnia. Abdominal pain and weight loss, agitation/restlessness, irritability, dyskinesia (tics), lethargy (drowsiness/fatigue), and dizziness.
- *Caution:* Avoid, if child is on MAO inhibitor or suffering from glaucoma and in <6 years of age.

PEMOLINE

Brand name: Cylert
- A schedule IV nonnarcotic (stimulant) controlled drug.
- *Available as:* Tablet 18.75, 37.5, and 75 mg.
- *Indication:* ADHD and narcolepsy.
- *Contraindication:* Simultaneous use of other stimulants and MAO inhibitors.
- *Dose:* Initial dose 1 mg/kg/day (PO), which may be built up in weekly increments of 0.5 mg/kg to a maximum of 3 mg/kg/day.

Chapter 27: Drugs for Attention-deficit Hyperactivity Disorder

- *Adverse drug reactions:* Insomnia, seizures, headache, movement disorder, hepatotoxicity, choreoathetosis, and precipitation attacks of Gilles de la Tourette syndrome.
- *Caution:* Avoid in liver disease.

NONSTIMULANTS

Atomoxetine

Brand names: Attentrol and Tomoxetin

- *Available as:* Tablet 10, 18, 25, 49, and 60 mg.
- *Indication:* ADHD not responding to stimulant drugs.
- *Dose:* 0.5 mg/kg/day (PO) as a single dose or in two divided doses. Through weekly increments, the nose may be increased to a maximum of 1.2 mg/kg/day, if needed.
- *Adverse drug reactions:* Insomnia, dryness of mouth, cough, decreased appetite, GI upset, Drowsiness, and irritability.
- *Caution:* Avoid <6 years.

Clonidine

See Chapter 16 (Antihypertensive Drugs).

Chapter 28

Drugs for Apnea of Prematurity

INTRODUCTION

Apnea of prematurity (AOP) is a condition in which *premature neonates:*
- *Have periods when they stop* breathing for 15–20 seconds.
- Develop oxygen saturation (SpO_2, 80% for over 4 seconds.
- Develop bradycardia (heart rate, two-thirds of baseline for over 4 seconds during sleep).

Why AOP? The brain and spinal cord regions that are responsible for normal breathing are not sufficiently mature in premature infants. In these babies, AOP may develop as a provocation from such adverse conditions as sepsis or idiopathic. Manifestations are the form of large bursts of breath followed by periods of shallow breathing or even stopped breathing.

For idiopathic apnea, common treatments include stimulation (usually tactile), methylxanthine, or assisted ventilation [e.g., nasal continuous positive airway pressure (CPAP) and mechanical ventilation].

CAFFEINE CITRATE

It is a central nervous system stimulant.

Brand names: Cafcit, Cafirate, Capnea, and Primicef
- *Available as:* Injection 20 mg/mL as 1, 2, 1.5, and 3 mL vials.
- *Indications:* Idiopathic apnea of prematurity.
- *Dose:* Start with a loading dose of 10–20 mg/kg (5–10 mg as base) as IV infusion over 30 minutes time span. Maintenance dose is 5 mg/kg (2.5 mg as base) in a single dose or two divided doses 24 hours after the loading dose.
- *Adverse drug reactions:* Tachycardia and tachypnea.
- *Caution:* Discontinue administration, if heart rate exceeds 180 minutes.

AMINOPHYLLINE

A methylxanthine that can be used for stimulating breathing.
- *Available as:* Injection 125 mg/mL (10 mL ampule).
- *Dose:* Loading dose 6 mg/kg/dose (IV)
  - Maintenance dose: 6 mg/kg/day divided q 6 h/q 8 h/q 12 h (IV)
  - Infuse slowly over a minimum of 20 minutes
- *Adverse drug reactions:* Rapid infusion may cause sudden death from cardiac arrhythmias.
- *Caution:* Administer very slowly to achieve a therapeutic level of 6–20 mg/mL. Level over 20 mg/mL is toxic.

Chapter 29: Drugs for Bleeding Control

INTRODUCTION

In children, a bleeding disorder may be inherited or acquired. The bleeding disorders include coagulation factor deficiencies, platelet deficiencies and/or dysfunctions. The workup of a child presenting with bleeding includes a detailed medical and bleeding history, family history, physical examination, and select laboratory tests.

AMINOCAPROIC ACID (6-AMINOHEXANOIC ACID)

A derivative and analog of the amino acid lysine; an effective inhibitor for enzymes that binds that particular residue, e.g., proteolytic enzymes like plasmin, the enzyme responsible for fibrinolysis.

Brand names: Amicar and Hemostat
- *Available as:* Tablet 500 mg and injection 250 mg/mL.
- *Indications:* Severe bleeding, systemic hyperfibrinolysis, traumatic ocular hyphema, and severe thrombocytopenia.
- *Dose:* Loading 100–200 mg/kg (PO and IV) followed by 100 mg/kg q 6 h with a maximum of 30 g.
- *Adverse drug reactions:* Headache, bradycardia, hypotension, nasal congestion, hypokalemia, and seizures.
- *Contraindication:* Disseminated intravascular coagulopathy (DIC) or consumptive coagulopathy.

- *Caution:* Avoid in upper urinary tract bleeding in which aminocaproic acid may cause intrarenal obstruction in the form of glomerular capillary thrombosis or clots in the renal pelvis and ureters.

ANTIHEMOPHILIC FACTOR

Brand names: Factor VIII, Fanhdi, Hemoctin Sdh, HemoRel-A, and Immunate.
- *Available as:* Injection 25 IU vial.
- *Dose:* 20–50 IU/kg/dose q 12 h.
- *Adverse drug reactions:* Transmission of some infections, e.g., hepatitis B and HIV.
- *Caution:* Do not mix this medicine with the liquid diluent until ready to give the injection. Do not use it in von Willebrand's disease.

ETHAMSYLATE

A hemostatic drug that enhances capillary endothelial resistance and promoting platelet adhesion. It also inhibits biosynthesis and action of those prostaglandins that cause platelet disaggregation, vasodilation, and increased capillary permeability.

Brand names: Dicynene, Ethasyl, and Sylate
- *Available as:* Tablet 250 and 500 mg and injection 125 mg/mL.
- *Indications:* Neonatal periventricular hemorrhage and menorrhagia.
- *Dose:* 12.5 mg/kg q 6 h
- *Adverse drug reactions:* Severe allergic reaction, high fever, headache, diarrhea, and skin rash.
- *Caution:* Avoid in pregnancy and lactation.

PROTAMINE SULFATE

Brand names: Newtain and Prota
- *Available as:* Injection 1% 10 mg/mL (ampule).
- *Indication:* Heparin overdose-induced hemorrhage.
- *Dose:* Loading dose 2.5–5 mg/kg (IV) over 5 minutes. Follow with 1–2.5 mg/kg q 4 h. 1 mg of protamine neutralizes 100 U of heparin.
- *Adverse drug reactions:* Increase in pulmonary artery pressure and decrease in peripheral blood pressure, myocardial oxygen consumption, cardiac output, and heart rate.
- *Caution:* Avoid overdose of protamine to safeguard against anticoagulation.

TRANEXAMIC ACID

It is an antifibrinolytic agent that tends to safeguard against breakdown of a clot, thereby stopping excessive bleeding.

Brand names: Clip, Pause, Tranexamic, and Tranfib
- *Available as:* Tablet 500 mg and injection 100 mg/mL.
- *Indications:* Major trauma, hemophilia, recurrent epistaxis, subconjunctival hemorrhage, tonsillectomy, tooth extraction, gastrointestinal bleed, and heavy menstruation.
- *Dose:*
  - PO 25 mg/kg/dose TDS
  - Injection 10 mg/kg/dose TDS
- *Adverse drug reactions:* Headache, backache, arthralgia, abdominal discomfort/pain, nasal sinus problem, abdominal pain, diarrhea, chills, fatigue, anemia; rarely pulmonary embolism, deep vein thrombosis, visual disturbances, anaphylaxis, and visual disturbances.
- *Contraindications:* Subjects on hormonal contraceptive, obesity, and cigarette smoking.
- *Caution:* Avoid in renal insufficiency.

Chapter 30

Drugs for Endocrinal Disorders/Hormones/Enzymes

INTRODUCTION

Endocrinal disorders warranting pharmacotherapy include pituitary, hypothalamus, thyroid, and pancreatic disorders. Anabolic steroids are indicated in some situations.

PITUITARY-RELATED DRUGS

Adrenocorticotropic Hormone

Adrenocorticotropic hormone (ACTH) stimulates the adrenal glands to release two hormones: (1) cortisol and (2) adrenaline.

Brand names: Acthar, Cosyntropin, and Synacthen
- *Available as:* Injection 60 IU/vial.
  - Gel 20 units, 40 units, and 60 units/mL.
- *Indications:* Sudden withdrawal of steroids after a prolonged course; infantile spasms, West syndrome, immunosuppression, as anti-inflammatory, muscle weakness in myasthenia gravis, as a substitute for steroids, for dynamic testing (ACTH test).[*]

---

[*]An *ACTH test* can help to diagnose adrenal or pituitary diseases.

- *Dose:*
  - *Infantile spasms:* 30 units/kg/day (IM and SC) in two divided doses, each dose not exceeding 100 units for 2 weeks.
  - *Immunosuppression/anti-inflammatory:* 0.8 unit/kg/day (IM, SC, and IV) as a single dose or in two divided doses/day.
- *Adverse drug reactions:* Acne, edema (from sodium and water retention), hypokalemia, electrolyte imbalance, obesity (Cushing syndrome), seizures, and osteoporosis.
- Cushing disease, fungal infection, and tuberculosis.
- Avoid administering live vaccine during the course of ACTH therapy.

Desmopressin Acetate

Brand names: D-Void and Desmospray

It is a vasopressin analog.
- *Indications:* A synthetic analog of vasopressin indicated in nocturnal enuresis and diabetes insipidus (central).
- *Available as:* Nasal spray 0.1 mg/mL, each dose = 10 µg.
- *Dose:* One intranasal spray in each nostril at bedtime initially; then two sprays in each nostril, if necessary.
- *Adverse drug reactions:* Headache, nausea, flushing, stomach pain, hypotension, overhydration, and hypernatremia.
- *Contraindications:* Habitual psychogenic polydipsia, hypotension, cardiac insufficiency, concomitant use of diuretics, and von Willebrand disease (type 2B).
- *Caution:* Avoid in nasal infection, rhinorrhea, cardiovascular disease, renal impairment, hypotension, cystic fibrosis, and hemophilia (hemophilia A with factor VIII levels <5%; hemophilia B; avoid using beyond 28 days at a stretch).

- *Drug interaction:* Chlorpromazine, indomethacin, tricyclic antidepressants, carbamazepine, and other pressor agents.

Growth Hormone (Somatropin)

Brand names: Genotropin, Saizen, and Norditropin

- *Available as:* Injection 4 units, 10 units, 12 units, 16 units/ampule or vial.
- *Indications:*
  - Definitive indication—growth hormone deficiency.
  - Relative indications—Turner syndrome, chronic renal failure, renal transplantation, and cranial irradiation causing neurosecretory dysfunction.
- *Dose:* 0.09–0.2 unit/kg/day (SC and IM) OD thrice a week till attainment of target height or bone fusion occurs.
- *Adverse drug reactions*: Premature bone fusion, gynecomastia, pseudotumor cerebri slipped capital femoral epiphysis, and worsening of scoliosis.
- *Caution:* Avoid >11 years age. Monitor bone fusion.

Somatostatin

Brand name: Sandostatin

- *Available as*: 50 and 100 µg/mL.
- *Indication*: Excess of growth hormone.
- *Dose*: 1–40 µg/kg/day. Repeat two to four times weekly.
- *Adverse drug reactions:* Nausea and diarrhea.

Vasopressin

This is already dealt within Chapter 23 (Cardiotonic Drugs). Besides diabetes insipidus (pituitary type), it is of value in catecholamine refractory shock and variceal bleeding in portal hypertension.

PANCREAS-RELATED DRUGS

Insulin

- *Available as:*
  - Soluble 40 IU/mL and 80 IU/mL (action about 6 hours).
  - Zinc suspension lente 40 IU/mL and 80 IU/mL (action about 24 hours).
  - Isophan (NPH) 40 IU/mL (action about 24 hours).
  - Protamine zinc 40 IU/mL (action about 24 hours).
- *Indication:* Diabetes mellitus.
- *Dose:*
  - 0.1 unit/kg/hour (soluble, by IV infusion).
  - 0.5 unit/kg/day in three divided doses.
- *Adverse drug reactions:* Hypoglycemic reactions, local or systemic allergic reactions, local infection, lipodystrophy, fibrous lipomata, and transient myopia.

Pancreatin

Brand names: Pancreatic enzyme, Pankreon, and Serutan

- *Available as:* Tablets and powder/granules of various strength.
- *Indications:* Dyspepsia and cystic fibrosis.
- *Dose:* 300–600 mg with each meal.
- *Adverse drug reactions:* Hypersensitivity reactions, impaction, rash, abdominal discomfort, constipation, and hyperuricemia.
- *Drug interactions:* H_2-receptor antagonists, omeprazol, and antacids.

THYROID-RELATED

Thyroxine

Brand names: Eltroxin, Thyrox, and Thyronorm

- *Available as:* Tablets 25, 50, 100, and 200 µg.

- *Indications:* Hypothyroid states, including congenital hypothyroidism.
- *Dose*—Start with 50–100 µg (PO). Increase every 3–4 weeks by increments of 25–50 µg to about 200–300 µg.
  - *Neonates:* 10–15 µg/kg/day (PO) OD.
  - *Later ages:* 5 µg/kg/day (PO) OD.
- *Adverse drug reactions:* Weight loss, arrhythmias, and congestive heart failure (CHF). Overdose may cause diarrhea, tachycardia, irritability, flushing, excessive sweating, headache, and cramps and advanced bone age followed by premature closure of epiphyses.
- *Caution:* Take special precautions in myocardial and adrenal insufficiency.

Thyroid (Desiccated)

- *Available as:* Tablets 15, 30, and 60 mg.
- *Dose:* 4 mg/day (PO) as single dose. Initially, 15 mg/day for infants and 30 mg/day in late years. Increase by increments of 15 mg every 1–3 weeks to 60–180 mg/day depending on child's age.
- *Adverse drug reactions:* Diarrhea, restlessness, excitability, sleeplessness, pain abdomen, vomiting, polyuria, and tremors.

Carbimazole

Brand name: Neomercazole
- *Available as:* Tablet 5 mg.
- *Indication:* Hyperthyroidism.
- *Dose:* 1–2 mg/kg/day (PO) q 8 hours.
- *Adverse drug reactions:* Nausea, loss of taste, sore throat, headache, skin problems such as urticaria, alopecia, and

pigmentation, bone marrow depression (agranulocytosis), nephritic syndrome, arthralgia, and rarely cholestatic jaundice.

ADRENALS-RELATED DRUGS

Beclomethasone

See Chapter 8 (Antiasthma Drugs).

Betamethasone

It is an adrenal corticosteroid and anti-inflammatory agent.

Brand names: Betnesol, Betacortril, Solubet, Celestone, and Walacort

- *Available as:* Drops 0.5 mg/mL. Tablets 0.5 and 1 mg. Injection 4 mg/mL.
- *Indications:* Antenatal use to enhance fetal lung maturity in preterm labor (labor starting before 34 weeks); congenital adrenal hyperplasia (CAH); cerebral edema, asthma collagenosis; and topical use to treat inflammatory conditions.
- *Dose:* Antenatal (to mother) 12 mg (IM) q 24 hours for two doses. Children 0.1–0.2 mg/kg/day (PO).
- *Adverse drug reactions*: Maternal pulmonary edema, headache, and hypertension.

Dexamethasone

It is an adrenal corticosteroid and anti-inflammatory agent.

Brand names: Decadron and Wymesone

- *Available as*: Tablet 0.5 mg. Injection 4 and 20 mg/mL.
- *Indications:* Inflammatory, allergic, autoimmune, and neoplastic disorders; cerebral edema; septic shock;

H. influenzae meningitis; and as antiemetic in chemotherapy as diagnostic agent.

- *Dose: Airway edema/extubation in neonates:* 0.25 mg/kg q 12 hours three to four doses.
  - Bronchopulmonary dysplasia 0.25 mg/kg/dose q 12 hours for six doses; thereafter taper over 1–6 weeks.
  - *Airway edema/extubation in infants and children:* 0.5–2 mg/kg/day divided q 6 hours.
  - *As antiemetic (in chemotherapy):* 10 mg/m^2 first dose followed by 5 mg/m^2/dose q 6 hours (IV).
  - *Anti-inflammatory:* 0.08–0.3 mg/kg/day divided q 6–12 hours (PO, IM, and IV).
  - *H. influenzae meningitis:* 0.6 mg/kg/day in divided q 6 hours for days 1–4 of antibiotics.
- *Adverse drug reactions:* Insomnia, nervousness, increased appetite, hypertension, hyperglycemia, GI hyperacidity and stress ulcers, cataracts, adrenal suppression, and growth retardation.
- *Caution*: Exercise special caution in its use in bronchopulmonary dysplasia in view of the enhanced risk of cerebral palsy.

Cortisone Acetate

Brand name: Cortin

- *Available as:* Tablet 25 mg.
- *Indications:* Physiologic replacement; stressful situations, say in adrenogenital syndrome; nephrotic syndrome, leukemia, lymphoma, rheumatic carditis, selected cases of tuberculosis, immunologic reactions; and autoimmune disease.
- *Dose:* 2.5–10 mg/kg/day (PO) in three divided doses. Half of this dose for IM or IV use.

- *Adverse drug reactions:* Cushingoid facies, hypertension, electrolyte disturbances, pseudotumor cerebri, acne, gastritis, increased appetite, peptic ulcer, activation of tuberculosis, poor resistance to infection, osteoporosis, glaucoma, cataract, growth retardation, myopathy, and adrenocortical atrophy.
- *Caution:* Special precautions are required in using the drug in peptic ulcer, diabetes, hypertension, and infection.

Table 1 lists the relative anti-inflammatory potency and sodium retaining potency of corticosteroids.

Hydrocortisone

Brand names: Efcorlin, Hydrocortone, and Hydrocortistab

- *Available as:* Tablets 10 and 20 mg. Injection 100 mg/vial.
- *Indications:* Acute severe asthma/status asthmaticus, endotoxic shock, acute adrenal insufficiency, congenital adrenal hyperplasia (CAH).
- *Dose:* Acute severe asthma/status asthmaticus: 25–50 mg/kg/dose (IV) 4–6 hours.

TABLE 1: Relative anti-inflammatory potency and sodium-retaining potency of different corticosteroids.

Corticosteroid	Anti-inflammatory potency (mg)	Sodium-retaining potency (mg)
Hydrocortisone	100	100
Cortisone	80	80
Prednisolone/Prednisone	20	100
Methylprednisolone	16	0
Triamcinolone	16	0
Dexamethasone	2	0
Desoxycorticosterone	0	2

- *Endotoxic shock:* 50 mg/kg to begin with, followed by 50–150 mg/kg/day in four divided doses as for 2–3 days.
- Acute adrenal insufficiency 50 mg/m^2/day.
- *Congenital adrenal hyperplasia:* 10–15 mg/m^2/day (one-fourth at noon and half at night). Maintenance dose 0.3–0.4 mg/kg/day (divided).
- *Adverse drug reactions*: Hypertension, hyperglycemia, hypokalemia, euphoria, insomnia, headache, Cushing syndrome, peptic ulcer disease, cataracts, immunosuppression, skin and muscle atrophy, acne, and edema.
- *Caution*: Avoid abrupt withdrawal which may cause acute adrenal insufficiency.

Prednisolone

It is a glucocorticoid for treating certain types of allergies, inflammatory conditions, autoimmune disorders, and cancers.

Brand names: Wysolone, Deltacortril, and Predone
- **Available as:** Tablets 5, 10, 20, and 40 mg.
- **Indications:** Treatment of inflammatory and allergic disorders, nephrotic syndrome, rheumatic carditis with congestive cardiac failure (CCF), immune/idiopathic thrombocytopenic purpura (ITP), certain encephalopathies and encephalitis, viral carditis, collagenosis, severe asthma, allergic skin conditions, and rheumatoid arthritis.
- **Dose:** 1–2 mg/kg/day (PO) in divided doses.
- **Adverse drug reactions:** Cushingoid facies, hypertension, euphoria, growth retardation, osteoporosis, myopathy, hyperglycemia, lowered resistance to infection, pseudotumor cerebri, activation of dormant tuberculosis, growth retardation, and edema from increased salt retention.

- *Caution:* Avoid prolong treatment course; titrate dose to obtain desired effect.

Methylprednisolone

It is an antiallergic, anti-inflammatory, and immunosuppressant glucocorticoid.

Brand names: Medrol, Depo-medrol, Solu-medrol, and Unidrol

- *Indications:* Immune/idiopathic thrombocytopenic purpura (ITP), chronic GBS, allergic, inflammatory, and neoplastic (as immunosuppressant) conditions; pulse therapy; and acute spinal cord injury.
- *Dose:*
    - Routine 0.5–2 (average 1) mg/kg/day (IM and IV)
    - Emergency 30 mg/kg (IV bolus) over 10–20 minutes; repeat after 4 hours if required.
    - Shock 30 mg/kg/dose q 6 hours × 2 days
    - Pulse therapy 30 mg/kg/day × 3–5 days
- *Caution:* Avoid in concurrent administration of live vaccine as also in presence of fungal or tuberculous infection.

Triamcinolone

It is a corticosteroid available in oral, topical, inhalation, and spray forms.

Brand names: Kenacort and Ledercort

- *Available as:* Tablet 4 mg.
- *Indications:* Inflammatory and allergic condition.
- *Dose*:
    - Up to 24 mg/day (PO) in divided doses.
    - 40 mg (deep IM).
    - 2.5–15 mg (Intra-articular).

- *Adverse drug reactions*: Tissue atrophy about injection site, fatigue, mental depression, myopathy (proximal), osteoporosis, cataracts, oral thrush, and growth retardation.
- *Caution:* Avoid <6 years of age.

ANABOLIC STEROIDS

Most common use (rather "abuse") is as performance-enhancing agents by competitive sportspersons and athletes. Increased muscle mass and strength appear to be related to the myotrophic action at androgen receptors, competitive antagonism at catabolism-mediating corticosteroid receptors and erythropoietic and psychological effects.

Adverse effects of anabolic steroids are listed in **Box 1**.

Methandienone

Brand name: Dianabol
- *Available as:* Tablets 1 and 5 mg. Drops 1 mg/30 drops.
- *Indications:* Weight loss and osteoporosis during steroid therapy.
- *Dose:* 0.04 mg/kg/day (PO).
- *Adverse drug reactions:* Nausea, edema, interference with menstruation, hepatic dysfunction, premature epiphyseal closure, gynecomastia, and virilization.
- *Contraindication:* Hepatic insufficiency.
- *Caution:* Do not use the drug for a period of >4 weeks at a time. However, the course may be resumed after an interruption of 6 weeks.

Nandrolone

Brand name: Durabolin
- *Available as:* Injection 10 and 25 mg/mL.

BOX 1: Common adverse effects of anabolic steroids.

- Increasing acneiform lesions
- Linear keloids, stria, oily hair, and hirsutism
- Males
  - Gynecomastia/breast pain
  - Testicular atrophy (irreversible)
  - Azoospermia (irreversible)
- Females
  - Breast atrophy (irreversible)
  - Clitoral enlargement
  - Menstrual abnormalities
- Serious psychologic effects
  - Uncontrolled rage
  - Depression
  - Mania
  - Mood fluctuations
  - Alteration in libido
- Fluid retention
- Growth retardation from accelerated epiphyseal closure (irreversible)
- IV use
  - HIV
  - HBV
- Liver
  - Acute hepatitis
  - Hepatomegaly
  - Hepatocellular carcinoma (irreversible)

(HBV: hepatitis B virus; HIV: human immunodeficiency virus)

- *Indications:* Weight loss; osteoporosis; during or after prolonged corticosteroid therapy; and uremia.
- *Dose:*
  - *Infants:* 5 mg once a week or 100 mg once a fortnight
  - *Children:* 10–12.5 mg once every 10 days.
- *Adverse drug reactions:* Nausea, edema, menstrual disturbance, hepatic dysfunction, premature epiphyseal

closure, gynecomastia, virilization, anorexia, epigastric pain, nausea, vomiting, diarrhea; transient rise of serum glutamic oxaloacetic transaminase (SGOT), serum glutamate pyruvate transaminase (SGPT), serum creatinine, bilirubin; anemia, thrombocytopenia, leukopenia, and agranulocytosis.
- *Contraindications:* Hypersensitivity to quinolones; epilepsy.
- *Caution:* Avoid in children below 12 years, except in desperate situations.

Oxymetholone

Brand names: Adroyed and Anadroyl
- *Available as:* Tablet 50 mg.
- *Indications:* Weight loss, osteoporosis, chemotherapy-induced anemia, HIV/AIDS wasting syndrome and during corticosteroid therapy.
- *Dose:* 0.1–0.8 mg/kg/day (PO).
- *Adverse drug reactions:* Nausea, edema, interference with menstruation, hepatic dysfunction, premature closure of epiphysis, virilization, and gynecomastia.

Ethylestrenol

Brand name: Orabolin
- *Available as:* Tablet 2 mg. Drops 1 mg/15 drops.
- *Indications:* Weight loss, osteoporosis, during steroid therapy.
- *Dose:* 0.06 mg (1 drop)/kg/day (PO).
- *Adverse drug reactions:* Nausea, edema, interference with menstruation hepatic dysfunction, premature closure of epiphysis, virilization, and gynecomastia.

31
Chapter

Drugs for Gout

INTRODUCTION

Gout is a sort of inflammatory arthritis resulting from high level of uric acid in blood. In a vast majority of cases, it results secondary to a kidney disease. It may be primary (without an obvious cause) or secondary to another disorder.

Primary juvenile gout, characterized by severe pain in big toe and joints such as knee, ankle, and hip, is rare. Children who are already suffering from diabetes, kidney disease, obesity, or certain blood cancers are at a high risk of developing gout.

ALLOPURINOL

Brand names: Aloric, Ciploric, and Zyloric
A xanthine oxidase inhibitor.

- *Available as:* Tablet 100 and 300 mg.
- *Indication:* To combat hyperuricemia and urate deposition in subjects on antimalignant therapy as an adjuvant; gout. Duchenn myopathy and Lesch-Nyhan syndrome (juvenile gout from an enzyme deficiency).
- *Dose:* 10–20 mg/kg/day in three divided doses.
- *Adverse drug reactions:* Hypersensitivity reactions (including Steven-Johnson syndrome), toxic epidermal necrosis, acute gout, fever, malaise, muscle aches, drowsiness leukopenia, leukocytosis, eosinophilia, bone

marrow depression, hepatomegaly, peripheral neuritis and cataract, and bone marrow depression. Undesirable reactions such as nausea, vomiting, diarrhea, headache, vertigo, and gastric irritation occur occasionally but do not warrant discontinuation of therapy.
- *Drug interaction:* Anticoagulants, azathioprine, chlorpropamide, mercaptopurine, vidarabine, ampicillin, amoxicillin, salicylates, cyclophosphamide, iron salts, cyclosporine, thiazide diuretics, high doses salicylates, and theophylline.
- *Contraindication:* Acute gout.
- *Caution:* Avoid in the presence of hypertension, cardiac insufficiency, renal insufficiency, hepatic dysfunction, etc. Ensure adequate fluid intake. At the time of starting treatment, administer colchicine for 1 month.

COLCHICINE

An alkaloid is used to prevent or treat gout attacks. Also, for preventing attacks of pain in the abdomen, chest, or joints caused by a certain inherited conditions (familial Mediterranean fever). Colchicine works by decreasing swelling and lessening the build-up of uric acid crystals that cause pain in the affected joints.

Brand names: Coljoy and Zycolchin
- *Available as:* Tablet 0.5 mg.
- *Indications:* Gout, both acute and chronic.
- *Dose:* Acute gout 0.5–0.6 (PO) mg q 2 hours as long as pain is there. The total daily dose must not exceed 8 mg.
- *Adverse drug reactions:* Nausea, vomiting, diarrhea, muscle cramping, abdominal pain; rarely bruising, and numbness.
- *Caution:* Avoid alcohol.

Probenecid

Brand names: Procid and Benocid

- *Available as:* Tablet 500 mg.
- *Indications:*
  - For competitive inhibition of tubular secretion and reabsorption of organic acids, e.g., in gout, hyperuricemia.
  - For cutting down excretion of penicillin in urine in order to build up very high blood level.
- *Dose:*
  - 250 mg twice daily for 1 week followed by 500 mg twice daily in gout and hyperuricemia.
  - 25 mg/kg as loading dose. Follow with 10 mg/kg 6–8 hourly for high-dose penicillin therapy.
- *Adverse drug reactions:* Frequency of micturition, headache, blood dyscrasia, GIT upset, flushing, hepatic necrosis, hemolysis, and nephrosis.
- *Contraindications:* Blood dyscrasias and renal uric acid stones.
- *Caution:* History of peptic ulcer disease and renal impairment.
- *Drug interaction:* Salicylates, pyrazinamide, sulfonylurea, sulfonamides, β-lactam antibiotics, indomethacin, and methotrexate.

Chapter 32

Drugs for Vertigo

INTRODUCTION

Vertigo is defined as a sensation of motion or spinning. It is a symptom, which is characterized by a feeling as if a person and/or objects around him are moving or spinning. Nausea, vomiting, sweating, or difficulties in walking may accompany it. The cause may be in inner ear (labyrinth) resulting in disturbance of balance, neck, or brain. When associated tinnitus, hearing loss, and a feeling of high pressure in the inner ear, it is termed "Ménière's disease".

BETAHISTINE DIHYDROCHLORIDE

Brand name: Vertin
- *Available as:* Tablet 8, 16, and 24 mg.
- *Indications:* Vertigo, tinnitus, and Ménière's disease.
- *Dose:* 8–16 mg (PO) TDS.
- *Adverse drug reactions:* Bloating, headache, heartburn or indigestion, nausea, and vomiting.
- *Caution:* Avoid <12 years in asthma.

CINNARIZINE

Brand names: Cinirone, Dizikind, Dizzigo, and Vertigon
- *Available as:* Tablet 25 and 75 mg (Forte).
- *Indications:* Vertigo, motion sickness, and Ménière's disease.

- *Dose:* 12.5–25 mg 1–2 hours before starting travel and 12.5 mg every 8 hours during course of travel.
- *Adverse drug reactions:* Drowsiness, sweating, dry mouth, headache, skin problems, lethargy, gastrointestinal upset, hypersensitivity reactions, movement disorder, and parkinsonism-like illness (both acute and chronic).
- *Caution:* Avoid concurrent administration of central nervous system (CNS) depressants.

Hematinics

INTRODUCTION
Hematinics are nutrient medications that tend to enhance the formation of blood cells in the process of hematopoiesis, resulting in increase in the hemoglobin content of the blood. The main hematinics are iron, vitamin B_{12}, and folate. Erythropoietin (EPO), a hormone that stimulates erythropoiesis, is sometimes used to increase the hemoglobin content of the blood. However, in actuality, EPO is not classified as a hematinic.

FERROUS SULFATE
Brand name: Fersolate (20% elemental iron)
- *Available as:* Tablet 200 mg providing 40 mg of elemental iron.
- *Indication:* Iron-deficiency anemia.
- *Dose:* 1 mg/kg/day (PO) for prophylaxis, 3–6 mg/kg (PO) for curative purposes (calculated in terms of elemental iron).
- *Adverse drug reactions:* Gastrointestinal tract (GIT) upset (both diarrhea and constipation are known to occur), hemochromatosis in cases of chronic hemolytic anemia.

FOLIC ACID
Brand names: Fol-5, Folet, Folum, and Folvite
- *Available as:* Tablet 5 and 10 mg.

- *Indications:* Megaloblastic anemia from folic acid deficiency, endemic tropical sprue, along with iron in iron-deficiency anemia, thalassemia, during course of phenytoin therapy; periconceptional therapy (1 month before and 2 months after conception) to prevent neural tube defects such as meningocele and meningomyelocele in the fetus.
- *Dose:* 5–20 mg/day (PO); 1 mg/day (IM) or 02 µg/kg/day.
- *Adverse drug reactions:* Rarely, hypersensitivity reactions, GI upset, sleep disturbances, rash, and bronchospasm.
- *Drug interaction:* Anticonvulsants, pyrimethamine, sulfasalazine, trimethoprim, oral contraceptives, methotrexate, alcohol, and pyrimethamine.
- *Contraindication:* Pernicious anemia.
- *Caution:* Folate-dependent tumors. Heavy doses camouflage manifestations from vitamin B_{12} deficiency other than neurologic complications.

IRON

- *Indication:* Iron-deficiency anemia.
- *Available as:*
  - Oral preparation **(Table 1)**.
  - *Injection:* Iron-dextran complex (IM and IV), iron sorbitol (IM). Iron sucrose.
- *Dose:* Prophylaxis/maintenance 0.5–1 mg/kg/day (PO), in terms of elemental iron, q 12 hours.
- *Therapeutic:* 3–6 mg/kg/day (PO), in terms of elemental iron, q 12 hours.
  - *Iron dextran complex:* Vide infra
  - *Iron sorbitrol:* Vide infra
  - *Iron sucrose:* Vide infra

TABLE 1: Element iron content of various oral iron salts.

Salt	Elemental iron (%)
Ferrous sulfate	20
Anhydrous ferrous sulfate	37
Ferrous fumarate	33
Ferrous fructose	25
Ferrous succinate	23
Ferrous lactate	19
Ferrous carbonate	16
Ferrous ammonium citrate	15
Ferrous choline citrate	20
Ferrous gluconate	12
Colloidal iron	50

Iron (III) hydroxide polymaltose complex 50 mg/5 mL or tablet

- *Adverse drug reactions:* GIT upset (nausea, vomiting, diarrhea, and abdominal pain) and staining of teeth.
- *Caution:* Accidental swallowing in large doses may cause iron poisoning with local irritative effects on GIT mucosa, hypoglycemia, metabolic acidosis, hepatic necrosis, pyloric stenosis, and even death.

IRON DEXTRAN

Brand name: Imferon

- *Available as:* Injection 50 mg/mL of elemental iron.
- *Indication:* Iron-deficiency anemia.
- *Dose:*

$$\text{Requirement (mg)} = \frac{0.3 \times \text{weight (lbs)} \times \text{Hb deficit (\%)}}{50}$$

or

$$= 4 \times \text{weight (kg)} \times \text{Hb deficit (g/dL)}$$

- The total requirements may be given intravenously as total dose infusion (TDI) or intramuscularly (daily 1–2 mL).
- *Adverse drug reactions:* Anaphylaxis, hypersensitivity reactions, fever, urticaria, nausea, vomiting, headache, arthralgia, and generalized lymphadenopathy.
- *Caution:* Always do sensitivity test before IV administration.

IRON SORBITOL

Brand name: Jectofer
- *Indication:* Iron-deficiency anemia.
- *Available as:* Injection 1.5 mL providing 50 mg/mL.
- *Dose:* 1.5 mg (0.33 mL)/kg/dose (IM).
- *Adverse drug reactions:* None observed so far.
- *Contraindications:* Severe liver or kidney damage, acute leukemia, and aplastic or hypoplastic anemia.

IRON SUCROSE COMPLEX

Brand name: Venofer
- *Indication:* Severe anemia in >2-year-old subjects with chronic kidney disease (CKD).
- *Available as:* IV injection 1 mL providing 20 mg elemental iron.
- *Dose:* Slow intravenous administration at a rate of 1 mL undiluted solution per minute and not exceeding 10 mL (200 mg iron) per injection.
- *Adverse drug reactions:* Hypersensitivity reactions including anaphylaxis (shock, hypotension, and circulatory collapse), muscle cramps, nausea, vomiting and diarrhea, disturbance of taste, and peripheral edema.

- *Contraindications:* <2 years age; iron overload.
- *Cautions:* Monitoring for hypersensitivity reactions at least for 30 minutes following completion of infusion. Also monitor BP.

VITAMIN B_{12} (COBALAMIN AND CYANOCOBALAMIN)

It is a water-soluble vitamin of B-complex group. It is available from meat, eggs, fish and milk (dairy) products (cheese and curd); also banana, mushroom, and potato.

Vitamin B_{12} is essential for the synthesis of DNA by the body, for the production of blood cells, and for maintaining the health of nerves. Its deficiency results in megaloblastic anemia and peripheral neuropathy manifesting as paresthesia (pricks and needles sensation, numbness, tingling, itching, skin crawling, burning sensation) and tremors. Normal blood level is >200 pg/mL. Ideally, it should be >300 pg/mL.

Brand names: Alkem, Bevidox, Cobex, Macraberin, Neurokind, and Triredisol

- *Available as:* Often, in combination with vitamin B_1 and B_6 or a neurofriendly molecule.
  - *Tablet:* 500, 1,500, and 5,000 µg.
  - *Injection:* 500 µg/mL.
- *Indications:* Nutritional supplement, megaloblastic anemia as such or in association with other conditions (say, infantile tremor syndrome, tropical sprue), paresthesia, enhanced requirements in hemorrhagic, renal, and liver disorders.
- *Daily requirement:* 0.3–2 µg.

- *Dose:* 250–1,000 µg (IM) on alternate days for 1–2 weeks followed by once a week until blood count returns to normal. Then, maintenance dose of 1,000 µg every 2–4 months.
- *Adverse drug reactions:* Very rare. Peripheral thrombosis, polycythemia vera, gout, and hypokalemia.
- *Drug interaction:* Alcohol and passive alcohol sensor (PAS).
- *Caution:* Since there is every chance of concurrent depletion of iron and folate stores as also hypokalemia, supplementation with these micronutrients is recommended.

34
Chapter
Immunoglobulins

INTRODUCTION

Immunoglobulins or antibodies are defined as proteins that the body's immune system produces in order to fight the invading bacteria or virus. When the body is exposed to invading microbes, it makes unique antibodies. These unique antibodies are specifically designed to fight and destroy only those microbes. The documented types of immunoglobulins are IgG, IgM, IgA, IgD, IgM, and IgE.

Immunoglobulin therapy is the use of a mixture of antibodies (immunoglobulins) to treat a number of health conditions, including primary immunodeficiency, idiopathic/immune thrombocytopenic purpura (ITP), chronic inflammatory demyelinating polyneuropathy, Kawasaki disease, and Guillain–Barré syndrome (GBS).

ANTI-RH (D) IMMUNOGLOBULIN

Brand names: Imogam and Matergam P.

- *Available as:* Intramuscular (IM) injection 100, 125, and 350 µg.
- *Indications:* Rh-negative mother, immediately after delivery, and chronic ITP
- *Dose:* Given to the Rh-negative mother 2 hours after delivery or abortion/MTP or latest 72 hours postpartum—
  - Without testing: Optimal standard dose 350 µg.

- With testing (up to 10 mL of fetal blood has entered the maternal circulation): 250 µg.
- For abortion and MTP cases (up to 10 weeks of conception): 100 µg.
- *Adverse drug reactions (ADRs):* Local reaction over the injection site, sensitization due to repeated injection.
- *Contraindications:* Rh (D) negative patient who has inadvertently received Rh (D) positive blood transfusion within 3 months before delivery
  - Patient earlier immunized to the Rh (D) blood factor.
- *Caution:* Protection given at delivery of first baby does not protect the mother from exposure to antigen received at a later time. Hence, the agent requires to be given immediately following each pregnancy.

ANTISNAKE VENOM

See Chapter 21 (Antitoxins).

DIPHTHERIA ANTITOXIN

See Chapter 21 (Antitoxins).

GAS GANGRENE ANTITOXIN

See Chapter 21 (Antitoxins).

HUMAN NORMAL IMMUNOGLOBULIN

Brand names: Bharglob, Gamafine, Gammalin, Globunal, and SII Gamma Globulin

- *Available as:* IM injection 10 and 16.5%, 1 mL vials.
- *Indications:* Prophylaxis/treatment of primary immune deficiency disorders, viral infections (measles, hepatitis, and HIV/AIDS), bacterial infections, burns, etc.

- *Doses:*
  - *Immunodeficiency disorders*: In order to maintain the serum IgG level >500 mg/dL, dose needs to be 300–400 mg/kg (IM) every 3–4 weeks.
  - *Attenuation of measles in close contacts:* 0.3 mL/kg of 10% sol (IM) within 5–6 days of exposure.
  - *Attenuation of hepatitis A (Preexposure prophylaxis):* 0.02–0.04 mL/kg of 10% sol (IM) within 14 days of likely exposure (preexposure prophylaxis for travelers from nonendemic areas).
  - *Attenuation of hepatitis A (postexposure prophylaxis):* 0.02 mL/kg of 10% solution plus hepatitis A virus (HAV) vaccine.

HUMAN HEPATITIS B SPECIFIC GLOBULIN/ HEPATITIS B IMMUNOGLOBULIN

Brand names: Gamma protect hepatitis, Hepabig, and Hepaglob

- *Indications:* Neonates of HbsAg positive mothers; accidental mucocutaneous exposure to Hep B-infected blood/blood products or accidental needle exposure.
- *Available as:* 0.5, 1, 3, and 5 mL ampules.
- *Doses:*
  - *Neonates of HbsAg positive mothers:* 0.5–1.0 mL (100–200 units) IM within 72 hours (within 12 hours is the best) of birth along with first dose of hepatitis B vaccine IM at a different site for active immunization.
  - *Accidental exposure:* 0.06–0.1 mL/kg (40 units/kg) IM within 24 hours (within 6 hours is the best) of exposure along with first dose of hepatitis B vaccine IM at a different site for active immunization.
- *Adverse drug reactions:* Anaphylactic reactions.

- *Contraindication:* Allergy or intolerance to human immunoglobulins.
- *Cautions:* Avoid giving immunoglobulin and vaccine at the same site.

HUMAN RABIES SPECIFIC IMMUNOGLOBULIN

Brand names: Berirab, Imogam Rabies, and Imorab.
- *Indications:* Category 3 bites
- *Available as:* 300, 750, 1,000 units vials.
- *Doses:*
  - *Human rabies immunoglobulin (HRIG):* 20 units/kg to be infiltrated into the wound and neighborhood. This is the preferred choice.
  - *Equine rabies immunoglobulin (ERIG):* 40 units/kg to be infiltrated into the wound and neighborhood.
- *Adverse drug reactions:* Rarely, anaphylaxis with ERIG.
- *Cautions:* Test hypersensitivity before administering the agent.

RABIES-SPECIFIC IMMUNOGLOBULINS

Respiratory Syncytial Virus Intravenous Immunoglobulin

Brand name: Raspi Gam
- *Available as:* Injection 50 mg/mL
- *Indications:* Prevention of serious respiratory syncytial virus (RSV) infection (bronchiolitis and pneumonia) in high-risk children (prematurity and bronchopulmonary dysplasia).
- *Dose:* 750 mg/kg (IV) once a month. The course should begin a month before and be ongoing during RSV season. For exact recommendations **(Box 1)**.

BOX 1: Recommendation for respiratory syncytial virus intravenous immunoglobulin.

- *Starting dose:* 1.5 mL/kg/h for 15 minutes
- Then, increase the rate to 3 mL/kg/h for 15 minutes
- If well-tolerated, increase the rate to a maximum of 6 mL/kg/h until a total of 750 mL/kg is administered

- *Adverse drug reactions:* Anaphylaxis, fever, headache, backache, arthralgia, skin reactions, and hypertension.
- *Contraindication:* Congenital heart disease (right-to-left shunt).

Human Tetanus Specific Immunoglobulin

Brand names: Equirab, ERIG, Carig, Tetagam P, Tetaglobulin, Tetglob, Tetanus Immunoglobulin, and Immunotetan

- *Indications:* Both prophylaxis and treatment of tetanus
- *Dose:* Prophylaxis: 250–500 units/kg (IM), high dose is for heavily contaminated wounds, presentation of wounded subject after a lapse of >24 hours.
- *Treatment:* 30–300 units/kg (IV). 250 units (intrathecal).

Varicella Zoster Immunoglobulin

Varicella zoster immunoglobulin (VZIG) provides passive immunity against varicella.

Brand name: Varitect

- *Available as:* Injection 125 units/5 mL ampule.
- *Indications:* All susceptible individuals **(Box 2)**.
  - Prophylaxis of varicella in neonates whose mothers suffer from varicella 5 days before delivery and up to 2 days following delivery.
  - Postexposure prophylaxis in immunocompromised children and pregnant women.

BOX 2: Susceptible individuals needing varicella zoster immunoglobulin (VZIG).

- All unvaccinated children who do not have a clinical history of varicella in the past
- All unvaccinated adults who are seronegative for anti-varicella IgG. Bone marrow transplant recipients are considered susceptible even if they had disease or received vaccinations prior to transplantation. A significant contact is defined as any face-to-face contact or stay within the same room for a period >1 hour with a patient with infectious varicella (defined as 1–2 days before the rash till all lesions have crusted) or disseminated herpes zoster.

The following groups meeting these two criteria and who are at high-risk of developing severe disease merit prophylaxis with VZIG.

- Neonates born to mothers who develop varicella 5 days before or 2 days after delivery. The risk of varicella related death in these infants as per older estimates is likely to be 30% but may be lower. Other full-term healthy newborns are not at increased risk for complications and do not merit prophylaxis if exposed to varicella.
- All neonates born at <28 weeks of gestation/with birth weight <1,000 g, exposed in the neonatal period
- All preterm neonates born at >28 weeks of gestation and exposed to varicella only if their mothers are negative for anti-varicella IgG, exposed to varicella
- Pregnant women exposed to varicella
- All immunocompromised children especially neoplastic disease, congenital or acquired immunodeficiency or those receiving immunosuppressive therapies
- Patients who received intravenous immunoglobulin @ 400 mg/kg in the past 3 weeks are deemed protected

- *Dose:*
  - *Infants:*
    - <10 kg 125 units (IM). For subsequent each 10 kg weight, dose is enhanced by 125 units.

- *Children:*
  - 10–20 kg 250 units (IM)
  - 20–30 kg 375 units (IM)
  - 30–40 kg 500 units (IM)
  - 40 kg 625 units (IM)
- *Adverse drug reactions:* Allergic reactions and anaphylaxis.
- *Precautions:* Best given within 48 hours and never after 96 hours of postexposure.
  - Maximum of 2.5 mL should be injected at one site.
  - Do not give in mothers actually suffering from herpes zoster.
- *Special remarks:* The cost of VZIG is prohibitive. If non-affordable/not available, other options with uncertain efficacy include intravenous immunoglobulin @ 200 mg/kg or oral acyclovir @ 80 mg/kg/day beginning from the 7th day of exposure and given for 7–10 days.

Tetanus Antitoxin

See Chapter 21 (Antitoxins).

Intravenous Immune Globulin

Brand names: Gamma IV, Isiven IV, Pentaglobin, Sandoglobulin, and ZY-IVGG.

- *Available as:* Injection 0.5, 1, 2.5, and 5.0 g vials.
- *Indications:* Immunodeficiency states, chronic ITP, Rh-isoimmunization, Kawasaki disease, GBS, hemolytic-uremic syndrome (HUS), and sepsis.
- *Doses:*
  - *Immunodeficiency state:* 100–400 mg/kg/dose (IV) every 2–4 weeks.

- *Kawasaki disease:* 2.0 g/kg IV infusion over 10-12 hours as a single dose.
  Or,
- 400 mg/kg/day (IV) for 4 days
- *Idiopathic thrombocytopenic purpura:* 800-1,000 mg/kg/dose (IV) for induction of response. Thereafter, 400-800 mg/kg/dose (IV) once every 4-6 weeks.

- *Adverse drug reactions:* Anaphylaxis, hypersensitivity reactions, fever, chills, hypotension, and transient tachycardia.
- *Contraindication:* IgA deficiency.
- *Cautions:* If adverse reaction, discontinue the infusion until the reaction is controlled. Resume at a slower rate in keeping with tolerance.

Scorpion Sting Antitoxin

See Chapter 21 (Antitoxins).

Chapter 35

Macrominerals

INTRODUCTION

The term, *macromineral*, denotes inorganic compounds in food that are proven to be essential for humans in quantities of >50 mg/day. Macrominerals of therapeutic value include calcium, magnesium, phosphorus, potassium, and sodium.

CALCIUM CHLORIDE

- *Indications:* Hypocalcemic states and cardiopulmonary resuscitation
- *Available as:* Oral solution of variable strengths. Injection 100 mg/mL
- *Dose:* 0.3 g/kg/day (PO and IV) in divided dose.
- *Adverse drug reactions (ADRs):* Bradycardia, gastric irritation, and necrosis at the site of IV injection.

CALCIUM GLUCONATE

- *Available as:* Tablet 0.5 and 1 g. Injection 100 mg/mL (10% solution).
- *Indications:* Hypocalcemic states and cardiopulmonary resuscitation.
- *Dose:* 0.5 g/kg/day (PO) in divided doses; 1–2 mL/kg/dose (IV).
- *Adverse drug reactions:* Bradycardia; gastrointestinal (GI) irritation with oral administration; necrosis at the site of IV injection.

- *Precaution:*
  - Avoid intramuscular administration.
  - Avoid in infants at risk of necrotizing enterocolitis (NEC).

CALCIUM PHOSPHATE

Brand names: Ostocalcium and Sovical
- *Available as:*
  - Tablet 125 mg (along with vitamin D and vitamin B_{12})
  - Syrup 25 mg, 200 mg/5 mL (along with vitamin D)
- *Dose:* 20–60 mg/kg/day.

MAGNESIUM SULFATE

- *Available as:* Injection (1 mL ampule) 1, 10, 25, and 50% solution **(Table 1)**.
- *Indications:* Severe protein-energy malnutrition (PEM), acute severe asthma refractory to conventional therapy, seizures, resuscitation, and arrhythmias.
- *Dose:* PEM 2–3 mEq (0.5–0.75 mL of 50% solution)/kg/day. Acute severe asthma (as adjunctive therapy)—25–75 mg/kg with a maximum of 2.5 g IV over 20 minutes. Resuscitation and arrhythmias—25–50 mg/kg (IV) over 10–30 minutes with a maximum dose of 2 g.
- *Adverse drug reactions:* Hypotension, flushing, central nervous system (CNS), respiratory, and cardiovascular (CV) depression.

TABLE 1: Magnesium content in various solutions.

50% solution	4 mEq/mL
25% solution	2 mEq/mL
10% solution	0.8 mEq/mL
1% solution	0.08 mEq/mL

- *Contraindication:* Acute renal failure.
- *Caution:* Monitoring of serum levels and cardiovascular status.

POTASSIUM CHLORIDE

Brand names: K-Gard, Keylyte, Potklor, and P-Lyte
- *Available as:* Injection 15% ampule; tablet 600 mg; and syrup 10%.
- *Indications:* Prevention and treatment of potassium depletion of whatsoever origin. Common electrocardiogram (ECG) changes associated with hypokalemia include loss of P waves, wide oral rehydration solution (ORS) complexes, decreased rate, and conduction disturbances.
- *Dose:*
  - 1–3 mEq/kg (PO) q 8–12 hours for prevention of hypokalemia during diuretic therapy.
  - 2–5 mEq/kg/day (PO) in kwashiorkor and marasmus with diarrhea
- *Adverse drug reactions:* Nausea, vomiting, flatulence, abdominal pain/discomfort and diarrhea, upper and lower GI conditions including obstruction, bleeding, ulceration, and perforation; skin rash; and hyperkalemia.
- *Caution*: Administer after the child has passed urine. Since GI symptoms are due to irritation of the GI tract, these are best prevented by taking the dose with meals or reducing the amount taken at a time.

SODIUM BICARBONATE

Brand name: Neut
- *Indications:* Documented metabolic acidosis, diabetic ketoacidosis, severe hyperkalemia, and cardiac arrest.

- *Available as*: Injection 75 mg/mL, i.e., 0.9 mEq/mL of 7.5% solution, and 10 mL ampule.
- *Dose:*
  - 7.5% solution of $NaCO_3$ (mEq or mL) = Base deficit × weight (kg) × 0.6
  - Roughly, $NaCO_3$ may be given in the dose of 1–2 mEq/kg/dose (IV). Rather than injection the neat solution, dilute it with equal volume of distilled water or double volume of glucose (5%).
- *Adverse drug reactions:* Tissue necrosis at the injection site, hypocalcemia, and hypernatremia.
- *Caution:* Do not administer a bolus dose in a neonate. Before administering IV infusion, make sure ventilation is adequate.

SODIUM CHLORIDE

- *Indications:* As an essential component of ORS in dehydration, hyponatremia; and moisturizer for nasal mucosa in rhinitis.
- *Available as:* ORS sachets; injection: 0.9 and 3%. Nasal spray: 0.9%; nasal gel: 0.9%.
- *Dose:*
  - Acute hyponatremia
  - Sodium (mEq) = Targeted sodium – actual sodium × weight (kg) × 0.6.

Chapter 36

Micronutrients

INTRODUCTION
Micronutrients are nutrients that are needed by the body in only minute quantities, say micrograms or milligrams/day rather than grams/day to perform various physiological functions. Strictly speaking, these include vitamins (dealt with in Chapter 43).

COPPER
"Iron twin" is also important for many enzymes.
- *Available as:* Oral as a part of multivitamins.
  - *Injection:* 0.4 mg/mL.
- *Indications:* Copper deficiency, prolonged zinc therapy, total parenteral nutrition (TPN), chronic therapy with a proton-pump inhibitor (PPI), and chronic severe malabsorption.
- *Dose:*
  - 2–5 mg PO with a maximum of 8 mg/day.
  - *TPN:* 0.3–1.5 mg/day IV.

CHROMIUM
It is involved in metabolism of blood glucose, regulation of insulin resistance, and metabolism of lipids.
- *Available as:* Tablets/capsules: 100, 150, and 200 mg.
- *Indications:* Prediabetics and diabetics, hyperlipidemia, chronic β-blocker use, and psychiatric conditions like bipolar disorder.

- *Dose:* 0.3–24 mg/day depending on age.
- *Adverse drug reactions (ADRs):* With high dose for prolonged period, GI upset, hypoglycemia, eczema, hepatotoxicity, nephrotoxicity, and cardiac arrhythmias.
- *Contraindications:* Kidney disease, aspirin, and non-steroidal anti-inflammatory drugs (NSAIDs).
- *Drug interactions:* Insulin, levothyroxine, and antacids.

IRON

See Chapter 33: Hematinics.

ZINC

Brand names: Zincolak, Zn-20, Zevit, and Zidust

- *Indications:* Zinc deficiency states, including diarrhea, acrodermatitis enteropathica, infantile tremor syndrome (ITS), and adolescent nutritional dwarfing; TPN supplement.
- *Available as:*
  - Suspension: 10 and 20 mg/mL
  - Capsules: 220 mg
- *Dose:*
  - *Maintenance/prophylaxis:* 0.01–0.04 mg/kg/day (daily needs)
  - *Therapeutic infants:* 0.5–1 mg/kg/day
  - *Diarrhea (both acute and chronic):* 10 mg/day for <6 months and 20 mg/day for >6 months for 2 weeks
  - *Acrodermatitis enteropathica:* 6 mg/kg/day
  - *ITS:* 6 mg/kg/day
  - *TPN supplement:* **Table 1**
- *Adverse drug reactions (ADRs):* Gastrointestinal tract (GIT) upset, drowsiness, dizziness, anemia, peripheral neuritis, paresthesia, malabsorption, and copper deficiency.

TABLE 1: Zinc supplements in total parenteral nutrition.

Preterm infants	400 μg/kg/24 hours
Infants <3 months	250 μg/kg/24 hours
Infants >3 months	100 μg/kg/24 hours
Children	50 μg/kg/24 hours

- *Caution:* Do not exceed a daily dose of 220 mg. Supplements of copper required in case of excessive doses of zinc.

Chapter 37

Muscle Relaxants

INTRODUCTION

Muscle relaxants are a group of drugs that reduce the excessive tone of the skeletal muscles. These are employed in clinical practice to alleviate symptoms such as muscle spasms, pain, and hyperreflexia. Two major therapeutic groups are—neuromuscular blockers and spasmolytics. Neuromuscular blockers act by interfering with transmission at the neuromuscular endplate and give temporary relief in emergency situations. Spasmolytics are centrally acting muscle relaxants that are used to alleviate musculoskeletal pain and spasms and to reduce spasticity in a variety of neurological condition such as spastic cerebral palsy.

BACLOFEN

It is a muscle-relaxant and antispasticity agent.

Brand names: Liofen, Lioresal, Riclofen, and Spinofen

- *Available as:* Tablet 10 and 25 mg.
- *Indications:* Muscle spasticity as in spinal disease (e.g., cerebral palsy) and cerebral disease; trigeminal neuralgia. Also for hiccup.
- *Dose:* 0.75–2 mg/kg/day (PO) in two to three divided doses. Depending on the response, initial dose may be enhanced by increments to the upper limit.

- *Adverse drug reactions (ADRs):* Drowsiness, dizziness, nausea, constipation, muscle weakness, fatigue, and insomnia.
- *Caution:* Avoid activity that needs alertness (say driving) and concurrent use of central nervous system (CNS) depressants.

BOTULINUM TOXIN

Brand name: Botox

Botulinum toxin (BTX) is a neurotoxic protein produced by the bacterium *Clostridium botulinum* and related species. It prevents the release of the neurotransmitter acetylcholine from axon endings at the neuromuscular junction, thereby reducing spasticity or causing flaccidity.
- *Available as:* Injection 100 units/vial.
- *Indications:* Spastic cerebral palsy. Also as a cosmetic application for removing facial wrinkles.
- *Dose:* 4 units/sitting. This total dose needs to be divided equally for the muscles to be injected. Repeat session after at least 2 months, if indicated.
- *Adverse drug reactions:* Paralysis of injected muscle.

DANTROLENE

Brand name: Dantrium
- *Available as:* Capsule 25, 50, and 100 mg.
- *Indications:* Spasticity in cerebral palsy, upper motor neuron lesions (stroke and spinal cord disease/injury). Also, prevention and attenuation of malignant hyperthermia.
- *Dose:* 1–6 mg/kg/day in two divided doses. Depending on the response, dose may be enhanced in weekly increments to the upper limit.

- *Adverse drug reactions:* Hepatotoxicity.
- *Contraindication:* Liver disease.
- *Caution:* Avoid activity that needs alertness (say driving) and concurrent use of CNS depressants.

METHOCARBAMOL

Brand names: Flexnol and Neuromol-MR

- *Available as:* Injection 100 mg/mL; tablet 500 and 750 mg.
- *Indications:* Spasticity from painful musculoskeletal conditions, tetanus.
- *Dose:* 10–15 mg/kg/dose (IV) every 6 hours and tablet 15 mg/kg/dose every 6–8 hours.
- *Adverse drug reactions:* Nausea, light headedness, headache, drowsiness, bradycardia, and hypotension.
- *Caution:* Avoid activity that needs alertness (say driving) and concurrent use of CNS depressants.

CHLORZOXAZONE

Brand names: Duodil, Myospas, and Parafon

- *Available as:*
  - Capsule 25, 50, and 100 mg.
  - *Combination:* Chlorzoxazone 250 mg + paracetamol 500 mg.
- *Indications:* Painful muscle spasm.
- *Dose:* 5–7 mg/kg/dose three to four times daily.
- *Adverse drug reactions:* Drowsiness, fever, rash, anorexia, and hepatitis.

Nasal Decongestants

INTRODUCTION

Nasal decongestants are agents used to relieve block or stuffiness (congestion) in the nose and rest of the upper respiratory tract. The opening up of the upper airway and the consequent relief, though short-term, assists in tiding over the acute illness. The active ingredient in most decongestants is either pseudoephedrine or phenylephrine. These medications may be available over the counter (OTC) in many countries. Saline nasal drops/sprays provide equally good relief in nasal congestion associated with upper respiratory infection, influenza, and other such conditions. Their safety and comfort of using as frequently as needed is a plus point.

PHENYLPROPANOLAMINE

Also termed norephedrine and norpseudoephedrine, it is a popular mucosal decongestant that is employed in various cold, flu, and cough preparations and as an appetite suppressant. Now, it stands condemned because of the risk of central nervous system (CNS) bleeding and stroke (ascribed to it in some young women). It is banned in some countries including the USA and the UK. In India, its use was banned on 27th January 2011. However, the ban was revoked by the Madras High Court on 13th September 2011.

PSEUDOEPHEDRINE HYDROCHLORIDE

Brand name: Sudafed
- *Available as:* Tablet 30 and 60 mg; syrup 30 mg/5 mL.
- *Indications:* Upper respiratory tract congestion including that of nasal mucosa and sinuses.
- *Dose:* 3–5 mg/kg/day in four divided doses.
- *Adverse drug reactions (ADRs):* Hypertensive reactions, palpitations, tachycardia, tremors, sweating, flushing, headache, nervousness, and insomnia.

OXYMETAZOLINE HYDROCHLORIDE

Brand names: Nasivion and Sinarest
- *Available as:* Nasal drops, 0.05%, 0.0250.01%
- *Indications:* Nasal congestion
- *Dose:* 1–2 drops into each nostril once or twice daily.
- *Adverse drug reactions:* Local stinging or burning, sneezing, dryness of mouth or throat, rebound congestion or rhinitis, headache, drowsiness, and palpitations.
- *Contraindications:* Rhinitis sicca and glaucoma.
- *Caution:* Avoid prolonged use (>1 week).

XYLOMETAZOLINE HYDROCHLORIDE

Brand names: Otrivin and Nasalin
- *Available as:* Nasal drops 0.05% for pediatric use.
- *Indications:* Congestion of upper respiratory mucosa especially that of nose and sinuses.
- *Dose:* 1–2 drops into each nostril once or twice daily.
- *Adverse drug reactions:* Local stinging or burning, sneezing, dryness of mouth or throat, rebound congestion or rhinitis, headache, drowsiness, and palpitations.
- *Contraindications:* Rhinitis sicca and glaucoma.
- *Caution:* Avoid prolonged use (>1 week).

Chapter 39

Nutritional Supplements

INTRODUCTION

Nutritional supplements, also termed dietary or food supplements, are dietary supplements providing vitamins, minerals, nutrients, botanicals, herbs, amino acids, and other substances that are intended to enhance human health. These are usually added to the diet or taken over and above the diet. These are indicated in deficiency states, when it becomes difficult to meet the requirement of the body from routine diet or routine dietary intake is partially or totally affected.

CARNITINE

Brand names: Carnitor and Carnivit

A quaternary ammonium compound involved in metabolism. It is sort of an amino acid that is naturally produced in the body.

- *Available as:* Tablet/capsule 330 and 500 mg; Syrup 200 mg/mL; Injection 500 mg/2.5 mL, 1 g/5 mL.
- *Indications:* Carnitine deficiency [both primary (genetic) and secondary (malnutrition, poor absorption, or access to only vegetables)], as supplement with total parenteral nutrition (TPN) and valproate therapy, prematurity, myopathy (including cardiomyopathy), and hemodialysis (long-term).

- *Dose:*
  - *Oral:* 50–100 mg/kg/day in two divided doses with a maximum of 3 g/day.
  - *Intravenous:* 50–100 mg/kg/day with a maximum of 1 g/day.
  - *For premature infants:* 10–20 mg/kg/day (IV) added to the TPN solution.
- *Adverse drug reactions:* Safe. High doses may cause nausea, vomiting, diarrhea, abdominal pain, muscle weakness; rarely seizures.
- *Caution:* Avoid in pregnancy, lactation, and seizures.

OMEGA-3 FATTY ACIDS

Brand names: Maxepa, Maxiguard, and Mega-3

Long-chain polyunsaturated fatty acids: (1) Eicosapentaenoic acid (EPA), (2) Docosahexaenoic acid (DHA), and (3) Arachidonic acid (AA). Also known as polyunsaturated fatty acids (PUFAs), these are health-friendly and essential for brain growth and development.

- *Available as:* Softgel, capsule, drops, usually providing DHA and EPA in combination with vitamin E and micronutrients.
- *Indications:* Infants and children at risk of neurologic disorder of cardiovascular disease, pregnancy, and lactation.
- *Adverse drug reactions:* Omega-3 supplements (DHA/EPA) can make bleeding more likely, especially when the child is simultaneously on nonsteroidal anti-inflammatory drugs (NSAIDs).
- *Caution:* Avoid in bleeding disorder and diabetes.

40
Chapter

Plasma Volume Expanders

INTRODUCTION

Plasma expanders are the hypertonic and/or hyperoncotic fluids that expand the circulating blood volume to a greater extent than isotonic and/or isooncotic fluids. These agents restore vascular volume, stabilizing circulatory hemodynamics and maintaining tissue perfusion in circulatory shock. Two general categories of expander are used, namely crystalloids and colloids. Crystalloids are aqueous solutions of mineral salts or other water-soluble molecules, and include normal saline (0.9% NaCl), Ringer lactate, and gelatine. Colloids include large insoluble molecules and include albumin and plasma-protein fraction.

CRYSTALLOIDS

Normal saline (NS) is the commonly used term for a solution of 0.9% w/v of NaCl, about 300 mOsm/L. Less commonly, this solution is referred to as *physiological saline* or *isotonic saline*, neither of which is technically accurate. NS is used frequently in intravenous drips (IVs) for patients who cannot take fluids orally and have developed or are in danger of developing dehydration or hypovolemia. NS is typically the first fluid used when hypovolemia is severe enough to threaten the adequacy of blood circulation, and has long been believed to be the safest fluid to give quickly in large volumes. However, it is now known that rapid infusion of NS can cause metabolic acidosis.

Ringer Solution

Lactated Ringer solution contains 28 mmol/L lactate, 4 mmol/L K^+, and 1.5 mmol/L Ca^{2+}. It is very similar—though not identical to—Hartmann solution, the ionic concentrations of which differ slightly.

Hypotonic saline is no longer recommended as a maintenance intravenous fluid in children.

Glucose (Dextrose)

IV glucose (also called dextrose) has the advantage of providing some energy and may thereby provide the entire or part of the energy component of parenteral nutrition.

Types of glucose/dextrose include:
- *D5W* (5% dextrose in water), which consists of 278 mmol/L dextrose.
- *D5NS* (5% dextrose in normal saline), which, in addition, contains normal saline.

COLLOIDS

Albumin

Brand names: Albudac, Albunol, Albumeon, and Albumin
- *Available as:* 5%, 25%, solution.
- *Indications:* Hypoproteinemia (severe) such as in nephrotic syndrome, severe PEM, protein-losing enteropathy, prolonged dysentery, cirrhosis, hookworm

Chapter 40: Plasma Volume Expanders

anemia, burns, cerebral edema, and preceding exchange transfusion in pathological neonatal hyperbilirubinemia.
- *Dose:* 5% solution, isotonic to total plasma, is given as continuous intravenous infusion at rate of 5-6 mL/min in all cases needing fast rise of blood volume; 25% solution is given by continuous intravenous infusion at the rate of 2 mL/min as follows:
  - 10-15 mL (IV), two to three times weekly in premature infants with hypoalbuminemia.
  - 50 mL (IV), two to three times, 5-6 hourly, followed by 100-200 mL in shock, collapses, and burns.
  - 50 mL daily in hypoalbuminemic edema. 100-150 mL every alternate day in nephrotic syndrome.
- *Adverse drug reactions:* Hypersensitivity reactions.
- *Contraindications:* CCF and severe anemia.
- *Caution:* Avoid high concentration albumin in neonates.
- *Special remarks*: Quite expensive. Hence, only infrequently used.

Dextran

Brand names: Lomodex-40 and Lomodex-70
- *Available as:* Lomodex-40 and Lomodex-70.
- *Indications:* Fluid replacement and plasma volume expander in shock, prevention of deep vein thrombosis, and pulmonary embolism.
- *Dose:*
  - First day 20 mL/kg
  - Second day and thereafter 10 mL/kg.
- *ADR:* Anaphylactic reaction.
- *Contraindications:* Bleeding disorder, congestive cardiac failure (CCF), and acute renal failure (ARF).
- *Caution:* Avoid use beyond 5 days.

Gelatin

Brand name: Haemaccel

- A colloid that is useful in hypovolemic shock
- *Available as:* Infusion of 500 mL
- *Indications:* Burns and shock (hypovolemic)
- *Dose:* 10-20 mL/kg IV bolus very rapidly
- *Adverse drug reactions:* By and large safe.
- *Caution:* Avoid its use in the presence of infection.

Chapter 41

Stool Softeners/Laxatives

INTRODUCTION

These are substances (oral or suppository forms) that loosen motions followed by increased bowel movements. They are used to treat and/or prevent constipation. Certain stimulant, lubricant and saline laxatives are used to evacuate the colon for rectal and bowel examinations, and may be supplemented with enemas under certain circumstances. High doses of laxatives may cause diarrhea. Being habit-forming, stool softeners should be used sparingly.

BISACODYL

A stimulant laxative, working by increasing the peristalsis.

Brand names: Conlax, Dulcolax, Julax, and Relax
- *Available as:* Tablet 5 mg, rectal suppository 5 and 10 mg.
- *Dose:* 5–15 mg once a day, higher dose being for adolescents.
- *Indications:* Constipation, before surgery, and before radiography of abdomen.
- *Adverse drug reactions:* Gastrointestinal upset, abdominal pain, and allergic reactions.
- *Contraindications:* Intestinal obstruction and appendicitis.
- *Caution:* Avoid using for >1 week.

DOCUSATE

Brand name: Laxicon
- *Available as:* Tablet 100 mg; Syrup 50 mg/5 mL.
- *Dose:* 20–60 mg as a single dose or in two divided doses.
- *Caution:* Avoid in infants <6 months and along with liquid paraffin.

LACTULOSE

A *nonabsorbable sugar* which is degraded to lactic acid and acetic acid, causing an acid pH and ammonia ion trapping.

Brand names: Duphalac, Evict, Lactulax, Livoluk, Looz, and Totalax
- *Available as:* Syrup 3.325 g/5 mL
- *Indications:* Constipation and hepatic dysfunction
- *Dose:*
  - 1–2 mL/kg/day in three to four divided doses
  - *Infants:* 2.5–10 mL/day in three to four divided doses (PO and PR)
  - *Children:* 40–90 mL/day in three to four divided doses (PO and PR)
  - Maximum single dose should not exceed 30–45 mL.
- *Adverse drug reactions:* Intestinal cramps, flatulence, and dehydration with dyselectrolytemia (hypokalemia and hypernatremia).
- *Contraindications:* Galactosemia, subjects on low galactose diets or on galactose-free or lactose-free diets, disaccharidase deficiency, and intestinal obstruction.
- *Drug interaction:* Neomycin, antacids and oral chemotherapy.
- *Caution:* Doses need to be adjusted to produce two to three loose motions/day.

Chapter 41: Stool Softeners/Laxatives

LIQUID PARAFFIN

It is a petroleum product—mixture of liquid hydrocarbons.

Brand names: Cremalax and Trulax
- *Indication:* As a lubricant laxative.
- *Available as:* Liquid paraffin 3.75 mL milk of magnesia 11.25/15 mL.
- *Dose:* 1–3 mL/kg
- *Adverse drug reactions:* Fat-soluble vitamin deficiency with prolonged use, rash, itching nausea, vomiting, abdominal discomfort; infrequently aspiration pneumonia.
- *Caution:* Avoid in children with chemical sensitivity.

SODIUM PICOSULFATE

Brand name: Cremalax
- *Available as:* Tablet 10 mg
- *Indications:* Constipation, including opium-induced; before radiologic procedure/bowel cleansing surgery.
- *Dose:* 2.5–5 mg at bedtime.
- *Adverse drug reactions:* Nausea, headache, and habit formation.
- *Caution:* Avoid its prolonged use; the dose should be taken at bedtime rather than during day; avoid alcohol use while taking this medicine.

Chapter 42

Vasodilators

INTRODUCTION

The term, *vasodilation*, denotes the widening of blood vessels from relaxation of smooth muscle cells within the vessel walls, in particular in the large veins, large arteries, and smaller arterioles. The process is the opposite of vasoconstriction which is the narrowing of blood vessels.

Quite a few drugs are available for vasodilation in clinical practice. These drugs relax the muscles in the wall of the arteries and veins. This effect prevents the muscles from contracting, thereby reducing tightening and narrowing of the vascular lumen. Consequent upon that, blood flows comfortably in the vasculature. The heart, therefore, does not have to pump as hard as, thereby decreasing the blood pressure.

CAPTOPRIL

See Chapter 16 (Antihypertensive Drugs).

DIAZOXIDE

See Chapter 16 (Antihypertensive Drugs).

HYDRALAZINE HYDROCHLORIDE

See Chapter 16 (Antihypertensive Drugs).

ISOSORBIDE DINITRATE

Brand names: Cardcap and Sorbtrate
- *Available as:* Tablet 5 and 10 mg; Capsule 20 and 40 mg.
- *Indications:* Intractable congestive cardiac failure (CCF) and angina pectoris.
- *Adverse drug reactions:* Dizziness/headache and lupus-like syndrome.
- *Dose:* 0.1 mg/kg/day (PO) q 6–8 hours; the dose must not exceed 2 mg kg/day.
- *Caution:* Avoid in infants and children.

ISOXSUPRINE HYDROCHLORIDE

Brand names: Duvadilan, Ipdilan, Perivalan, and Udlan
- *Available as:* Tablet 10 and 20 mg; Injection 5 mg/mL (2 mL ampule).
- *Indications:* Premature labor.
- *Dose:* 0.5–1 mg/kg/day (IM and IV infusion) q 8 hours.
- *Caution:* Not recommended in children but can be used in teen-aged pregnant girls.

MINOXDIL

See Chapter 16 (Antihypertensive Drugs).

NIFEDIPINE

See Chapter 16 (Antihypertensive Drugs).

NITROGLYCERINE

Brand names: NIG, Nitrocin, and Nitroject
- *Available as:* Injection 5 mg/mL.
- *Indications:* Shock, hypertensive emergency, CCF, and portal hypertension.

- *Dose:* To begin with, 0.25–0.5 μg/kg/min (IV infusion). This needs to be treated by 0.5 μg/kg/min q 3–5 minutes to as high as 5 μg/kg/min.
- Dilution should be normal saline or 5% dextrose (50–100 μg/mL).
- *Adverse drug reactions:* Flushing, tachycardia, hypotension, and dizziness/headache.

PHENOXYBENZAMINE

See Chapter 16 (Antihypertensive Drugs).

PRAZOSIN

See Chapter 16 (Antihypertensive Drugs).

SODIUM NITROPRUSSIDE

See Chapter 16 (Antihypertensive Drugs).

TOLAZOLINE HYDROCHLORIDE

Brand name: Priscol
- *Available as:* Injection 25 mg/mL (4 mL vial).
- *Indications:* Persistent pulmonary arterial hypertension, especially in respiratory distress syndrome.
- *Dose:* 1–2 mg/kg (IV through a peripheral or central vein draining into superior vena cava) in 10 minutes. In case, it leads to improvement in arterial oxygenation, continue as IV infusion in dose of 0.2 mg/kg/h.
- *Adverse drug reactions:* Hypotension, tachycardia, flushing, thrombocytopenia, gastrointestinal bleed, pulmonary bleed, and oliguria.
- *Caution:* Monitor and maintain vital signs, as oxygenation, acid-base status, fluid, and electrolytes.

Chapter 43

Vitamins

INTRODUCTION

Vitamins are a sort of micronutrients that are essentially required by the body though in small amounts. Vitamins play an important role in the healthy growth and development of the body. As a rule, a balanced diet with a variety of foods is usually good enough to obtain required quantity of vitamins.

These may be of two types:
1. Water-soluble (B-complex including B_{12} and C)
2. Fat-soluble (A, D, E, and K).

BIOTIN

Brand names: H-Vit and Oltin
- *Available as*: Tablet 5 mg.
- *Indications:* Biotin deficiency, primary biotinidase deficiency, premature hair loss, and periconceptional for prevention of facial dysmorphism in the fetus
- *Dose*:
  - Nutritional deficiency of biotin 5–20 mg OD
  - Biotinidase deficiency 5–10 mg OD.

VITAMIN A

Brand names: Aquasol and Arovit
- *Available as:* Oral suspension 50,000 IU/2 mL ampule; Tablet/capsule 25,000 IU and 50,000 IU.

- *Indications:* Vitamin A deficiency (VAD) states (both prophylactic and therapeutic); measles, diarrhea; occasionally respiratory infections and iron deficiency anemia (IDA).
- *Dose*: Prophylaxis: <6 months 50,000 IU; 6–12 months 100,000 IU; >1 year 200,000 IU.
- The dose should be repeated every 6 months for a total of nine doses by 5th birthday.
- *Treatment:* **Table 1** gives the WHO/UNICEF schedule.
- *Adverse drug reactions:* Anorexia, growth failure, headache, irritability, painful swelling of long bones (hyperostosis), pseudotumor cerebri, and neural tube defects.

VITAMIN B$_1$ (THIAMINE)

Brand names: Benalgis, Beneuron, and Berin
- *Available as*: Tablet 75 and 100 mg; Injection 100 mg/mL.
- *Indications:* Beriberi, neuropathy, cardiomyopathy, and inborn errors of metabolism.

TABLE 1: WHO/UNICEF treatment schedule of xerophthalmia.

Children 1–6 years and above	
Immediately on diagnosis	200,000 IU vitamin A (PO)
The following day	200,000 IU vitamin A (PO)
4 weeks later	200,000 IU vitamin A (PO)
Children under 1 year and under 8 kg weight at any age	
Half the doses as indicated for children 1–6 years and above	
For night blindness or Bitot spot	
Treat with a daily dose of	10,000 IU of vitamin A (PO) for 2 weeks

Note: If there is a persistent vomiting or profuse diarrhea, then an intramuscular injection of 100,000 IU of water-miscible vitamin A (but not an oil-based preparation) may be substituted for the first dose.

- *Daily requirement:* 0.1–1.0 mg or 0.5 mg/1,000 kcal diet.
- *Dose:*
  - *Beriberi:* 10–25 mg/day (IM and IV). 10–50 mg/day (PO)
  - Inborn errors of metabolism 100 mg every 8 hours
  - Collapse from cardiomyopathy 25 mg (IV) slowly.

VITAMIN B$_2$ (RIBOFLAVIN)

Brand names: Lipobal
- *Available as:* Tablet 20 mg
- *Indications:* Deficiency states like angular stomatitis/cheilosis; metabolic disease.
- *Daily requirement:* Recommended dietary allowance (RDA) 0.6 mg/1,000 kcal dietary consumption/day (1–3 mg/day).
- *Dose:*
  - 2.5–10 mg/day in two or three divided doses
  - In metabolic disease, dose is high, i.e., 50–150 mg once or twice daily.
- *Adverse drug reactions:* Infrequently, diarrhea and polyuria.
- *Caution:* Prepare the parents/child for yellow discoloration of urine that is harmless.

VITAMIN B$_3$ (NIACIN AND NICOTINIC ACID)

Brand names: Nialip, Nicocin, and Beplex Forte
- *Available as:* Tablet 375 and 500 mg. In combination with other vitamins (Beplex Forte) 45 mg.
- *Indications:* Nutritional supplement, pellagra, and hyperlipidemia.
- *Daily requirement:* 5–15 mg/day.
- *Dose:*
  - Pellagra 50–100 mg thrice daily
  - Hyperlipidemia 5–10 mg/kg/day.

PANTOTHENIC ACID (VITAMIN B$_5$)

Brand names: Calpan, D-Pantothenic acid

- *Available as:* In combination with other vitamins.
- *Indications:* Burning feet syndrome, attention deficit hyperactivity disorder (ADHD), and hyperlipidemia
- *Dose:* Though the RDA is just 1–7 mg/day, high dose (100–300 mg twice or thrice daily) is recommended for therapeutic benefit.
- *Adverse drug reactions:* Rarely, allergic reactions.

VITAMIN B$_6$ (PYRIDOXINE)

Brand names: Benadon, Bevidox, and Neurobion

- *Available as:* In combination with vitamins B$_1$ and B$_{12}$ and, in some preparations, with additional vitamins/micronutrients.
- *Indications:* Pyridoxine dependent seizures and anemia, sideroblastic anemia, pyridoxine-deficiency neuropathy, isoniazid (INH)-induced neuropathy, and penicillamine-induced neuropathy.
- *Doses:*
  - 0.3–3 mg/kg/day (PO and IV)
  - Seizures 100 mg (IV) in 1 minute followed by 50–100 mg/day
  - Neuropathy 50 mg (PO) TDS
- *Adverse drug reactions:* Rarely, sedation, and respiratory depression.

VITAMIN B$_{12}$ (COBALAMIN AND CYNOCOBALAMINE)

It is a water-soluble vitamin of B-complex group, it is available from meat, eggs, fish milk, and milk (dairy) products (cheese and curd); also banana, mushroom, and potato.

- It is essential for the synthesis of DNA by the body, for the production of blood cells, and for maintaining the health of nerves. Its deficiency results in megaloblastic anemia and peripheral neuropathy. Manifestations include paresthesia and movement disorder (as in infantile tremor syndrome). Normal blood level is >200 pg/mL though, Ideally, it should be >300 pg/mL.

Brand names: Alkem, Bevidex, Cobex, Macraberin, Neurokind, and Triredisol.

- *Available as:* Often, in combination with vitamin B_1 and B_6. Tablets 500, 1,500, and 5,000 µg. Injection 500 µg/mL.
- *Indications:* Nutritional supplement, megaloblastic anemia as such or in association with other conditions (say, infantile tremor syndrome, and tropical sprue), paresthesia (pins and needles sensation), enhanced requirements in hemorrhagic, renal, and liver disorders.
- *Daily requirement:* 0.3–2 µg.
- *Dose:* 250–1,000 µg (IM) on alternate days for 1–2 weeks followed by once a week until blood count returns to normal. Then, maintenance dose of 1,000 µg every 2–4 months.
- *Adverse drug reactions:* It is very rare. Peripheral thrombosis, polycythemia vera, gout, and hypokalemia.
- *Drug interaction:* Alcohol and passive alcohol sensor (PAS)
- *Caution:* Since there is every chance of concurrent depletion of iron and folate stores as also hypokalemia, supplementation with these micronutrients is recommended.

VITAMIN C (ASCORBIC ACID)

Brand names: Redoxon, Sorvicin, Chewcee, Succee, and Limcee
- *Available as:* Tablets 50, 100, and 500 mg; Drops 100 mg/20 drops; Injection 500 mg/5 mL.

- *Indications:* Vitamin C deficiency states, especially scurvy; as antioxidant and hemostatic agent; methemoglobinemia; iron-deficiency anemia; transient tyrosinemia of newborn; and Chédiak–Higashi syndrome.
- *Dose:* 100–500 mg/day (PO and IV)
- *Adverse drug reactions:* Vomiting, flushing, diarrhea, hyperoxaluria; and gastritis with overdose.

VITAMIN D (CHOLECALCIFEROL)

A nutrient as well as a hormone or prohormone, essential for bone formation, maintenance, and strength, may support the immune system and other body functions. Sources include sunlight and such foods as salmon fish, egg yolk, milk and its products, and supplements. Normal levels 20–60 ng/mL.

Brand names: Arachitol and Calcirol

- *Indications:* Prophylaxis of vitamin D deficiency and therapy of Vitamin D deficiency rickets.
- *Available as:* Injection 300,000 and 600,000 IU/1 mL ampule; Granules 60,000 IU/sachet; Tablet 60,000 IU; Drops 400 and 800 IU/mL.
- *Dose:* A daily oral dose of 400 IU during the whole first year of life is now a standard recommendation for all infants.

  As per Stross regimen, a massive dose of 600,000 IU (IM and PO) to be repeated after 3–4 weeks gap, once or twice, if indicated. In infants, a dose of 300,000 IU suffices. Alternatively, 30,000–60,000 units/day (PO) may be given for 10 days. For prevention of rickets, the same dose may be given every 6 months.
- *Adverse drug reactions:* Hyperostosis or Caffey's disease in the form of irritability, anorexia, hypotonia, constipation, anemia, calciuria, metastatic calcification, fever, and high

erythrocyte sedimentation rate (ESR). Affected bones develop soft swellings over them. X-ray shows hyperplasia of the subperiosteal bone. Pseudotumor cerebri and nephrocalcinosis may also occur.

- *Caution:* Ensure adequate intake of oral calcium (through diet or supplements) when vitamin D is being given. Else osteoporosis may occur.
- *Antidote:* Sodium sulfate, 0.5% solution in milk (PO). Increase to 1–2% until diarrhea shows up.

VITAMIN E (TOCOFEROL)

It is an antioxidant; 1 mg = 1.5 units.

Brand names: Evit, Evion, and Tocofer

- *Available as:* Drops 50 mg/mL; Pearls 30, 100, 200, 400, and 600 mg.
- *Indications:* Anemia of prematurity, sickle cell anemia, cystic fibrosis, β-thalassemia, retinopathy of prematurity (ROP), bronchopulmonary dysplasia, Rett syndrome, abetalipoproteinemia, cholestasis; and muscle cramps.
- *Daily requirement:* 25–100 IU
- *Dose:*
  - *Neonates*: 25–50 IU/day (PO)
  - *Children:* 1 mg/kg/day (PO)
  - *Adolescents:* 60–75 mg/day (PO)
  - *Sickle cell anemia:* 450 mg/day (PO)
  - *Cystic fibrosis:* 100–400 mg/day (PO)
  - *β-thalassemia:* 750 mg/day (PO)
- *Adverse drug reactions:* Rarely, diarrhea, lethargy, cramps, and muscles weakness
- *Contraindication:* None recorded so far.
- *Caution:* Avoid giving simultaneously with iron since it reduces iron absorption.

VITAMIN K

Brand names: Kapilin, Kenadon, and Menadione sulfate

- *Available as:* Injection 0.5 mg, 10 mg/mL; Tablet 1 mg.
- *Indications:* Hemorrhagic disease of the newborn (HDN), liver disorders causing bleeding tendency, vitamin K-dependent clotting factor(s) deficiency, and cholestasis.
- *Doses:*
  - Prophylaxis of HDN (within 1 hour of birth)
  - Premature neonates 0.5 mg (IM)
  - Term neonates 1 mg (IM)
- *Therapy:*
  5–10 mg/dose (IM, SC, and IV)
- *Adverse drug reactions:* Rare. Anaphylaxis (when given rapidly IV), hyperbilirubinemia when dose >20 mg, severe hemolytic anemia.
- *Caution:* Monitoring prothrombin time and partial thromboplastin time (PTT).

Section 3

Drugs for Infectious Diseases

44. Antibacterial Drugs (Antibiotics)
45. Antimycobacterial Drugs
46. Antiviral Drugs
47. Antifungal Drugs
48. Antiparasitic (Intestinal) Drugs
49. Antiparasitic (Extraintestinal) Drugs

Chapter 44

Antibacterial Drugs (Antibiotics)

INTRODUCTION

Antibiotics, employed in treatment and prevention of bacterial infections, act by either killing the bacteria (bactericidal) or by inhibiting their growth (bacteriostatic). Their effectiveness and easy access have also led to their overuse, rather abuse, prompting bacteria to develop resistance (*antibacterial or antibiotic resistance*). Today, antibacterial resistance has emerged as a serious public health threat globally. Hence, rational use of antibacterial drugs is a "must" to meet this challenge. In this context, antibiotic stewardship and work on antibiotic alternatives and adjuncts such as antibodies, probiotics, phages, etc. merits priority of attention. Additionally, development of new antibiotics to combat the nearly dry antibiotic space is mandatory to cover serious multidrug-resistant pathogens, including the superbugs.

AMINOGLYCOSIDES

Aminoglycosides, natural or semisynthetic antibiotics derived from actinomycetes, are potent, broad-spectrum, bactericidal antibiotics which exert their action through inhibition of protein synthesis. Streptomycin was among the earliest discovered antibiotics and spearheaded the treatment of tuberculosis over several decades.

Amikacin

First semisynthetic aminoglycoside; derivative of kanamycin A; effective against gram-positive as well as gram-negative organisms—just like tobramycin.

Brand names: Amicin, Mikacin, Mikastar, and Omnikacin
- *Available as:* Injections 100, 250, and 500 mg/vial
- *Indications:* Fulminant gram-negative infections (septicemia, pneumonia, meningitis, peritonitis, infected burns, and postoperative sepsis), and gram-positive infections resistant to other aminoglycosides, e.g., nosocomial infections as in burns, in intensive care unit (ICU), and in immunocompromised subjects.
- *Dose:* 15–25 mg/kg/day divided q 8–12 hours
- *Adverse drug reactions (ADRs):* Nephrotoxicity, ototoxicity (mainly cochlear), neuromuscular blockade, hypersensitivity reactions such as drug fever, rash, eosinophilia, tremors, nausea, vomiting, headache, and overgrowth of nonsusceptible microorganisms.
- *Contraindications:* Known hypersensitivity to aminoglycosides.
- *Caution:* Suitable reduction in dose must be made in renal insufficiency depending on creatinine clearance and blood urea nitrogen (BUN).

Gentamicin Sulfate

It is an aminoglycoside and binds to 30S subunit of bacterial ribosome; induces translation misreading, freezing of initiation complex.

Brand names: Garamycin Genta, Genticare, Genticyn, and Ranbiotic
- *Available as:* Injections 40 and 80 mg/mL.
- *Indications:* Life-threatening fulminant gram-negative infections, e.g., septicemia, meningitis, and urinary tract infection (UTI)
- *Dose:*
  - 3–5 mg/kg/day (IV and IM) in first week of life and up to 7.5 mg/kg/day later in two to three divided doses in life-threatening situations
  - 0.8–1.2 mg/kg/day (IV and IM) in two to three divided doses for UTIs
- *Adverse drug reactions:* Nephrotoxic, hepatotoxic, ototoxic, fever, rash, convulsions, joint pains, hypotension, purpura, anemia, and granulocytopenia.
- *Drug interactions:* Frusemide, ethacrynic acid, vitamin K, nephrotoxic and ototoxic drugs, cephalosporins, penicillins, anesthetics, and neuromuscular blocking agents.
- *Contraindications:* Myasthenia gravis, previous toxic reaction in the form of nephrotoxicity or ototoxicity.
- *Caution:* Reduce frequency in renal impairment.

Kanamycin Sulfate

Brand name: Kancin
- *Available as:* Injection 0.5 g and 1.0 g vials.
- *Indications:* Neonatal septicemia, urogenital, respiratory, central nervous system (CNS), soft tissue and gastro-intestinal tract (GIT) infections due to *Staphylococcus*; a reserve drug for resistant tuberculosis.
- *Dose:* 15 mg/kg/day (IM and IV) in two to three divided doses. Intravenous (IV) administration should be slow over 30 minutes to 1 hour.

- *Tuberculosis (MDR):* 15–30 mg/kg (IM).
- *Adverse drug reactions:* Nephrotoxic, ototoxic, rash, fever, headache, and paresthesia.
- *Drug interaction:* Frusemide, ethacrynic acid, neuromuscular blocking agents, and anesthetics.
- *Contraindications:* Pregnancy and lactation.
- *Caution:* Myasthenia gravis, parkinsonism; monitor serum creatinine in renal impairment, as also auditory and vestibular functions.
- *Remarks:* With the availability of more potent and relatively safe aminoglycosides, use of kanamycin is considerably diminished.

Neomycin

Brand names: Mycifradin, Neo-Fradin, Neo-Tab, Neosporin, and Nebasulf

- *Available as:* Topical-skin and ophthalmic powder/cream/ointment in varied combinations with bacitracin, sulfacetamide, polymyxin B, etc. Capsule/Tablet: 350 and 500 mg.
- *Indications:* Infrequently, in selected cases of enteritis; hepatic coma and abdominal surgery (for sterilization of the gut); skin and ophthalmic infections.
- *Drug interaction:* Decreases absorption of digoxin.
- *Dose:*
  - Infants 50 mg/kg/day (PO) in three divided doses
  - Children 50–100 mg/kg/day (PO) in three to four divided doses
- *Adverse drug reactions:* Nephrotoxicity, ototoxicity, malabsorption, hepatic dysfunction, muscle weakness, wheeze, rash, superinfection with *Candida* secondary to suppression of normal gut flora.

- *Contraindications:* Impaired renal function.
- *Caution:* Avoid for routine use as an antidiarrheal antibiotic and even in hepatic encephalopathy.
- *Special remarks:* Neomycin-containing antidiarrheal formulations for children stand banned in India. Systemic use of neomycin is nearly a story of the past. The agent is almost limited to topical use in combination with other agents.

Netilmicin

Brand name: Netromycin

- *Available as:* Ampules—10, 25, 50, and 100 mg/mL. Vials: 50, 200, and 300 mg/vial.
- *Indications:* Infections caused by gram-negative bacilli (*E. coli*, *Pseudomonas*, and *Klebsiella*); employed usually in combination with one of the penicillins or cephalosporins but not through the same syringe or infusion.
- *Dose:* 5–7.5 mg/kg/day (IM and IV) q 8 h. In infants, up to 10 mg/kg/day may be given.
- *Adverse drug reactions:* Nephrotoxicity (renal tubular dysfunction with loss of sodium, calcium, and magnesium), ototoxicity, and neuromuscular blockade with pancuronium.
- *Drug interactions:* Frusemide, ethacrynic acid, cephalosporins, citrated blood, neuromuscular blocking drugs, and anesthetics.
- *Contraindications:* Renal insufficiency, pregnancy, and lactation.
- *Caution:* Myasthenia gravis, parkinsonism, dehydration, infant botulism, hypocalcemia; requires monitoring.

Sisomicin Sulfate

Brand names: Ensamycin, Sisomin, Sisonest, Sisoptin, Sisowill, Somicin

- *Available as:* Injection 10 mg/mL in 1 mL ampule, 50 mg/mL in 1 mL ampule.
- *Doses:*
  - *4 weeks to 1 year:* 4.5–6 mg/kg/day in three divided doses
  - *Above 1 year:* 3–4.5 mg/kg/day in three divided doses
- *Indications:* Serious pyogenic infections, including gram-negative septicemia
- *Adverse drug reactions:* Nephrotoxicity, neurotoxicity in the form of dizziness, vertigo, tinnitus, noises in the ear, deafness, and muscle weakness.
- *Drug interaction:* Ototoxic, neurotoxic, and nephrotoxic agents, other aminoglycosides, cephalosporins, vancomycin, cisplatin, amphotericin B, methoxyflurane, diuretics, and anesthetics.
- *Contraindication:* Hypersensitivity/toxic reaction to any of the aminoglycosides.
- *Caution:* Monitor renal and eighth cranial nerve function during therapy. Use particular caution in subjects with neuromuscular disorders like myasthenia gravis.

Streptomycin Sulfate

Brand name: Ambistryn-S

- *Available as:* Injection—1 g vial; Syrup—0.28 g/5 mL; and Tablet—0.2 g
- *Indications:* Tuberculosis; occasionally, pathogens susceptible to this drug only.
- *Dose:* 20–50 mg/kg/day (IM); 1–2 mg/kg/day (IT); and 100 mg/kg/day (PO) in divided doses

- *Adverse drug reactions:* Deafness, renal damage, allergic reactions, eosinophilia, fever, rash, CNS depression, and blood dyscrasia.
- *Drug interaction:* Frusemide, ethacrynic acid, mannitol, other aminoglycosides, polymyxin B, colistin sulfate, cyclosporine, neuromuscular blocking drugs, and anesthetics.
- *Contraindications:* Disease of ear, especially suppurative otitis media (SOM), and labyrinthitis.
- *Cautions:* Impaired liver or kidney function, prematurity, impaired vestibular and auditory functions, pregnancy, lactation, and myasthenia gravis.

Tobramycin Sulfate

An aminoglycoside closely related to gentamicin, including antimicrobial spectrum, except that it is two to three times more active in vitro against *Pseudomonas aeruginosa*.

Brand name: Tobraneg

- *Available as:* Injection 20, 60, and 80 mg vials. Ophthalmic solution/ointment.
- *Indications:* Fulminant gram-positive and gram-negative infections under aerobic conditions, including *Pseudomonas aeruginosa* in which this is the aminoglycoside of choice.
- *Dose:*
  - *Neonates under 7 days:* 4 mg/kg/day (IV and IM) in two doses
  - *Neonates above 7 days:* 6 mg/kg/day (IV and IM) in three doses
- *Adverse drug reactions:* Anemia, granulocytopenia, thrombocytopenia, fever, rash, urticaria, gastrointestinal (GI) upset, headache, and lethargy liver dysfunction.

- *Drug interactions:* Likely to potentiate other nephrotoxic and ototoxic drugs.
- *Contraindications:* Known allergy to aminoglycosides, pregnancy, and lactation.
- *Caution:* Avoid its administration in conjunction with heparin, penicillin, and cephalosporins; control blood levels and dosage in renal impairment.

B-LACTAMS

β-lactams Group 1: Penicillins

Penicillins are a group of antibiotics derived from *Penicillium fungi*. Penicillin antibiotics are historically significant because they were the first effective medicines against many previously serious diseases such as syphilis and *Staphylococcus* infections.

Penicillinase-sensitive Penicillins

Procaine Penicillin
- *Available as:* Injection 4 lakhs units/vial.
- *Indications:* Moderately severe infections with gram-positive organisms.
- *Doses:*
  - *Under 4 years:* 2 lakhs (IM) daily or twice a day
  - *Over 4 years:* 4 lakhs (IM) daily or twice a day
- *Adverse drug reactions:* β-lactam safety profile (rash and eosinophilia), allergy, hypersensitive reactions in the form of rash, fever, bronchospasm, vasculitis, serum sickness, Stevens–Johnson syndrome, and anaphylaxis. The clinical picture of anaphylaxis consists of sudden hypotension, bronchospasm with asthma, skin eruptions, diarrhea, nausea, and vomiting.

Chapter 44: Antibacterial Drugs (Antibiotics)

Benzyl (Crystalline) Penicillin

- *Indications:* Severe infection with gram-positive organisms.
- *Dose:* 50 thousands to 4 lakhs units/kg/day (IM and IV) in four divided doses. Higher limit is for severe infections like pyogenic meningitis or septicemia. For bacterial endocarditis, as much as 100,00,000 units/day.
- *Adverse drug reactions:* β-lactam safety profile (rash and eosinophilia) and allergy. Hypersensitive reactions in the form of rash, fever, bronchospasm, vasculitis, serum sickness, Stevens–Johnson syndrome, and anaphylaxis. The clinical picture of anaphylaxis consists of sudden hypotension, bronchospasm with asthma, skin eruptions, diarrhea, nausea, and vomiting. Excessive dose may cause seizures.

Benzathine Penicillin
Brand names: Longacillin, Penidure LA-6, 12, and 24

- *Available as:* Vials 12 lakhs (1.2 mega) units.
- *Indications:* Rheumatic fever prophylaxis, syphilis, streptococcal infections, pyoderma, and post-traumatic tetanus.
- *Dose for secondary prophylaxis in rheumatic fever:*
  - >27 kg weight 12 lakhs units every 3 weeks
  - <27 kg weight 6 lakhs units every 3 weeks
- *Adverse drug reactions:* β-lactam safety profile (rash and eosinophilia) and allergy
  Hypersensitive reactions in the form of rash, fever, bronchospasm, vasculitis, serum sickness, Stevens–Johnson syndrome, and anaphylaxis. The clinical picture of anaphylaxis consists of sudden hypotension, bronchospasm with asthma, skin eruptions, diarrhea, nausea, and vomiting.
- *Remarks:* Penidure LA-6, which was available earlier, stands withdrawn now. Only Penidure LA-12 is available currently.

Oral Penicillin: Penicillin V (Phenoxymethyl Penicillin)
This is an acid-resistant penicillin administered orally.

Brand names: Kaypen and Penivoral
- *Available as:* Tablets 2, 4, and 8 lakhs units.
- *Indications:* Mild-to-moderate gram-positive infections; also, some gram-negative (*N. gonorrhoeae* and *N. meningitidis*) infections.
- *Dose:* 50 thousands units/kg/day in two divided doses.
- *Adverse drug reactions:* β-lactam safety profile (rash and eosinophilia) and allergy. Hypersensitive reactions in the form of rash, fever, bronchospasm, vasculitis, serum sickness, Stevens–Johnson syndrome, and anaphylaxis. Clinical picture of anaphylaxis consists of sudden hypotension, bronchospasm with asthma, skin eruptions, diarrhea, nausea, and vomiting. Seizures with overdose.

Penicillinase-resistant (Semisynthetic) Penicillins

The noteworthy feature of these semisynthetic penicillins is the side chains that protect the β-lactam ring from the onslaught of enzyme, and penicillinase. These are the drug of choice for penicillinase-producing *Staphylococcus aureus*, provided that the pathogens are not methicillin-resistant. The most important member of this class is cloxacillin. Others, say oxacillin, nafcillin, dicloxacillin, flucloxacillin, etc. are not marketed in India.

Cloxacillin

Brand name: Bioclox
- *Available as:* Capsules 250 and 500 mg; suspension 125 mg/measure; Injections 250 and 500 mg/vial.
- *Indications:* Staphylococcal infections.

- *Doses:* 50–200 mg/kg/day (PO and IV) in four divided doses. The higher limit is in case of staphylococcal meningitis.
- *Adverse drug reactions:* GIT upset, rash, rise in serum glutamic oxaloacetic transaminase (SGOT), superadded infections with gram-negative bacteria and fungi.
- *Contraindications:* Hypersensitivity to penicillins, asthma, hay fever, and urticaria.
- *Precaution:* Oral administration 1 hour before or 2 hours after food.

Extended-spectrum (Modified or Amino) Penicillins

Amoxicillin

Brand names: Novamox, Flemoxin, and Wymox

- *Available as:* Capsules 250 and 500 mg; Tablets 125 and 250 mg; Syrup 125 and 250 mg/5 mL; Drops 100 mg/mL.
- *Indications:* Respiratory, genitourinary, GI, soft tissue, ENT, etc. infections caused by pneumococci, streptococci, *H. influenzae*, *E. coli*, and gonorrhea.
- *Dose:* 20–50 mg/kg/day, divided q 8–12 h.
- *Adverse drug reactions:* Diarrhea, vomiting, maculopapular rash, urticaria, and rise in SGOT.
- *Drug interaction:* Probenecid.

Amoxicillin-clavulanate (Coamoxiclav)

Brand names: Augmentin and Acuclav

- *Available as:*
  - *Tablet:* 375 mg (amoxicillin 250 mg and clavulanate 125 mg); 625 mg (amoxicillin 500 mg and clavulanate 125 mg); 1,000 mg (amoxicillin 875 mg and clavulanate 125 mg).

- *Syrup:* Amoxicillin 200 mg, clavulanate 28.5 mg/5 mL
- *Injection (IV):* 300 mg (amoxicillin 250 mg and clavulanate 50 mg); 600 mg (amoxicillin 500 mg and clavulanate 100 mg); 1.2 g (amoxicillin 1,000 mg and clavulanate 200 mg).
- *Indications:* Beta-lactam (amoxicillin), β-lactamase inhibitor (clavulanate or clavulanic acid as potassium salt) for boosting amoxicillin activity against penicillinase producing bacteria such as *S. aureus*, *Streptococcus pneumoniae*, *H. influenzae*, *M. catarrhalis*, *E. coli*, *Klebsiella*, and *B. fragilis*.
- *Doses:*
  - 20–45 mg/kg/day (PO) divided q 8–12 h
  - In AOM, give higher dose 80–90 mg/kg/day
  - 30 mg/kg (IV) every 8 hours; may give 6 hours in more serious infections (Calculations are based on amoxicillin).
- *Adverse drug reactions:* Diarrhea, vomiting, maculopapular rash, urticaria, and rise in SGOT.
- *Drug interaction:* Probenecid.
- *Contraindication:* Hypersensitivity.
- *Caution:* Reduce dose and frequency in renal impairment.

Ampicillin

Brand names: Roscillin, Campicillin, and Synthocilin

- *Available as:* Tablets—125 and 250 mg; Capsule— 250 and 500 mg; and Syrup—125 and 250 mg/mL. Injection (IM, IV, and IT) 250 mg and 500 mg.
- *Indications:* Respiratory, genitourinary, GI, soft tissue, ENT, etc. infections due to gram-negative as well as gram-positive organisms.

- *Dose:* 50–400 mg/kg/day in four divided doses, the upper limit being the recommendation for very severe infections such as pyogenic meningitis and septicemia.
- *Adverse drug reactions:* Hypersensitivity reactions, rash, GIT upset, convulsions, eosinophilia, superadded infection with *Pseudomonas* and *Candida* due to change in the normal flora of the GIT, mild hepatic dysfunction, and agranulocytosis.
- *Contraindication:* Hypersensitivity.
- *Drug interactions:* Probenecid, anticoagulants, allopurinol, and urine glucose determinations.
- *Caution:* Monitor blood, liver, and kidney function when therapy exceeds 10 days. Avoid in infectious mononucleosis, renal impairment, and lymphatic leukemia.

Ampicillin-Sulbactam

It is a combination of a β-lactam, ampicillin, a β-lactamase inhibitor, and sulbactam.

Brand name: Sulbacin

- *Available as:* Injection ampicillin 1 g, sulbactam 500 mg/vial.
- *Indications:* Beta-lactam (ampicillin) + β-lactamase inhibitor (sulbactam) for boosting ampicillin activity against penicillinase-producing bacteria such as *S. aureus*, *Streptococcus pneumoniae*, *H. influenzae*, *M. catarrhalis*, *E. coli*, *Klebsiella*, and *B. fragilis*.
- *Dose:* 100–200 mg/kg/day (IM and IV) divided q 4–8 h. Calculations are based on ampicillin component.
- *Adverse drug reactions:* Diarrhea, especially pseudomembranous colitis (PMC), *C. difficile*-associated diarrhea (CDAD), skin, rash, and hypersensitivity.

- *Contraindication:* Hypersensitivity.
- *Drug interaction:* Probenecid.

Extended-spectrum Penicillins

Piperacillin

Brand name: Zosyn

- *Available as:* Injection (IV and IM) 1, 2, and 4 g. Also, in combination with β-lactamase inhibitor, and tazobactam.
- *Indications:* Many gram-positive and gram-negative infections, including infections caused by *E. coli*, *Enterobacter*, *Serratia*, *Pseudomonas*, and *Bacteroides*.
- *Doses:* Generally, 50–300 mg/kg/day (IV and IM) in three to four divided doses (upper limit for serious infections).
  - *Neonates:* <7 days 150 mg/kg/day (IV) q 8–12 h, 7 days 200 mg/kg/day q 6–8 h
  - *Infants and children:* 200–300 mg q 4–6 h
  - *Cystic fibrosis:* 350–500 mg/kg/day (IV)
- *Adverse drug reactions:* β-lactam safety profile (rash, eosinophilia, and transient rise in liver enzymes).
- *Drug interaction:* Probenecid.
- *Caution:* Renal excretion; inactivated by penicillinase.

Ticarcillin

Brand names: TICAPLUS, Ticar, Ticarnic, and Ticoplus

- *Available as:* Injection 3 g. Also, in combination with clavulanic acid (ticarcillin 3 g and clavulanic acid 100 mg)
- *Indications:* Severe infections caused by *E. coli*, *Enterobacter*, *Serratia*, *Pseudomonas*, and *Bacteroides*.
- *Dose:* 200–300 mg/kg/day (in terms of ticarcillin) q 6–8 h (IV and IM)

- *Neonates:*
  - <7 days/>2,000 g 150 mg/kg/day (IV) q 8–12 h (two to three divided doses)
  - >7 day/>2,000 g 225 mg/kg/day (IV) q 8 h
  - 7 days/<1,200 g 150 mg/kg/day (IV)
  - 7 days 1,200–2,000 g 225 mg/kg/day
- *Cystic fibrosis:* 400–600 mg/kg/day (IV).
- *Adverse drug reactions:* β-lactam safety profile (rash and eosinophilia)
- *Drug interaction:* Probenecid
- *Caution:* Renal excretion; inactivated by penicillinase. Monitor liver function test (LFT).

Antipseudomonas (Carboxy and Ureido) Penicillins

Carbenicillin
Brand name: Carbelin
- *Available as:* Injection 1 g vial.
- *Indications: Pseudomonas* and indole-positive *Proteus* infections.
- *Dose:* 400–600 mg/kg/day (IM and IV) in four to six divided doses, the higher range being for *Pseudomonas* infections.
  - *Neonates:*
    - <7 days and 2,000 g 225 mg/kg/day (IM and IV) in three divided doses
    - >2,000 g 300 mg/kg/day (IM and IV) in four divided doses
    - >7 days 300–400 mg/kg/day (IM and IV) in four divided doses
- *Adverse drug reactions:* These are generally on the same lines as in case of injectable penicillin. Others include local pain, local phlebitis, abnormalities of coagulation leading to bleeding, and hypokalemia.

- *Contraindication:* It is known as penicillin allergy.
- *Precaution:* The vials should be stored in a cool dry place below 5°C temperature. Do not mix in the same syringe with gentamicin to prevent inactivation of the latter.

Piperacillin

Brand name: Zosyn

- It is far more (around eight times) active than carbenicillin in its pseudomonal potency.
- Details are available under "Extended Spectrum Penicillins".

Ticarcillin

Brand name: Ticar

- Its pseudomonal activity is greater than carbenicillin.
- Details are available under "Extended Spectrum Penicillins".

β-lactams Group 2: Cephalosporins

Cephalosporins are semisynthetic broad-spectrum antibiotics.

Cephalosporins are divided into five generations. Higher the generation, greater the activity against gram-negative pathogens with simultaneous fall in activity against gram-positive pathogens **(Box 1)**. Adverse drug reactions common to cephalosporins are given in **Box 2**.

Cefaclor

It is a semisynthetic broad-spectrum second generation cephalosporin; and bactericidal.

Brand name: Keflor

- *Available as:* Capsule 250 mg; suspension 125 g/5 mL; and drops 100 mg/mL

Chapter 44: Antibacterial Drugs (Antibiotics)

BOX 1: Five generations of cephalosporins.

First generation: These are active against most gram-positive cocci with the exception of enterococci and methicillin-resistant *S. aureus*, some strains of *E. coli, K. pneumoniae,* and *P. mirabilis*. These agents do not cross the blood–brain barrier and, hence, are ineffective in treating central nervous system infections:
- Cefadroxil
- Cefazolin
- Cephalexin
- Cephalothin
- Cephapirin
- Cephradine

Second generation: These are more active against gram-negative bacteria, e.g., *H. influenzae* (type B), *N. gonorrhoeae* and enteric gram-negative bacteria. Certain members of this group (cefaclor) cross blood–brain barrier and are effective in treating bacterial meningitis:
- Cefaclor
- Cefuroxime
- Cefuroxime axetil
- Cefpodoxime

Third generation: These are relatively less effective against gram-positive cocci but more effective against most strains of enteric gram-negative bacilli with the exception of *Clostridium difficile*, significantly effective against *P. aeruginosa* and very effective against *H. influenzae* and *N. gonorrhoeae*: This is the group that stands most prescribed presently.
- Ceftriaxone
- Cefotaxime
- Ceftazidime
- Ceftibuten
- Cefixime
- Cefoperazone
- Ceftizoxime

Fourth generation: These are similar to third generation cephalosprins with the extended action against gram-negative pathogens such as *Pseudomonas, Proteus, Enterobacter,* and *Klebsiellas:*
- Cefpirome
- Cefepime
- Cefpodoxime

Fifth generation: These have powerful pseudomonal activity and are less prone to resistance. These are effective against methicillin-resistant *Staphylococcus aureus (MRSA)*—and community-acquired pneumonia.
- Ceftobiprole
- Ceftaroline

BOX 2: Adverse reactions of cephalosporins in general.

- *Hypersensitivity:* Rash, urticaria, serum sickness, and anaphylaxis
- *Gastrointestinal tract:* Nausea, vomiting, and diarrhea
- *Hepatic:* Biliary sludge and transient transaminase elevation
- *Renal:* Interstitial nephritis
- *Central nervous system:* Seizures
- *Hematologic:* Eosinophilia, neutropenia, thrombocytopenia, impaired platelet aggregation, and hemolytic anemia
- *Miscellaneous:* Drug fever, phlebitis, superinfection, disulfiram-like reaction, false-positive Coombs, glycosuria, and serum creatinine

- *Indications:* Particularly useful in β-lactamase producing organisms like *H. influenzae* and *B. catarrhalis* causing upper and lower respiratory infections (LRIs).

    Otitis media is caused by *Streptococcus pneumoniae, H. influenzae, B. catarrhalis, Streptococcus pyogenes,* and *Staphylococcus aureus.*
- Upper respiratory tract infection (URTI), including pharyngitis and tonsillitis, is caused by *Streptococcus pyogenes*. Other ENT infections like rhinosinusitis, acute laryngitis, epiglottitis, otitis externa caused by *Streptococcus pneumoniae, Staphylococcus aureus,* and *Streptococcus pyogenes.*
- Lower respiratory infection caused by *Streptococcus pneumoniae, H. influenzae, B. catarrhalis, Staphylococcus aureus,* gram-negative bacilli like *E. coli, Klebsiella,* and *Proteus.*
- Skin infections caused by *Staphylococcus aureus* and *Streptococcus pyogenes*
- UTI caused by *E. coli, Proteus mirabilis, Klebsiella spp.,* and *Staphylococcus aureus*
- Gonococcal urethritis

- *Dose:* 20–40 mg/kg/day (maximum 1 g) in three divided doses.
- *Adverse drug reactions:* Infrequent and minor.
  - *Hypersensitivity reaction:* Morbilliform eruptions, pruritus, urticaria, serum sickness-like reactions, Stevens–Johnson syndrome, toxic epidermal necrolysis, and anaphylaxis.
  - *CNS:* Reversible hyperactivity nervousness, insomnia, confusion, hypertonia, dizziness, and somnolence.
  - *GIT:* Nausea, vomiting and diarrhea, PMC, and transient hepatitis.
  - *Kidneys:* Reversible interstitial nephritis.
  - *Hemopoietic:* Transient lymphocytosis, leukopenia, neutropenia, thrombocytopenia, and eosinophilia.
  - *Renal:* Raised BUN and serum creatinine.
  - *Liver:* Raised SGOT, serum glutamic pyruvic transaminase (SGPT), and alkaline phosphatase.
- *Drug interaction:* Probenecid.
- *Contraindication:* Known allergy to cephalosporins.
- *Precaution:* Avoid in preterm infants and infants <1 month of age, and in penicillin allergy.

Cefadroxil

First generation cephalosporin active against *Staphylococcus aureus, Streptococcus, E. coli., Klebsiella,* and *Proteus.*

Brand names: Bludrox, Cefadrox, Cefadur, Droxyl, and *Odoxil*

- *Available as:* Dry syrup 125 and 250 mg/5 mL. Tablets/Capsules 250, 500, and 1,000 mg.
- *Indications:* Majority of gram-positive and gram-negative, penicillin-sensitive as well as penicillin-resistant

pathogens: UTI, skin infections. URI, including tonsillitis and pharyngitis.
- *Dose:* 30 mg/kg/day in two divided doses.
- *Adverse drug reactions:* Nausea, vomiting, diarrhea, dysuria, PMC, hypersensitivity reactions, allergies, genital pruritus/moniliasis, vaginitis, and moderate neutropenia (transient).
- *Drug interactions:* Probenecid, false-positive Coombs test or ClinTest.
- *Contraindications:* Known allergy to cephalosporins/penicillin group of antibiotics.
- *Cautions:* Exercise restraint in penicillin-allergic subjects. Observe for idiosyncrasy. Use caution in renal impairment; modify dose according to creatinine clearance.

Cefazolin Sodium

It is first generation cephalosporin active against *Staphylococcus aureus*, *Streptococcus*, *E. coli*, *Klebsiella,* and *Proteus*; not effective in *Pseudomonas*.

Brand name: Azolin
- *Indications:* Most serious gram-positive and -negative infections, including penicillin-resistant ones, but excluding *Pseudomonas*.
- *Available as:* Injection 500 mg, 1 g.
- *Dose:* 25–100 mg/kg/day (IM and IV) in two to four divided doses.
- *Adverse drug reactions:* Hypersensitivity reactions such as drug fever, rash, pruritus, eosinophilia, and rarely, anaphylaxis and bronchospasm, vomiting, anorexia, hepatotoxicity with transient rise in SGOT, SGPT, and alkaline phosphatase, nephrotoxicity (transient rise in

BUN), pain over injection site, thrombophlebitis, and oral thrush.
- *Drug interactions:* Loop diuretics, probenecid, and aminoglycosides.
- *Contraindication:* Known hypersensitivity to cephalosporin.
- *Caution*: Reduce dose in impaired renal function. In mild, moderate, and severe impairment, the dose should be 60% and 10% of the usual dose. Only one dose may be given.
- Avoid in premature infants under 1 month.

Extended-spectrum Semisynthetic Cephalosporin

Cefdinir
Brand name: Sefdin
- *Available as:* Capsule 300 mg; suspension 125 mg/5 mL.
- *Indications:* Community-acquired pneumonia (CAP), acute exacerbation of chronic bronchitis, acute bacterial sinusitis, and uncomplicated skin infections.
- *Dose:* 14 mg/kg/day (maximum 600 mg/day) in one or two daily doses
- *Adverse drug reactions:* Nausea, diarrhea, including CDAD or constipation, indigestion, anorexia, headache, abdominal pain, superinfection, PMC; dizziness, drowsiness; weakness, rash, serum sickness-like reactions, and anaphylaxis.
- *Drug interaction:* Probenecid, antacids, and iron supplements.
- *Contraindication:* Hypersensitivity to cephalosporins.
- *Caution:* Avoid under 6 months of age. Reduce dosage in renal insufficiency, i.e., when creatinine clearance <60 mL/min.

Administer at least 2 hours apart consumption of antacids and iron-containing products which are known to remarkably cut down its absorption.

Cefditoren Pivoxil
Brand names: Proxecef and Spectracef
- *Available as:* Tablets (dispersible) 30 and 50 mg.
- *Indications:* Respiratory infections, tonsillitis, pharyngitis, especially when Group A *Streptococcus* (GAS) haemolyticus.
- *Dose:* 3 mg/kg/dose q 9 h × 5–7 days.
- *Adverse drug reactions:* Allergic reaction, diarrhea, anorexia, asthma-like symptoms, coagulation time increased, constipation, dizziness, dry mouth, eructation, facial edema, fever, flatulence, and fungal infections.
- *Contraindications:* Carnitine deficiency and inborn errors of metabolism.
- *Caution:* Reduce dose or avoid in significant renal insufficiency.

Cefixime

It is third generation cephalosporin active against most bacteria (including *Salmonella typhi*), except *Staphylococcus* and *Pseudomonas*. CNS penetration is inadequate.

Brand names: Cemax and Suprax
- *Available as:* Tablets 50, 100, and 200 mg; suspension 50 and 100 mg/5 mL.
- *Indications:* Most bacteria (including *Salmonella typhi*), except *Staphylococcus* and *Pseudomonas*.
- *Dose:* Usually, 8 mg/kg/day in two divided doses. In enteric fever, double the dose if required.
- *Adverse drug reactions:* GIT upset. Also, *see* **Box 2**.
- *Drug interaction:* Probenecid.
- *Contraindication:* Known cephalosporin allergy.
- *Caution:* Avoid in CNS infections and known penicillin allergy.

Cefoperazone

It is third generation cephalosporin effective against gram-positive and gram-negative bacteria, including *Pseudomonas* (weak antipseudomonal activity).

Brand name: Magnamycin
- *Available as:* Injections 250 and 500 mg, 1 g, and 2 g.
- *Indications:* Serious gram-positive and gram-negative bacterial infections, including *Pseudomonas*.
- *Dose:* 100–150 mg/kg/day (IM and IV) divided q 8–12 h
- *Adverse drug reactions:* GI upset, rash, urticaria, fever, and reversible neutropenia.
- *Drug interaction:* Disulfiram-like reaction with alcohol.
- *Caution:* Avoid in severe biliary obstruction, hepatic disease, and coexisting renal dysfunction.

Cefoperazone-sulbactam

It is a combination of the third-generation cephalosporin (cefoperazone) and the potent β-lactamase inhibitor (sulbactam) in 1:1 ratio.

Brand name: Magnex
- *Available as:* Injections 1 and 2 g vial (half cefoperazone and half sulbactam).
- *Indications:* Most serious infections caused by gram-positive, gram-negative, and anaerobic organisms, including septicemia and meningitis.
- *Dose:* 50–80 mg/kg/day with reference to cefoperazone (IM and IV) in two to four divided doses. The neonates should receive the lower limit of dose in two divided doses.
- *Adverse drug reactions:* GI upset, rash, urticaria, fever, reversible neutropenia, and transient abnormality of LFTs.
- *Contraindication:* Known hypersensitivity to cephalosporins.

- *Drug interactions:* Disulfiram-like reaction with alcohol.
- *Caution:* Avoid in significant biliary obstruction, hepatic dysfunction, and renal dysfunction.

Cefotaxime Sodium

It is a third generation cephalosporin and resistant to β-lactamase.

Brand names: Claforan and Omnatax

- *Available as:* Injection 250 mg, 1 g vial.
- *Indications:* Fulminant and life-threatening infections (gram-positive and -negative, anaerobes), especially where inactivation by β-lactamases is suspected.
- *Dose:* 50–200 mg/kg/day (IM and IV) in two to four divided doses. In preterm infants, do not exceed 50 mg/kg/day.
- *Adverse drug reactions:* Hypersensitivity reactions such as anaphylaxis, bronchospasm, urticaria, rash, fever, and eosinophilia, adenopathy, and PMC.
- *Contraindication:* Allergy to penicillin.
- *Cautions:* Never dissolve the drug in soda bicarbonate solution. Do not store above 25°C. In renal impairment (creatinine clearance <5, reduce dose by half.

Cefpodoxime Proxetil

It is third generation cephalosporin active against most bacterial infections, except *Pseudomonas*.

Brand names: Cepodem and Monocef-O

- *Available as*: Tablets 100 and 200 mg; suspension 50 and 100 mg/5 mL.
- *Indications*: Most bacterial infections, except *Pseudomonas.*
- *Dose:* 10 mg/kg/day in two divided doses.

- *Adverse drug reactions: See* **Box 2**.
- *Contraindication:* Known cephalosporin allergy.
- *Drug interaction:* Probenecid; antacids, and H-2 receptor antagonists are likely to cut down its absorption.
- *Caution:* Avoid in CNS infections and known penicillin allergy.

Cefprozil

It is second generation cephalosporin active against *Staphylococcus aureus*, *Streptococcus*, *H. influenzae*, *E. coli*, *M. chalis*, *Klebsiella*, and *Proteus*. No effect of food on bioavailability.

Brand name: Refzil
- *Available as:* Tablets 250 and 500 mg; Suspension 125 and 250 mg/5 mL.
- *Indications:* Susceptible bacterial infections (vide infra).
- *Dose:* 30 mg/kg/day in two to three divided doses.
- *Adverse drug reactions: See* **Box 2**.
- *Caution:* β-lactam safety profile (rash and eosinophilia). Monitor renal parameters.

Ceftaroline

Fifth generation IV cephalosporin both for serious gram-negative and gram-positive infections with a spectrum that is similar to the other fifth generation cephalosporin, i.e., ceftobiprole.

Brand names: Teflaro and Zinforo
- *Available as:* IV injections 400 and 600 mg/vial.
- *Indications:* Complicated skin and other soft-tissue infections and CAP caused by gram-negative and gram-positive pathogens.

- *Dose:* 10–20 mg/kg/day (IV infusion) in two divided doses for 5–7 days in CAP and up to 14 days in complicated soft-tissue infections. IV infusion should be given over 1 hour.
- *Adverse drug reactions:* Nausea, vomiting, constipation, diarrhea, dizziness, and itching; hypokalemia, elevation of transaminases; phlebitis; rarely hypersensitivity reactions.
- *Contraindication:* Hypersensitivity to cephalosporins
- *Drug interactions:* Probenecid
- *Cautions:* Reduce the dose in renal impairment.

Ceftazidime

Brand name: Fortum

- *Available as:* Injections 250, 500, and 1,000 mg/vial.
- *Indications:* Serious gram-negative hospital infections and most gram-positive infections, including *Pseudomonas*.
- *Doses:*
    - Under 2 months 25–60 mg/kg/day (IM and IV) in two divided doses.
    - Above 2 months 30–100 mg/kg/day (IM and IV) in two to three divided doses.
- *Adverse drug reactions:* Pain over injection site, phlebitis/thrombophlebitis, rash, fever, pruritus, anaphylaxis, thrombocytopenia, and slight increase in hepatic enzymes.
- *Contraindication:* Known hypersensitivity to cephalosporins.
- *Caution:* Impaired renal failure, when glomerular filtration rate is below 50 mL/min, reduce dose.

Ceftibuten

Brand name: Procadex

- *Available as:* Dry powder 90 mg/5 mL. Capsule 400 mg.
- *Indications:* A third generation cephalosporin indicated in a wide range of infections, except Group B *Streptococcus*

(GBS), *Staphylococcus, Enterococcus, Listeria spp., Bacteroides spp.* and *Clostridium spp.*; also, effective in enteric fever.

- *Dose:* 9 mg/kg once a day.
- *Adverse drug reactions:* GI disturbances, rash, headache, dizziness, blood dyscrasias, enzyme abnormalities, colitis, and seizures.
- *Contraindications:* Known allergy to cephalosporins.
- *Precaution:* Avoid in infants under 6 months, penicillin hypersensitivity, renal impairment, and GI disease.

Ceftizoxime

Brand names: Cefizox and Eldcef

- *Available as:* Injections 250 and 500 mg, 1 g vials.
- *Indications:* Severe infections, including sepsis, CNS infections, and anaerobes; effective in immunocompromised states.
- *Dose:* 100–200 mg/kg/day (IM and IV) in three to four divided doses.
- *Adverse drug reactions:* Pain at injection site, GI upset, superinfection (candidiasis), eosinophilia, neutropenia, leukopenia, thrombocytopenia, high blood urea and liver enzymes, and positive Coombs test.
- *Contraindications:* Known hypersensitivity to cephalosporins.
- *Drug interactions:* Aminoglycosides and loop diuretics.
- *Caution:* Avoid in known penicillin allergy.

Ceftobiprole

Fifth generation cephalosporin that is highly broad-spectrum (covers a variety of different bacteria) effective against both gram-positive and gram-negative pathogens; now successfully completed phase III clinical trials.

Brand names: Zeftera/Zevtera
- *Available as:* IV injection for infusion.
- *Indications:* Activity in the test tube against gram-positive cocci, including methicillin-resistant *Staphylococcus aureus* (MRSA) and methicillin-resistant *Staphylococcus epidermidis* (MRSE), penicillin-resistant *Streptococcus pneumoniae (PRSP)*, *Enterococcus faecalis* as well as many gram-negative bacilli including Amp C producing *E. coli* and *Pseudomonas aeruginosa*. Major indications include complicated soft-tissue infections as well as nosocomial pneumonia caused by resistant strains of MRSA, enterococci, and *S. pneumoniae*, especially ventilator-associated pneumonia (VAP) and CAP
- *Dose:* 8–16 mg/kg/day in two divided doses as IV infusion administered in 2 hours for 5–14 days (longer duration is for soft-tissue infections).
- *Adverse drug reactions:* Nausea, vomiting, caramel-like taste disturbance, headache, *Clostridium difficile*-associated diarrhea; rarely anaphylactic reactions.
- *Drug interactions:* Oral contraceptives and warfarin.
- *Contraindications:* Hypersensitivity to cephalosporins.
- *Caution:* Monitor the dose in renal impairment.

Ceftriaxone
It is a third generation cephalosporin with coverage of life-threatening infections, including *Pseudomonas*.

Brand name: Monocef IV
- *Available as:* Injections 250, 500, and 1,000 mg/vial.
- *Indications:* Life-threatening gram-positive and gram-negative infections, including penicillin-resistant *Staphylococcus* and many strains of *Pseudomonas aeruginosa*, and some anaerobic bacteria.

- *Dose:* 20–80 mg/kg/day (IM and IV) in one or two doses.
- *Adverse drug reactions:* Pain, induration, and tenderness at the injection site, thrombophlebitis at IV site, pruritus, fever chills, eosinophilia, thrombocytosis, leukopenia, anemia, neutropenia, lymphopenia, thrombocytopenia, diarrhea, nausea, vomiting, alkaline phosphatase, bilirubin, SGOT and SGPT rise, BUN rise, creatinine elevation, casts in urine, headache, dizziness, moniliasis, and vaginitis PMC.
- *Contraindication:* Known allergy to cephalosporins.
- *Cautions:* Give cautiously to subjects with known penicillin allergy. Do not mix with other antimicrobial agents. Give cautiously in subjects with GI disease.

Ceftriaxone with Sulbactam

It is a third generation cephalosporin empowered with β-lactamase inhibition via sulbactam.

Brand names: Magnex, Sulbacef, and Zocef

- *Available as:* Injection 500, 1 g vials (ceftriaxone and sulbactam in 1:1 ratio).
- *Indications:* For providing extended spectrum for β-lactamase pathogens.
- *Dose:* Ceftriaxone, 20–40 mg/kg/day (IV and IM) in two to four divided doses.
- *Adverse drug reactions:* Pain, induration, and tenderness at injection site, thrombophlebitis when given IV, fever with chills, pruritus, diarrhea, nausea, vomiting, headache, dizziness, moniliasis, vaginitis, PMC, eosinophilia, thrombocytopenia, raised alkaline phosphatase, bilirubin, SGOT and SGPT, raised BUN, raised creatinine, and casts in urine.
- *Contraindication:* Known allergy to cephalosporins.

- *Caution:* Avoid/give cautiously in subjects with known penicillin allergy and GI disease. Do not mix with other antimicrobial agents.

Cefuroxime

It is a second generation cephalosporin, and resistant to gram-negative β-lactamase.

Brand name: Supacef

- *Available as:* Injections 250 and 750 mg/vial.
- *Indications:* Life-threatening gram-positive and gram-negative infections, including penicillin-resistant *Staphylococcus aureus* strains.
- *Dose:* 15–150 mg/kg/day (IM and IV) in two or three divided doses.
- *Adverse drug reactions:* Rash, GI upset, anemia, eosinophilia, transient rise in serum bilirubin in liver disease, and pain at IM injection site.
- *Contraindication:* Known allergy to cephalosporins.
- *Caution:* Take special care in subjects with known anaphylaxis to penicillin, or when the drug is needed to be given in higher doses in conjunction with frusemide or some other potent diuretic.

Cefuroxime Axetil

It is an oral prodrug of cefuroxime.

Brand names: Altacef and Ceftum

- *Available as:* Tablets/Capsules 125, 250, and 500 mg; suspension 125 mg/5 mL.
- *Indications:* Useful in a wide range of gram-positive and gram-negative infections, including β-lactamase producing organisms.
- *Dose:* 25–50 mg/kg/day in two divided doses.

- *Adverse drug reactions:* See cefuroxime.
- *Contraindications:* See cefuroxime.
- *Caution:* See cefuroxime.

Cephalexin

It is a first generation cephalosporin active against *Staphylococcus aureus, Streptococcus, E. coli, Klebsiella,* and *Proteus.*

Brand names: Sporidex and Sepexin

- *Available as:* Capsules 250 and 500 mg; dry syrup 125 mg/5 mL.
- *Indications:* Respiratory, genitourinary, skin, and soft tissue, ENT infections, osteomyelitis, septicemia, and bacterial endocarditis.
- *Dose:* 50–100 mg/kg/day in two to four divided doses.
- *Adverse drug reactions:* Nausea, vomiting, diarrhea, allergic skin reactions, eosinophilia, positive Coombs test, overgrowth of nonsusceptible organisms.
- *Drug interaction:* Probenecid
- *Precaution:* β-lactam safety profile (rash and eosinophilia).

β-lactams Group 3: Nonpenicillin, Noncephalosporin β-lactams

Aztreonam

Brand name: Azenam

- *Available as:* Injection 500 mg, 1 g, and 2 g vial.
- *Indications:* Gram-negative infections of lower respiratory tract, including pulmonary infections in cystic fibrosis; septicemia, meningitis caused by *H. influenzae* type b (Hib) and *N. meningitidis*, pyelonephritis, cystitis, asymptomatic bacteriuria, gonorrhea, adjunct to surgery in management of infections.

- *Dose:* 30–50 mg/kg/dose (IM and IV) every 6–8 hours.
- *Adverse drug reactions:* Vomiting, diarrhea, skin rash, injection site reactions, PMC, CDAD, superinfection, blood dyscrasias, elevation in liver enzymes (aminotransferases), and serum creatinine.
- *Drug interactions:* Frusemide, probenecid, aminoglycosides, cefoxitin, and imipenem.
- *Contraindications:* Pregnancy and lactation.
- *Cautions:* Monitor renal and hepatic function, particularly in high-dose or prolonged therapy.
- *Special remarks:* In view of absence of cross-reactivity with, by and large, all other β-lactams (ceftazidime may well be excluded), it can be employed in subjects with allergy to penicillins or cephalosporins.

Imipenem-cilastatin

Brand name: Cilanem-500

- *Available as:* Injection 500 mg each of imipenem and cilastatin
- *Indications:* A broad-spectrum β-lactam antimicrobial for aerobic as well as anaerobic extended-spectrum β-lactamase-producing (ESBL) bacterial infections (both gram-positive and gram-negative).
- *Dose:* 15 mg/kg/dose (IV infusion) every 6 hourly with a maximum of 2 g/day.
- *Adverse drug reactions:* Local and allergic reactions, phlebitis, GI upset, rash, fever, blood dyscrasias, hepatic dysfunction, renal dysfunction, CNS disturbances, hearing loss, seizures, confusion, dizziness, somnolence, hypotension, perverted taste, superinfections, PMC, and CDAD.
- *Drug interaction:* Probenecid, valproic acid, ganciclovir, divalproex sodium, and estrogen contraceptives.

- *Contraindications:* <3 months, lactation.
- *Precautions:* Penicillin, cephalosporin or other allergy, colitis, concomitant use with valproic acid, CNS disorders, renal impairment, meningitis, brain abscess, granulocytopenia, prolonged use, and pregnancy.

Meropenem

It is an ultra-broad-spectrum parenteral antibiotic of the carbapenem group.

Brand names: Meroza, Merotrol, Morocrit and Valupenem

- *Available as:* Injection 500 mg and 1 g.
- *Indications:* Anaerobic, aerobic, and facultative gram-positive and gram-negative microorganisms, e.g., pneumonia, septicemia, bacterial meningitis, febrile neutropenia; skin and soft tissue, GI and urinary tract, and other intra-abdominal infections; cystic fibrosis with superimposed bacterial infections.
- *Dose:*
  - *Complicated skin infections:* 10 mg/kg/dose IV every 8 hourly.
  - *Sepsis and intra-abdominal infections:* 20 mg/kg/dose IV every 8 hourly.
  - *Bacterial meningitis:* 40 mg/kg/dose IV every 8 hourly.
- *Adverse drug reactions:* Injection site inflammation and pain; nausea, vomiting, diarrhea/constipation, rash, and headache; rarely, neuropathy; hepatic and renal dysfunction; thrombocytosis/thrombocytopenia, anemia, and eosinophilia; and CDAD.
- *Contraindications:* Known hypersensitivity.
- *Drug interactions:* Probenecid and valproic acid; nephrotoxic agents.

- *Cautions:* Lactating mothers and hepatic/renal impairment; seizure disorder, pretreatment skin test in penicillin-allergic children. Monitor hepatic, renal, and hemopoietic function during long-term use.

MACROLIDES

Macrolides are antibiotics with a complex cyclic structure. They exert bacteriostatic action.

Macrolides are indicated for the treatment of gram-positive cocci and intracellular pathogens (*Mycoplasma* and *Chlamydia*). They are considered to be safe antibiotics as far as ADRs are concerned.

Azithromycin

It is a macrolide with very long half-life, thereby imparting it the uniqueness of once daily dosing.

Brand names: Azee, Aziwok, and Azithral

- *Available as:* Tablets 200 and 500 mg; suspension 100 and 200 mg/5 mL.
- *Indications:* Infections with *S. aureus*, *Streptococcus*, *H. influenzae*, *V. cholerae*, *Campylobacter*, *Mycoplasma*, *Legionella*; *Salmonella typhi*, *Chlamydia trachomatis*; nontuberculous *Mycobacterium* disease [especially *M. avium complex* (MAC)], in combination with other antibiotics.
- *Dose:*
  - Routine–10 mg/kg as a single dose on first day followed by 5 mg/kg OD for next 4 days or 10 mg/kg/day OD for only 3 days, 30 mg/kg as single-dose therapy.
  - In case of GAS pharyngitis: 12 mg/kg/day OD for 5 days.

- In case of cholera, 20 mg/kg as a single dose once only
- In case of enteric fever, 20 mg/kg/day for 1–2 weeks
- In nontuberculous mycobacterial (NTM) infection such as MAC, 5 mg/kg/day. The duration of therapy is not yet clearly specified. But, it has got to be a prolonged therapy, usually for 1 year. More experience is needed in this respect.

- *Adverse drug reactions:* Mild GIT upset, reversible rise in liver enzymes, allergic reactions, PMC, photosensitivity and other dermatosis, and exacerbation of myasthenia gravis.
- *Drug interaction:* Antacids, digoxin, carbamazepine, phenytoin, theophylline, fluconazole, cyclosporine, and anticoagulants.
- *Caution:* Renal and hepatic dysfunction.

Clarithromycin

Brand name: Claribid

- *Available as:* Tablets 250 and 500 mg; suspension 75 mg/5 mL.
- *Indications:* A macrolide antibiotic indicated in treatment of upper and LRIs (mild to moderate) and skin infections due to susceptible bacteria, say *H. influenzae, M. catarrhalis, M. pneumoniae, S. aureus, S. pneumoniae, C. trachomatis,* and *Legionella* spp.; nontuberculous mycobacteria.
- *Dose:* 15 mg/kg/day in two divided doses.
- In NTM infection such as MAC, 7.5 mg/kg/day. The duration of therapy is not yet clearly specified. But, it has got to be a prolonged therapy, usually 1 year. More experience is needed in this respect.
- *Adverse drug reactions:* GI upset, allergic reactions, and rise in intraocular pressure (IOP).

- *Drug interactions:* Theophylline, digoxin, rifampicin, carbamazepine, phenobarbital, phenytoin, midazolam, sodium valproate, oral anticoagulants, cisapride, primazole, ergot derivatives, drugs metabolized by P450, statins, warfarin, colchicines, quinidine, cyclosporine, bromocriptine, and zidovudine.
- *Contraindications:* Hepatic dysfunction, hypersensitivity to clarithromycin, erythromycin, azithromycin or clarithromycin, and raised IOP (glaucoma).
- *Cautions:* Renal/hepatic impairment, arrhythmias, QT interval prolongation, pregnancy, and lactation.

Erythromycin

It is a bacteriostatic antimicrobial most active against gram-positive pathogens, *Corynebacterium diphtheriae*, and *Mycoplasma pneumoniae*.

Brand name: Althrocin

- *Available as:* Tablets 100 and 250 mg; suspension 100 mg/5 mL.
- *Indications:* Respiratory infections, especially pharyngitis, tonsillitis, sinusitis, pneumonia; *M. pneumoniae*; soft tissue and wound infections; pertussis; diphtheria carriers. Also employed for promoting GI motility and feeding intolerance in preterms; cholera, *Campylobacter jejuni* infection.
- *Dose:* 30–50 mg/kg/day (PO) in divided doses.
- *Adverse drug reactions:* GIT upset, abdominal pain, hypersensitivity reactions, eosinophilia, and hepatic dysfunction.
- *Drug interaction:* Astemizole, terfenadine, carbamazepine, theophylline, cyclosporine, digoxin, tacrolimus; antagonizes hepatic CYP450,344 activity.

- *Contraindications:* Impaired liver function; concomitant cisapride, pimozide, and porphyria.
- *Caution:* Renal impairment; cholestatic jaundice: Immediately, the drug must be discontinued.

Roxithromycin

Brand names: Roxeptin and Roxid
- *Available as:* Tablets 50 and 150 mg; Syrup 50 mg/5 mL.
- *Indications:* Respiratory infections, sinusitis, pharyngitis, tonsillitis, and genital infections.
- *Dose:* 5 mg/kg/day (PO) q 12 h.
- *Adverse drug reactions:* Nausea, vomiting, diarrhea, PMC, superinfection, rash, and transient rise in liver transaminase.
- *Drug interactions:* Theophylline, digoxin, warfarin, ergot alkaloids, midazolam, cyclosporine, and disopyramide.
- *Contraindications:* Severe liver dysfunctions and ergotamine-like agents.
- *Precaution:* Renal or hepatic insufficiency, pregnancy, and lactation.

Spiramycin

Brand name: Rovamycin
- *Available as:* Tablet 1.5 and 3.5 mIU. Syrup 0.375 mIU/5 mL.
- *Indications:* Respiratory infections, urethritis, and toxoplasmosis.
- *Doses:*
  - Congenital toxoplasmosis 0.15–0.3 mIU/kg BD.
  - Toxoplasmosis in pregnant women 6–8 mIU/day in two to four divided doses for 3 weeks. Repeat 3-week course after 2-week intervals till parturition.
  - Other infections: 1.5–2.5 mIU BD.

- *Adverse drug reactions:* Nausea, vomiting, diarrhea, and skin allergy.
- *Contraindication:* Lactation and hypersensitivity.
- *Cautions:* Hypersensitivity and lactation.

Telithromycin

It is a structural derivative of macrolide and erythromycin, and is the first ketolide antibiotic to enter clinical use. A ketolide antibiotic blocks bacterial protein synthesis. It is uniquely designed to combat DRSP. *Streptococcus pneumoniae*, *Haemophilus influenzae*, *Streptococcus pyogenes*, and *Moraxella catarrhalis* are susceptible to telithromycin. It also is active against some of the atypical respiratory pathogens such as *Chlamydia pneumoniae*, *Legionella pneumophila*, and *Mycoplasma pneumoniae*. However, it does not cover MRSA, GRE, or any enteric gram-negative bacteria.

Brand name: Ketek
- *Available as:* Tablet 300 and 400 mg.
- *Indications:* It is indicated for treating upper and LRIs, such as acute sinusitis, chronic bronchitis, and CAP.
- *Dose:* 10–15 mg/kg with a maximum of 800 mg/day administered in two divided doses for 5 days for chronic bronchitis or sinusitis. For CAP, same dose should be administered daily for 7–10 days. Dosage of telithromycin has not been established for patients with severe renal impairment.
- *Adverse drug reactions:* Diarrhea, nausea, vomiting, headache, dizziness, and persistent unpleasant taste. Antibiotic-associated PMC due to *Clostridium* overgrowth in the bowel, and prolongation of QT interval, and transient vision disturbances.

- *Contraindications:* Myasthenia gravis, liver and renal dysfunction, and QTc prolongation.
- *Drug interaction:* Phenobarbital, phenytoin, and carbamazepine may cause subtherapeutic levels of telithromycin. Digitalis, theophylline, metoprolol, and oral contraceptive levels may also be affected by telithromycin.
- *Cautions:* Because telithromycin is metabolized mainly by the liver, dosage adjustment may be necessary in patients with liver impairment. Special attention is needed when ketoconazole, itraconazole, antilipidemic statins, midazolam, and cisapride are administered concomitantly with telithromycin because these drugs have direct hepatic effects.

LINCOSAMIDES

Lincomycin HCl

Brand name: Lynx

- *Available as:* Capsule 250 and 500 mg; syrup 125 mg/5 mL. Injection 300 mg/mL.
- *Indications:* Serious infections due to susceptible strains of streptococci, pneumococci, and staphylococci.
- *Dose:*
    - 30–60 mg/kg/day (PO) in three divided doses
    - 10–20 mg/kg/day (IM and IV) in two or three divided doses. IV dose needs to be administered as 10 mg/mL solution over a span of 1–4 hours.
- *Adverse drug reactions:* Vomiting, persistent diarrhea, altered taste or smell, overgrowth of yeast, urticaria, superadded infection, abdominal pain, muscle pain, pruritus, hepatotoxicity, and CDAD/colitis.
- *Drug interactions:* Neuromuscular blocking drugs.

- *Contraindications:* Hypersensitivity to lincomycin or clindamycin.
- *Cautions:* Asthma, allergy, and GI disease.

Clindamycin

It is a semisynthetic derivative of lincomycin, effective in serious staphylococcal infections involving bones and joints, peritonitis, and endocarditis prophylaxis.

Brand names: Dalacin and Dalcap

- *Available as:* Injection 150 mg/mL. Capsules 75, 150, and 300 mg; suspension 75 mg/5 mL topical.
- *Indications:* Gram-positive aerobes and anaerobes; serious infections caused by MRSA; invasive GAS infections in combination with a β-lactam; anaerobic infections; and acne (topical preparation).
- *Doses:*
  - Under 7 days and weight under 2,000 g—10 mg/kg/day in three divided doses.
  - Under 7 days and over 2,000 g—15 mg/kg/day in three divided doses.
  - Children 20–45 mg/kg/day in three to four divided doses.
- *Adverse drug reactions:* Nausea, diarrhea, CDAD, PMC (infrequent in children but common in adults), rash, liver dysfunction, neutropenia, eosinophilia, agranulocytosis, thrombocytopenia, and abscess at injection site.
- *Drug interaction:* Neuromuscular-blocking agents.
- *Contraindications:* Diarrheal state.
- *Cautions:* Renal or hepatic dysfunction. Discontinue therapy in case of development of persistent diarrhea or colitis. Administer slowly IV over 30–60 minutes.

Chapter 44: Antibacterial Drugs (Antibiotics)

QUINOLONES AND FLUOROQUINOLONES

Ciprofloxacin

A high-performance quinolone active against *Pseudomonas aeruginosa, Serratia, Enterobacter, Shigella, Salmonella, Campylobacter, Neisseria gonorrhoeae, H. influenzae, M. catarrhalis, Staphylococcus aureus* (selected), and *Streptococcus*.

Brand names: Cifran, Ciplox, and Ciprobid

- *Available as:* Tablets 250 and 500 mg; Injections 1 mg and 2 mg/mL.
- *Indications:* Infections of the urinary tract, GIT, respiratory tract, bones and joints, and skin; serious life-threatening infections, e.g., septicemia and resistant enteric fever; hospital-acquired infections; prevention of sepsis in immunocompromised hosts.
- *Dose:* 15–30 mg/kg/day (PO) in two divided doses, 5–10 mg/kg/day (IV) in two divided doses.
- *Adverse drug reactions:* Tendonitis, GI intolerance (nausea, vomiting, and diarrhea), anorexia, abdominal pain, flatulence, and PMC; dizziness, headache, insomnia, confusion agitation, tremors, ataxia, seizures, hallucinations, visual disturbances, migraine, and deafness; rash, pruritus, drug fever, anaphylaxis, Stevens-Johnson syndrome, photosensitivity, eosinophilia; hepatitis, raised SGOT, SGPT, alkaline phosphatase, and serum bilirubin; crystalluria, nephritis, transient renal failure, raised blood urea, creatine, crystalluria, hematuria, anemia, thrombocytopenia, and thrombocytosis; thrombophlebitis and superinfections.

The joint destruction (encountered in juvenile animals) is not seen in humans.

- *Drug interactions:* Antacids (containing Mg, Ca, and Al), carbamazepine, theophylline, digoxin, oral anticoagulants, terfenadine, cyclosporine, tacrolimus, and astemizole (same as in case of erythromycin; operates by antagonizing hepatic CYP450 activity).
- *Contraindications:* Hypersensitivity to quinolones; children and growing adolescents, except when benefits overweigh risk, tendon disorders, and concurrent use of tizanidine.
- *Cautions:*
  - Avoid the drug 1–2 hours before and 4 hours after the antacids.
  - Avoid with theophylline and nonsteroidal anti-inflammatory drugs (NSAIDs)
  - Avoid in epileptics.
  - Monitor drug dose in case of renal disease, creatinine clearance under 30 mL/min.

Levofloxacin

A levo-isomer of ofloxacin.

Brand names: Levoflox, Leeflox, and Lomflox

- *Available as:* Tablets 250 and 500 mg; Injection 500 mg/100 mL IV infusion.
- *Indications:* Gram-positive and gram-negative infections; MDR-TB.
- *Dose:* 10–15 mg/kg OD or in two divided doses
- *Adverse drug reactions:* Nausea, diarrhea, dizziness, headache, photosensitivity, peripheral neuropathy (paresthesia, hypoesthesia, and weakness), and rupture of tendons.
- *Drug interactions:* Antacids, sucralfate, and probenecid.

- *Contraindications:* <8 years, hypersensitivity, lactation, and pregnancy.
- *Caution:* Avoid in children <8 years, severe renal impairment; avoid exposure to sunlight; discontinue in case of hypersensitivity, photosensitivity, and neuropathy.

Nalidixic Acid

It is a first generation quinolone effective against gram-negative pathogens, e.g., *E. coli, Enterobacter, Klebsiella, and Proteus.*

Brand name: Negadix
- *Available as:* Tablets 125 and 500 mg.
- *Indications:* Lower UTI; dysentery due to gram-negative organisms.
- *Dose:* 50 mg/kg/day (PO) in four divided doses.
- *Adverse drug reactions:* GIT upset, vertigo, dizziness, rash, photosensitivity, eosinophilia, mental disturbances, convulsions, raised intracranial tension (pseudotumor cerebri), hepatotoxicity, and nephrotoxicity.
- *Drug interaction:* Antacids (liquid).
- *Contraindications: <3 months*, seizure disorder, and porphyria; concomitant therapy with melphalan or other related cancer chemotherapeutic alkylating agents.
- *Cautions:* Exercise special care while using it in patients with liver disease, epilepsy, and severely impaired kidney function. It must not be used in systemic infections.

Norfloxacin

Brand names: Norbactin, Normax and Noroxin
- *Available as:* Tablets 200, 400, and 800 mg.
- *Indications:* Serious GI infections, UTI, and gonococcal infection.

- *Doses:* 4–12 mg/kg/day for 5 days in GI infection and 7–21 days for UTI in single or two divided doses; gonorrhea needs a single high dose.
- *Adverse drug reactions:* Hypersensitivity reactions, vasculitis, edema face, glottis or tongue, dyspnea, shock, sleeplessness, headache, hallucinations, visual, smell, and taste disturbances; psychotic reactions; anorexia, epigastric pain, nausea, vomiting, and diarrhea; transient rise of SGOT, SGPT, serum creatinine, and bilirubin; anemia, thrombocytopenia, leukopenia, and agranulocytosis.
- *Drug interactions:* Antacids, probenecid, nitrofurantoin, anticoagulants, and caffeine.
- *Contraindication:* Hypersensitivity to quinolones; <3 months of age, epilepsy, and porphyria.
- *Caution:* Avoid in children below 12 years, except in desperate situations.

Ofloxacin

It is a fluorinated quinolone.

Brand name: Tarivid
- *Available as:* Tablets 200 and 400 mg.
- *Indications:* Infections of lower respiratory tract, genitourinary tract, GIT (especially typhoid fever), skin, and soft tissue; peritonitis and gonorrhea.
- *Dose:* 4–16 mg/kg/day as a single dose or in two divided doses.
- *Adverse drug reactions:* Anorexia, epigastric pain, nausea, vomiting, and diarrhea; transient rise of SGOT, SGPT, serum creatinine, and bilirubin; anemia, thrombocytopenia, leukopenia, and agranulocytosis.

- *Drug interactions:* Antacids (magnesium and aluminum), iron, sucralfate, NSAIDs, theophylline, warfarin, insulin, oral hypoglycemic, drugs metabolized by CYP450, probenecid, cimetidine, furosemide, methotrexate, anticoagulants, steroids, phenobarbital, anesthetics, and hypotensive drugs.
- *Contraindications:* Hypersensitivity to quinolones; epilepsy. Hypersensitivity reactions; vasculitis, edema face, glottis or tongue, dyspnea, and shock; sleeplessness, headache, hallucination, visual disturbances, smell and taste disturbances, and psychotic reactions.
- *Caution:* Avoid in children below 12 years of age except in desperate situations.

Pefloxacin

Brand names: Pefbid and Pelox
- *Available as:* Tablet 400 mg; IV infusion 400 mg/100 mL.
- *Indications:* Severe infections in adolescents caused by sensitive gram-negative bacteria and staphylococci.
- *Dose:* 12 mg/kg/day (PO) q 12 h or IV infusion.
- *Adverse drug reactions:* Epigastric discomfort, nausea, vomiting, tendinitis (even rupture of tendon), muscular pains, articular pains, headache, vigilance disorders, and thrombocytopenia.
- *Drug interaction:* Antacids; enhances risk of theophylline toxicity; and chloride solutions.
- *Contraindication:* Allergy to quinolones.
- *Precaution:* Avoid in respiratory infections, exposure to ultraviolet light.

Sparfloxacin

Brand name: Sparx
- *Available as:* Tablets 100 and 200 mg

- *Indications:* Gram-positive and gram-negative pathogens.
- *Dose:* 4 mg/kg/day (PO) OD or two divided doses.
- *Adverse drug reactions:* Nausea, diarrhea, heartburn, anorexia, rash, tendinitis/ruture, eosinophilia, thrombocytopenia, fall in hemoglobin, WBC, and RBC.
- *Drug interactions:* Erythromycin, phenothiazines, digoxin, tricyclic antidepressants, etc.
- *Contraindications:* Hypersensitivity, G6PD deficiency, pregnancy, and lactation.
- *Cautions:* Avoid sunlight exposure; avoid in hypokalemia, hypomagnesemia, seizure disorder, and arrhythmias.

TETRACYCLINES

Doxycycline

Brand names: Biodoxi and Doxypal

- *Available as:* Tablet 100 mg.
- *Indications:* Several bacterial, protozoal, and rickettsial infections; malaria prophylaxis, treatment of complicated malaria in conjunction with other antimalarials.
- *Dose:* 2–5 mg/kg/day (maximum 200 mg) as a single dose or in two divided doses.
- *Adverse drug reactions:* Nausea, vomiting, abdominal pain, dryness of mouth, and CDAD; photosensitivity, pruritus, Stevens–Johnson syndrome; hemolytic anemia; superimposed infections, e.g., vaginitis; pseudotumor cerebri (on withdrawal); infrequently, esophagitis; in young children (<8 years), tooth discoloration (permanent staining), enamel hypoplasia, and retarded growth of fibula.
- *Contraindications:* Known hypersensitivity; children <8 years.

- *Drug interactions:* Antacids, laxatives, oral iron, oral anticoagulants; carbamazepine, phenytoin, and barbiturates reduce its half-life.
- *Cautions:*
  - Monitor hepatic and renal parameters.
  - Avoid exposure to sunlight/ultraviolet rays during therapy.
  - Avoid in children <8 years in the wake of risk of staining of teeth and growth retardation.

Oxytetracycline

Brand name: Terramycin

- *Available as:* Capsule 250 mg; Injection 50 mg/mL.
- *Indications:* Systemic infections (respiratory, genitourinary, ENT, venereal, soft tissue, etc.). brucellosis, *Chlamydia*, *Mycoplasma*, *Rickettsia*; acne vulgaris.
- *Doses:*
  - 25–50 mg/kg/day (PO) in four divided doses
  - 15–25 mg/kg/day (IM) in two divided doses
  - 10–15 mg/kg/day (IV) in two divided doses
- *Adverse drug reactions:* Dental discoloration and enamel hypoplasia, retardation of bone growth rate, especially in fibula, photosensitivity, GI upset, pseudotumor cerebri, allergic reactions, and superinfections; rarely hepatotoxicity and blood dyscrasias.
- *Drug interactions:* Antacids, milk, mineral supplements, and oral contraceptives.
- *Contraindications:* Children <8 years, hypersensitivity, renal impairment, pregnancy, and lactation.
- *Cautions:* Hepatic impairment, myasthenia gravis, systemic lupus erythematosus (SLE), and porphyria.

Tetracycline Hydrochloride

Brand names: Hostacycline and Resteclin
- *Available as:* Tablet/Capsule 100 mg; suspension 25 mg and 50 mg/5 mL.
- *Indications:* Systemic infections (respiratory, genitourinary, ENT, venereal, soft tissue, etc.) brucellosis, *Chlamydia*, *Mycoplasma*, *Rickettsia*; acne vulgaris.
- *Dose:* 5 mg/kg/day (PO) on divided doses on first day. Then, 2.5 mg/kg/day once daily.
- *Adverse drug reactions:* Dental discoloration and enamel hypoplasia, retardation of bone growth rate, especially in fibula, photosensitivity, GI upset, pseudotumor cerebri, allergic reactions, superinfections, CDAD; rarely hepatotoxicity and blood dyscrasias.
- *Drug interactions:* Antacids, milk, mineral supplements, and oral contraceptives.
- *Contraindications:* Children <8 years, hypersensitivity, renal impairment, pregnancy, and lactation.
- *Cautions:* Hepatic impairment, myasthenia gravis, SLE, porphyria; avoid exposure to sunlight/UV rays.

Minocycline

Brand name: Cynomycin
- *Available as:* Capsules 50 and 100 mg.
- *Indications:* Meningococcal carrier state, exacerbation of chronic bronchitis, brucellosis, *Chlamydia*, *Mycoplasma*, and *Rickettsia*, pleural effusion secondary to cirrhosis or malignancy; acne vulgaris.
- *Dose:* Initially 4 mg/kg (PO) followed by 4 mg/kg/day in two divided doses.
- *Adverse drug reactions:* Hypersensitivity reactions, GI upset, vestibular disorders, impaired hearing,

Chapter 44: Antibacterial Drugs (Antibiotics)

pseudotumor cerebri, superinfections, rise in BUN, blood dyscrasias, autoimmune hepatitis, buccal mucosal discoloration, CDAD; rarely pericarditis, myocarditis, vasculitis, hepatotoxicity, renal failure, pancreatitis, interstitial nephritis, SLE, and hyperpigmentation.

- *Drug interactions:* Antacids, mineral supplements, penicillins, ergot alkaloids, digoxin, urinary alkalinizers, methoxyflurane, and oral anticoagulants.
- *Contraindications:* Children <8 years, lactation, pregnancy, and renal failure.
- *Cautions:*
  - *Renal impairment:* Monitor serum creatine and blood urea levels.
  - *Hepatic impairment:* Monitor for hepatitis, SLE or unusual pigmentation every 3 months in long-term therapy. Continue therapy for 2 days after symptomatic control.

Tigecycline

Tigecycline, a broad-spectrum glycylcycline antibiotic resembling tetracyclines, has the Food and Drug Administration (FDA) approval for IV administration only. It is a semisynthetic derivative of minocycline.

Antibacterial spectrum includes a broad range of gram-positive, gram-negative, atypical, anaerobic, and antibiotic-resistant bacteria including MRSA, vancomycin-resistant enterococci (VRE), and PRSP. Unlike conventional tetracyclines, it is bacteriostatic, being effective against tetracycline-resistant gram-positive and gram-negative microorganisms, including MRSA and VRE. However, *Pseudomonas* is not covered by it.

Brand name: Tygacil

- *Available as:* Each single-dose vial containing 50 mg of tigecycline as an orange lyophilized powder for reconstitution.
- *Indications:* It is most effective for complicated skin and soft-tissue infections and intra-abdominal infections acquired either in the hospital or the community.
- *Dose:* 1–2 mg/kg with a maximum of 100 mg for the first dose over 30–60 minutes followed by a 0.5–1 mg with a maximum of 50 mg dose every 12 hours for 5–14 days. No dosage adjustment is needed in patients with renal or liver impairment.
- *Adverse drug reactions:* Photosensitivity and GI effects, such as nausea, vomiting, and diarrhea. Use in children will cause permanent discoloration of teeth. Pain and swelling at the injection site can occur.
- *Drug interaction:* Warfarin, oral contraceptive, amphotericin B, chlorpromazine, methylprednisolone, and voriconazole.
- *Contraindications:* Pregnancy and lactation.
- *Precautions:* Severe live four dysfunction, cholestasis, hypersensitivity, sepsis/shock, and intestinal perforation; avoid ultraviolet rays.
- *Special remarks:* Very expensive, a vial costing over INR 3,000.

GLYCOPEPTIDE ANTIBIOTICS

Vancomycin

It is a first generation complex glycoprotein antibiotic, the glycopeptide inhibiting synthesis of cell wall in gram-positive bacteria.

Brand name: Vancocin

- *Available as:* Injection 500 mg vial.
- *Indication:* Life-threatening methicillin-resistant staphylococcal (MRSA) infections. Oral administration is of value in PMC caused by such bacteria as *Clostridium difficile* and *Staphylococcus aureus*.
- *Dose:* Severe infections.
  - Children: 45–60 mg/kg/day in two to three divided doses (IV slow).
  - Adolescents: 0.5 g 6 hourly or 1 g 12 hourly (IV slow).
  - Neonates:
    - <1,200 g <7 days—15 mg/kg/day OD (Slow IV)
    - >1,200 g <7 days—30 mg/kg/day in 2 divided doses (IV slow)
    - <1,200 g >7 days—15 mg/kg/day OD (IV slow)
    - >1,200 g >7 days—30–45 mg/kg/day in two to three divided doses
- *Adverse drug reactions:* Anaphylactoid reaction, flushing, nephrotoxicity, ototoxicity, neutropenia, nausea, chills, pyrexia, rash, eosinophilia, and phlebitis. Rapid infusion may lead to sudden, profound fall in blood pressure, flushing, and itching (the so-called "red man syndrome").
- *Drug interaction:* Neurotoxic and nephrotoxic agents and anesthetics.
- *Contraindication:* Renal and auditory diseases.
- *Cautions:* Avoid combining with aminoglycoside since the combination is likely to boost the nephrotoxicity of each drug. Reduce dose in renal insufficiency. Monitor blood levels.

Teicoplanin

It is a newer first-generation glycopeptide antibiotic.

Brand name: Targocid

- *Available as:* Injections 200 and 400 mg/vial for reconstitution.
- *Indications:* Resistant gram-positive bacteria only but more than vancomycin against enterococci (enterococcal endocarditis) and equally active against MRSA. Secondly, it may be effective in some VRSA.
- *Doses:*
  - *Children ≥2 months:*
    - *Severe infection or neutropenic:* 10 mg/kg IV 12 hourly for first three doses then 10 mg/kg daily IV/IM.
    - *Moderate infection:* 10 mg/kg 12 hourly IV for first three doses then 6 mg/kg daily IV/IM.
  - *Neonate single loading dose:* 16 mg/kg. Maintenance—8 mg/kg IV infusion over 30 minutes daily.
- *Adverse drug reactions:* GI upset in the form of nausea, vomiting, and diarrhea, anaphylaxis, rashes, urticaria, fever, granulocytopenia; rarely hearing loss and histamine—release reactions.
- *Drug interactions:* Nephrotoxic drugs such as aminoglycosides, frusemide, cyclosporine, and amphotericin B.
- *Contraindications:* Hypersensitivity, pregnancy, and lactation.
- *Cautions:* Renal insufficiency; concurrent administration with drug having ototoxicity and nephrotoxicity.

Dalbavancin (Daptomycin)

The first-generation glycopeptides are vancomycin and teicoplanin which are prototypes. Now, the second-generation glycopeptides have been synthesized.

- Dalbavancin and oritavancin, the two members of the second-generation glycopeptides, have bactericidal activity against MRSA, vancomycin-resistant *Staphylococcus aureus* (VRSA), vancomycin-resistant *E. coli* and drug-resistant *Streptococcus pneumoniae (DRSP), and Streptococcus pyogenes*, i.e., GAS.
- It has a long half-life of 6–10 days, allowing for a long-spaced dosing schedule.
- It exerts its antibacterial activity through effect on membrane permeability and nanoscale lipid membrane organization.
- Antibacterial spectrum includes serious gram-positive hospital infections, particularly MRSA and teicoplanin-resistant strains.

Brand name: Cubicin
- *Available as:* Single-use vials, each containing 500 mg as a sterile and lyophilized powder. The contents of the vial should be reconstituted, using aseptic technique, to 50 mg/mL.
- *Indications:* Skin and soft-tissue infections. It has not shown efficacy in pneumonia. Currently, it is undergoing clinical trials for treatment of bacteremia and endocarditis.
- *Dose:* 4 mg/kg in 0.9% sodium chloride over a 30-minute period once every 24 hours for 7–14 days. Due to the drug's long half-life of 9–12 days, a dalbavancin treatment regimen consists of a once-a-week IV dose. The pharmacokinetics of this drug allows an intermittent dosing schedule which could be suitable for home IV therapy. A once-a-week dose schedule could obviate the need for continuous IV lines and decrease risk of iatrogenic local or bloodstream infections.

- *Adverse drug reactions:* Unusual muscle pain, tenderness, and weakness; numbness or tingling; dysuria; diarrhea (watery or bloody); anemia; easy bruising or bleeding; and chest pain or swelling. Minor side-effects include constipation, nausea, diarrhea, and vomiting; redness, discomfort, or irritation over injection site; cough and sore throat; back pain; anorexia; headache; anxiety, confusion, and insomnia; and mild skin rash.
- *Drug interaction:* Dextrose IV solutions.
- *Caution:* Dosage modification is needed in patients with renal impairment.

Oritavancin

Like dalbavancin, that was developed as a replacement for vancomycin, this novel lipoglycopeptide (derived from vancomycin with phospholipid bilayer) too has by and large crossed the clinical trials stage and holds promise for use in serious gram-positive bacterial infections.

It has a powerful bactericidal activity against vancomycin-resistant *Staphylococcus aureus* and *Enterococcus* species.

- *Indications:* Complicated skin and soft-tissue infections from susceptible pathogens.
- *Special remarks:* Oritavancin is awaiting for FDA approval.

OXAZOLIDINONE ANTIBIOTICS

Linezolid

This is the first commercially available oxazolidinone antibiotic. It is usually reserved for the treatment of serious gram-positive bacterial infections where older antibiotics have failed due to antibiotic resistance, i.e., methicillin or penicillin resistance. It is very expensive. It was approved by the FDA for clinical use in 2000. Repeated studies have shown that linezolid is superior to vancomycin in treating MRSA infections. Linezolid has outperformed glycopeptides in both HA-MRSA and CA-MRSA infections. However, reports of resistance and treatment failures have appeared.

Its mechanism of action is unique in as much as that it is the first synthesized antibiotic that acts by inhibiting the initiation of bacterial protein synthesis.

Antibacterial spectrum, in addition to MRSA, includes other gram-positive pathogens like *E. faecium*, *S. agalactiae*, *S. pyogenes*, and *Streptococcus pneumoniae*. It is only bacteriostatic against most *Enterococcus* species. Against gram-negative pathogens, it is ineffective.

Brand name: Linox
- *Available as:* Tablets 400 and 600 mg; oral suspension powder (after reconstitution 100 mg/5 mL). Injection in an inactive medium for IV administration, 200 mg/100 mL, 400 mg/200 mL, 600 mg/300 mL.
- *Indications:* MRSA, VRE, coagulase-negative staphylococci, and penicillin-resistant pneumococci. It is recommended for pneumonia (both community-acquired and nosocomial) caused by drug-resistant *Streptococcus pneumoniae* (DRSP), surgical site infections, complicated skin and soft-tissue infections, and diabetic foot infections; septicemia, osteomyelitis, and endocarditis.
- *Dose:* 10 mg/kg (PO and IV) q 12 hours for 10–14 days. IV administration should be through infusion over a period of 30–120 minutes.
- *Adverse drug reactions:* Rash, anorexia, diarrhea, nausea, constipation, headache, and fever. Occasionally, severe allergic reaction, or tinnitus, or PMC, and lactic acidosis;

anemia, thrombocytopenia, and myelosuppression may occur.
- *Drug interaction:* Probenecid.
- *Contraindications:* Known hypersensitivity to linezolid, concurrent administration with phenelzine, and isocarboxazid; lactation.
- *Caution:* Its administration with pseudoephedrine and foodstuffs containing tyramine should be avoided since it is a monoamine oxidase inhibitor (MAOI).

Dalfopristin-Quinupristin

This dual drug is a prototype of the group streptogramins which is highly useful for resistant gram-positive infections. Quinupristin and dalfopristin are both streptogramin antibiotics, derived from pristinamycin. Quinupristin is derived from pristinamycin IA and dalfopristin from pristinamycin IIA. They are combined in a weight-to-weight ratio of 30% quinupristin to 70% dalfopristin.

Brand name: Synercid
- *Available as:* IV Injection 150 mg quinupristin and 350 mg dalfopristin.
- *Indications*: MRSA, coagulase-negative *Staphylococcus*, penicillin-susceptible and penicillin-resistant *Pneumococcus*, vancomycin-resistant *E. faecium* (not *E. faecalis*).
- *Dose:*
  - VRE 7.5 mg/kg q 8 h IV, preferably through central catheter to prevent venous irritation and phlebitis.
  - Skin infections 7.5 mg/kg q 12 h IV.
- *Adverse drug reactions:* Local pain, edema, phlebitis, nausea, diarrhea, arthralgia, and myalgia.

- *Contraindications:* Known hypersensitivity to the two components or to other streptogramins (e.g., pristinamycin or virginiamycin).
- *Drug interactions:* A potent inhibitor of cytochrome P450 (CYP3A4), thereby enhancing the effects of terfenadine, astemizole, indinavir, midazolam, Ca channel blockers, warfarin, cisapride, and cyclosporine.
- *Cautions:* Use in children >12 years, preferably >16 years, for which it stands approved. Avoid in CNS infections for which it is not yet approved.

SULFONAMIDES

Sulfadiazine

Brand name: Zad-G

- *Available as:* Tablet 500 mg; injection 250 mg/mL; and cream 2.5 and 5%.
- *Indications:* UTI, toxoplasmosis, meningococcal meningitis; bacterial skin infections; and alternative prophylaxis against acute rheumatic fever.
- *Doses:*
  - 100–150 mg/kg/day (PO) in divided doses; 100 mg/kg/day (IV) in divided doses.
  - 500 mg to 1 g daily for alternative prophylaxis (patients allergic to penicillin) in rheumatic fever.
- *Adverse drug reactions:* Allergic reactions including Stevens–Johnson syndrome, crystalluria, cyanosis, jaundice, and purpura hemolytic anemia in G6PD deficiency.
- *Contraindication:* Hypersensitivity.
- *Caution:* Generous intake of water needed during therapy; avoid in G6PD deficiency subjects.

Sulfamethoxazole with Trimethoprim

Brand names: Septran and Bactrim

- *Available as:*
  - Adult tablet
    - 80 mg trimethoprim and 400 mg sulfamethoxazole
    - 160 mg trimethoprim and 800 mg sulfamethoxazole
  - *Pediatric tablet:* 20 mg trimethoprim and 100 mg sulfamethoxazole
  - *Suspension:* 40 mg trimethoprim and 200 mg sulfamethoxazole/5 mL
  - *Injection (5 mL):* 80 mg trimethoprim and 400 mg sulfamethoxazole
- *Indications:* Respiratory, GIT, urinary tract, ENT, and skin/soft tissue infections; typhoid and paratyphoid fevers; nontuberculous *Mycobacteria*; *Pneumocystis carinii* superinfection in HIV/AIDS.
- *Dose:* 4–10 mg/kg/day (O and IV) in terms of trimethoprim.
- *Adverse drug reactions:* Gastric upset, nausea, vomiting, glossitis, anorexia, malaise, skin rash, crystalluria, and rarely blood dyscrasias.
- *Drug interactions:* SMZ–protein displacement with warfarin, phenytoin, methotrexate. TMP–phenytoin, cyclosporine, rifampicin, and warfarin.
- *Contraindications:* Sulfonamide allergy and neonatal period; also, any individual with G6PD deficiency; premature infants for first 3 months.
- *Caution:* The injectable cotrimoxazole should never be given directly. The drug should be diluted in normal saline or 5% dextrose in a proportion of its 5 mL (1 ampule) to 125 mL of infusion. The rate of infusion should be about 2–6 mL/min. Infusion solution must be used within 6 hours of preparation.

Chapter 44: Antibacterial Drugs (Antibiotics)

Sulfasalazine

Brand name: Salazopyrin
- *Available as:* Tablet 500 mg.
- *Indications:* Inflammatory bowel disease (IBD), i.e., ulcerative colitis and Crohn's disease, and rheumatoid arthritis.
- *Dose:*
  - *Starting dose:* 50–75 mg/kg/day (PO) div q 4 to 6 h with a maximum of 6 g/day
  - *Maintenance dose:* 25–50 mg/kg/day (PO) div q 6 to 8 h with a maximum of 2 g/day
- *Adverse drug reactions:* Drug rash, dizziness, headache, GI disturbances, nephrotoxicity (crystalluria); rarely blood dyscrasias.
- *Drug interactions:* Protein displacement with warfarin, phenytoin, and methotrexate.
- *Contraindications:* Sulfonamide allergy; G6PD deficiency.
- *Precaution:* Avoid <2 years age. Drink plenty of water.

Sulfisoxazole

Brand name: Gantrisin
- *Available as:* Tablet 500 mg; suspension 500 mg/5 mL.
- *Indications:* Otitis media, chronic bronchitis, lower UTI due to susceptible pathogens.
- *Dose:* 5–60 mg/kg/day in two divided doses
- *Adverse drug reactions:* Nausea, vomiting, crystalluria, rash, Stevens–Johnson syndrome, renal, and hepatic impairment.
- *Drug interaction:* Protein displacement with warfarin, phenytoin, and methotrexate.
- *Contraindications:* Hypersensitivity to sulfonamides or chemically-related drugs (e.g., sulfonylureas, thiazide and

loop diuretics, carbonic anhydrase inhibitors, sunscreens containing p-aminobenzoic acid, and local anesthetics); hypersensitivity to salicylates; porphyria; children younger than 2 months of age; and pregnancy at term.
- *Precaution:* Avoid in renal disease.

MISCELLANEOUS ANTIBACTERIAL DRUGS

Chloramphenicol

It was originally obtained from *Streptomyces venezuelae* in 1947, now it is entirely a synthetic product.

Brand names: Chloromycetin and Paraxin
- *Available as:* Capsule/Dragee/tablet 250 and 500 mg; suspension 125 mg/5 mL; and injection 250 mg/mL.
- *Indications:* Typhoid fever; *H. influenzae* and other severe infections.
- *Dose:* 50–100 mg/kg/day (O, IM, and IV) in divided doses, 25 mg/kg/day (O, IM, and IV) in first 2 weeks of life when it is best avoided on account of the risk of developing gray baby syndrome.
- *Adverse drug reactions:* Bone marrow depression (parenteral chloramphenicol is relatively less dangerous than oral chloramphenicol as regard bone marrow depression), allergic reaction, GIT upset, peripheral neuritis, and retrobulbar neuritis.

In preterm newborns, it may rarely cause *gray baby syndrome* which is a cardiovascular collapse characterized by appearance of symptoms like vomiting or regurgitation, and refusal to suck and abdominal distention. These occur after 2–3 days of continued therapy. In another day or so the infant develops ashen-gray color, cyanosis, and becomes limp. Prognosis is extremely poor with very high fatality.

This condition is due to a lack of glucuronidation reactions occurring in the baby, thus leading to an accumulation of toxic chloramphenicol metabolites.

The uridine diphosphate (UDP)-glucuronyl transferase enzyme system of infants, especially premature infants, is immature and incapable of metabolizing the excessive drug load. Insufficient renal excretion of the unconjugated drug makes its own contribution.

- *Drug interactions:* It inhibits metabolism of tolbutamide, chlorpropamide, warfarin, cyclophosphamide, and phenytoin. Such drugs as phenobarbital, phenytoin, and rifampicin enhance its metabolism, thereby contributing to failure of adequate response.
- *Contraindications:* Hematologic disorders.
- *Caution:* Monitor blood counts; avoid in minor infections that can be treated with other antimicrobials.
- *Special remarks:* Having had only limited prescriptions over the past couple of decades on account of emergence of resistance, antimicrobial sensitivity to chloramphenicol is now bouncing back.

Metronidazole

Brand names: Flagyl and Metrogyl

- *Available as:* Tablets 200, 400, and 600 mg; suspension 100 and 200 mg/5 mL; and injection 2 mg/mL.
- *Indications:* Anaerobic infections; also in giardiasis, amebiasis, trichomoniasis, acute ulcerative gingivitis, and PMS dracunculiasis.
- *Doses:*
  - Newborns:
    - <1,200 g 7.5 mg/kg (O and IV) 48 h
    - <7 days 1,200–2,000 g 7.5 mg/kg/24 h (O and IV) q 24 h

- >2,000 g 15 mg/kg/24 h (O and IV) divide 12 h
- >7 days 1,200–2,000 g 15 mg/kg/24 (O and IV) h divided q 12 h
- >2,000 g 30 mg/kg/24 h (O and IV) divided q 12 h
- Children:
  - 30 mg/kg/day (IV) for anaerobic infections
  - 21 mg/kg/day (IV) severe amebic dysentery
  - 10–20 mg/kg/day (PO) for 5–7 days in divided doses for giardiasis
  - 20–50 mg/kg/day (PO) for 10 days in divided doses for amebiasis
- *Adverse drug reactions:* Metallic taste lasting for some days, nausea, vomiting, headache, diarrhea, dizziness, rash, itching, furred tongue, incoordination, leukopenia, hypotension, and poor tolerance with alcohol.
- *Drug interactions:* Phenobarbital, phenytoin, hepatic enzyme inducers, alcohol, oral anticoagulants, cimetidine, and disulfiram.
- *Contraindications:* Active CNS disease, blood dyscrasias, first trimester of pregnancy, and lactation.
- *Caution:* Avoid in children weighing <15 kg.

Rifampicin

This drug acts through inhibition of bacterial RNA polymerase.

Brand names: Coxid, Macox, R-cin, Rifampin, and Rifamycin

- *Available as:* Capsules 150, 300, 450, and 600 mg; syrup 100 mg/5 mL.
- *Indications:* Second agent (synergistic) for *S. aureus* infections; elimination of nasopharyngeal colonization in carriers of *H. influenzae* type B and *N. meningitidis* resistant to penicillin and sulfas; tuberculosis and leprosy.

- *Dose:* 10–20 mg/kg/day (PO) as a single daily dose before food.
- *Adverse drug reactions:* Nausea, hypersensitivity reactions, hepatic dysfunction, orange-red staining of saliva, sputum, sweat, urine and stool, GIT upset, heartburn, rash, drowsiness, headache, confusion, numbness, cramps, visual disturbances, eosinophilia, and thrombocytopenia.
- *Drug interactions:* Phenytoin, steroids, narcotics, alcohol, digoxin, hypoglycemic, oral contraceptives, and disulfiram.
- *Contraindications:* Optic neuritis and jaundice.
- *Caution:* Impaired liver and renal function.

Chapter 45: Antimycobacterial Drugs

INTRODUCTION

Major members of the *Mycobacterium* genus are tuberculosis, nontuberculous mycobacteriosis (NTM), and leprosy.

Antimycobacterial drugs are usually employed in combination chemotherapy to kill heterogeneous populations of bacterial cells located in different conditions within the host, and to prevent drug resistance. Currently available chemotherapeutic agents are highly effective in managing drug-sensitive tuberculosis. As a result of the global HIV epidemic and the emergence drug resistance in case of tuberculosis, efforts to control tuberculosis are getting undermined. There is a need to develop new safe, effective, and affordable antimycobacterial drugs to manage both drug-sensitive and drug-resistant disease. Mercifully, the combination therapy has been effective in controlling leprosy.

ANTITUBERCULOUS DRUGS

Antituberculous drugs are conventionally categorized in three groups (**Box 1**).

BOX 1: Categories of antituberculous drugs.

Group 1: First-line drugs
- Isoniazid
- Rifampicin
- Streptomycin
- Pyrazinamide
- Ethambutol

Group 2: Second-line drugs
- Cycloserine
- Ethionamide
- Para-aminosalicylic acid (PAS)
- Kanamycin
- Capreomycin

Group 3: Reserve drugs
- Quinolones (Ciprofloxacin)
- Amikacin
- Ampicillin
- Imipenem

Now tendency to categorize antituberculous drugs in terms of efficacy and experience of use is on the increase **(Box 2)**.

FIRST-LINE DRUGS

Isoniazid (Isonicotinic Acid)

Brand names: Ipcazide, Isokin, Isonex, Siozide, and Solonex

- *Available as:* Tablets 50, 100, and 300 mg; Syrup 50 and 100 mg/5 mL.
- *Dose:* 5–10 mg/kg/day (PO) as a single dose or in two to three divided doses
- *Adverse drug reactions:* Weight gain, constipation, euphoria, pellagra-like dermatosis, peripheral neuritis, convulsions, and hepatotoxicity.
- *Contraindication:* Liver disease

BOX 2: Categories of antituberculous drugs based on efficacy and experience of use.

Group 1: First-line drugs
- Isoniazid (H)
- Rifampicin (R)
- Pyrazinamide (Z)
- Ethambutol (E)
- Streptomycin (S)

Group 2: Second-line drugs (Injectable)
- Kanamycin (Km)
- Amikacin (Am)
- Capreomycin (Cm)

Group 3: Fluoroquinolones
- Ofloxacin (Ofx)
- Levofloxacin (Lfx)
- Moxifloxacin (Mfx)
- Gatifloxacin (Gfx)

Group 4: Oral second-line drugs
- Ethionamide (Eto)
- Prothionamide (Pto)
- Cycloserine (Cs)
- Terizidone (Trd)
- Para-aminosalicylic acid (PAS)

Group 5: Drugs with unclear efficacy
- Clofazimine (Cfz)
- Linezolid (Lzd)
- Amoxycillin-clavulanic acid (Amx/Clv)
- Thiacetazone (Thz)
- Imipenem/cilastatin (Ipm/Cln)
- High-dose isoniazid (High dose H)
- Clarithromycin (Clr)

- *Drug interactions:* Alcohol, antacids, carbamazepine, ketoconazole, phenytoin, rifampicin, and valproate.
- *Caution:* Monitor hepatic and ocular function.

Ethambutol

Brand name: Combutol

- *Available as:* Tablets 200, 400, 500, and 800 mg.
- *Dose:* 15–25 mg/kg/day (PO) in a single dose.
- *Adverse drug reactions:* Drowsiness, gastrointestinal tract (GIT) upset, rash, headache, dizziness, euphoria, swelling of tongue, hepatic and renal dysfunction, leukopenia, bone marrow depression, aggravation of grand mal attacks, and visual disturbances.
- *Caution:* Avoid in preschoolers in view of difficulty in evaluating their vision.

Pyrazinamide

Brand names: PZA-Ciba, P-Zide, and Pyzina

- *Available as:* Tablet 500 and 750 mg, 1 g; Syrup 250 mg/5 mL.
- *Dose:* 20–35 mg/kg/day (PO) as a single dose; maximum dose 2 g daily.
- *Adverse drug reactions:* Nausea, vomiting, hepatotoxicity (especially in diabetics and alcoholics), hyperuricemia, gout, anorexia nervosa, arthralgia, myalgia, rash, dysuria, sideroblastic anemia; rarely blood dyscrasias and photosensitivity.
- *Drug interactions:* Uricosurics, probenecid, and sulfinpyrazone.
- *Contraindications:* Gout and hepatic dysfunction; lactation.
- *Caution:* Monitor liver function test (LFT), blood uric acid estimation regularly.

Rifampicin

Brand names: R-cin, Rifamycin, and Siticox

- *Indications:* Tuberculosis; leprosy; carriers of *N. meningitidis* resistant to penicillin and sulfa.
- *Available as:* Capsule 150, 300, 450, and 600 mg; Syrup 100 mg/5 mL.
- *Dose:* 10–20 mg/kg/day (PO) as a single daily dose before food.
- *Adverse drug reactions:* Nausea, hypersensitivity reactions, hepatic dysfunction, orange-red staining of saliva, sputum, sweat, urine and stool, GIT upset, heartburn, rash, drowsiness, headache, confusion, numbness, cramps, visual disturbances, eosinophilia, and thrombocytopenia.
- *Drug interactions:* Phenytoin, steroids, narcotics, alcohol, digoxin, hypoglycemic, oral contraceptives, and disulfiram.
- *Contraindication:* Optic neuritis and jaundice.
- *Caution:* Caution patients/parents about orange-red staining of saliva, sputum, sweat, urine, and stool.

Streptomycin

Brand name: Ambistryn-S

- *Available as:* Injection 750 mg, 1 g/vial.
- *Dose:* 15–20 mg/kg/day (IM) for 3 months.
- *Adverse drug reactions:* Ototoxicity, nephrotoxicity, anaphylaxis, fever, rash, urticaria, angioneurotic edema, esosinophilia, hemolytic anemia, blood dyscrasias, azotemia, muscle weakness, and amblyopia.
- *Drug interactions:* Diuretics (especially frusemide), mannitol, other aminoglycosides, ethacrynic acid, polymyxin B, colistin, cyclosporine, anesthetics, and neuromuscular blocking agents.

- *Contraindications:* Hypersensitivity, vestibular damage, and suppurative otitis media (SOM).
- *Cautions:* Impaired hepatic and kidney function, prematurity, impaired vestibular/auditory function, myasthenia gravis, pregnancy, and lactation.

SECOND-LINE DRUGS

Capreomycin

Brand name: Capreo
- *Available as:* Injection 500 mg vial.
- *Indication:* Multidrug-resistant tuberculosis (MDR-TB).
- *Dose:* 15–30 mg/kg/day (IM) with a maximum of 1 g.
- *Adverse drug reactions:* Allergic reactions (rash, itching, swelling, and breathing problem) local pain, dizziness, and electrolyte disturbances.
- *Caution:* Avoid activity needing alertness (say driving).

Ethionamide

Brand names: Ethide, Ethocid, Myobd, and Mycotuf
- *Available as:* Tablet 250 mg.
- *Indication:* Tuberculosis when other drugs are ineffective or contraindicated.
- *Dose:* 10–20 mg/kg/day with a maximum of 500–750 mg daily (PO) in two to three divided doses.
- *Adverse drug reactions:* Nausea, vomiting, diarrhea, anorexia, salivation, abdominal pain, icterus, rash, acne, alopecia, mental changes, peripheral neuritis, and photosensitivity.
- *Contraindications:* Hepatic damage and pregnancy.
- *Caution:* Monitor liver function test (LFT) periodically.

Cycloserine

Brand name: Cyclorine
- *Available as:* Capsule 250 mg.
- *Indication:* Second-line drug for resistant TB; in combination with other antituberculosis therapy (ATT).
- *Dose:* 10 mg/kg/day in two divided doses; may be increased to 15–20 mg/kg/day in two divided doses after 2 weeks.
- *Adverse drug reactions:* Headache, dizziness, vertigo, drowsiness, depression, tremors, seizures, psychosis, rash, liver dysfunction, and megaloblastic anemia.
- *Drug interaction:* Alcohol.
- *Contraindications:* Severe renal impairment, epilepsy, alcohol dependence, psychotic states, and porphyria.
- *Caution:* Reduce dose in impaired renal function; discontinue in case of allergic rash or CNS toxicity; monitor blood, and renal and liver function status periodically.

Kanamycin

Brand name: Kancin
- *Available as:* Injection 0.5 and 1.0 g vials.
- *Indications:* Tuberculosis as a second-line drug. Also, neonatal sepsis, urogenital, respiratory, central nervous system (CNS), soft tissue and GIT infections due to *Staphylococcus*.
- *Dose:* 15–39 mg/kg/day (IM) in one or two divided doses.
- *Adverse drug reactions:* Nephrotoxic, ototoxic, rash, fever, headache, and paresthesia.
- *Contraindications:* Pregnancy and lactation.
- *Drug interaction:* Furosemide, ethacrynic acid, neuromuscular blocking agents, and anesthetics.
- *Precaution:* Myasthenia gravis, Parkinsonism, and monitor in renal impairment.

Para-aminosalicylic Acid

It is a structural analog of para-aminobenzoic acid (PABA), acting by competitively inhibiting the synthesis of folic acid as do the sulfonamides.

- *Available as:* Generic sodium para-aminosalicylic acid (PAS) 80 g/100 g granules; 4 g packets.
- *Indication:* Resistant tuberculosis as a second-line drug in combination with other ATT.
- *Dose:* 200–300 mg/kg/day (PO) in three to four divided doses, essentially after food. The granules are best mixed with a liquid and swallowed whole.
- *Adverse drug reactions:* Gastrointestinal (GI) disturbances, weight loss, hepatotoxicity, hypersensitivity; hypokalemia, hematuria, albuminuria, and crystalluria.
- *Drug interaction:* It may decrease the absorption of rifampicin; on the other hand, its adverse effects are potentiated when given along with ethionamide.
- *Caution:* Liver insufficiency; monitor for weight loss and liver and renal function.

Prothionamide

It is a thioamide derivative.

Brand names: Mycotuf, Pethide, Prothiocid, and Protomid

- *Available as:* Tablet 250 mg.
- *Indications:* Multidrug-resistant (MDR) tuberculosis.
- *Dose:* 15–20 mg/kg/day (PO) in two to three divided doses.
- *Adverse drug reactions:* Nausea, vomiting, depression, and hallucinations. Rarely, jaundice, menstrual disturbances, and peripheral neuropathy.
- *Contraindication:* Pregnancy as it has been shown to be teratogenic in animal studies.

- *Caution:* Avoid in severe liver disease. Blood sugar levels need to be monitored in diabetics.

Ciprofloxacin

A high-performance quinolone active against *Pseudomonas aeruginosa, Serratia, Enterobacter, Shigella, Salmonella, Campylobacter, Neisseria gonorrhoeae, Haemophilus influenzae, Moraxella catarrhalis, Staphylococcus aureus* (selected), and *Streptococcus*.

Brand names: Cifran and Ciplox
- *Available as:* Tablets 250 and 500 mg; Injection 1 and 2 mg/mL.
- *Indications:* Resistant tuberculosis as a reserve drug in combination with other ATT. Also, infections of the urinary tract, GIT, respiratory tract, bones and joints, skin; serious life-threatening infections, e.g., septicemia, resistant enteric fever; hospital-acquired infections; and prevention of sepsis in immunocompromised hosts.
- *Dose:* 15–30 mg/kg/day (PO) in two divided doses, 5–10 mg/kg/day (IV) in two divided doses.
- *Adverse drug reactions:* Tendonitis, gastrointestinal intolerance (nausea, vomiting, and diarrhea), anorexia, abdominal pain, flatulence, pseudomembranous colitis; dizziness, headache, insomnia, confusion agitation, tremors, ataxia, seizures, hallucinations, visual disturbances, migraine, and deafness; rash, pruritus, drug fever, anaphylaxis, Stevens–Johnson syndrome, photosensitivity, and eosinophilia; hepatitis and raised aspartate aminotransferase [AST or serum glutamic-oxaloacetic transaminase (SGOT)], alanine aminotransferase [ALT or serum glutamic pyruvic transaminase (SGPT)],

Chapter 45: Antimycobacterial Drugs

alkaline phosphatase, serum bilirubin; crystalluria, nephritis, transient renal failure, raised blood urea, creatine, hematuria, anemia, thrombocytopenia, and thrombocytosis; thrombophlebitis and superinfections.

The joint destruction (encountered in juvenile animals) is not seen in humans.

- *Drug interactions:* Antacids (containing Mg, Ca, and Al), sucraflate, theophylline, probenecid, warfarin, and cyclosporine.
- *Contraindication:* Hypersensitivity to quinolones.
- *Cautions:*
  - Avoid the drug 1–2 hours before and 4 hours after the antacids.
  - Avoid with theophylline and nonsteroidal anti-inflammatory drugs (NSAIDs).
  - Avoid in epileptics.

Levofloxacin

It is a levo isomer of ofloxacin.

Brand names: Levoflox, Leeflox, and Lomflox

- *Indications:* MDR-TB as a reserve drug in combination with other ATT. Gram-positive and gram-negative infections.
- *Available as:* Tablet 250 and 500 mg. Injection 500 mg/100 mL IV infusion.
- *Dose:* 10–15 mg/kg OD or in two divided doses.
- *Adverse drug reactions:* Nausea, diarrhea, dizziness, headache, photosensitivity, peripheral neuropathy (paresthesia, hypoesthesia, and weakness), and rupture of tendons.
- *Drug interactions:* Antacids, sucralfate, and probenecid.

- *Contraindications:* <8 years, hypersensitivity, lactation, and pregnancy.
- *Caution:* Avoid in children <8 years, severe renal impairment; avoid exposure to sunlight; discontinue in case of hypersensitivity, photosensitivity, and neuropathy manifestations.

Amikacin

First semisynthetic aminoglycoside; derivative of kanamycin A; effective against gram-positive as well as gram-negative organisms—just like tobramycin.

Brand names: Amicin and Mikicin
- *Available as:* Injection 100, 250, and 500 mg/vial.
- *Indications:* Tuberculosis (third line, i.e., reserve drug) in combination with other ATT. Also, fulminant gram-negative infections (sepsis, pneumonia, meningitis, peritonitis, infected burns, and postoperative sepsis), and gram-positive infections resistant to other aminoglycosides, e.g., nosocomial infections like in burns, in ICU, and in immunocompromised subjects.
- *Dose:* 15–25 mg/kg/day divided 8–12 hours.
- *Adverse drug reactions:* Nephrotoxicity, ototoxicity (mainly cochlear), neuromuscular blockade, hypersensitivity reactions such as drug fever, rash, eosinophilia, tremors, nausea, vomiting, headache, and overgrowth of non-susceptible microorganisms.
- *Contraindications:* Known hypersensitivity to aminoglycosides.
- *Caution:* Suitable reduction in dose must be made in renal insufficiency depending on creatinine clearance and blood urea nitrogen (BUN).

Imipenem/Cilastatin

Brand name: Cilanem-500

- *Available as:* Injection 500 mg each of imipenem and cilastatin.
- *Indications:* Multidrug-resistant tuberculosis (MDR-TB) as reserve/third-line drug along with other ATT. Being a broad-spectrum β-lactam antimicrobial, also employed for serious aerobic as well as anaerobic extended spectrum β-lactamase (ESBL)-producing bacterial infections (both gram positive and gram negative).
- *Dose:* 15 mg/kg/dose (IV infusion) every 6 hourly with a maximum of 2 g/day.
- *Adverse drug reactions:* Local and allergic reactions, phlebitis, GI upset, rash, fever, blood dyscrasias, hepatic dysfunction, renal dysfunction, CNS disturbances, hearing loss, seizures, confusion, dizziness, somnolence, hypotension, perverted taste, superinfections, pseudo-membranous colitis, and *Clostridium difficile*-associated diarrhea (CDAD).
- *Drug interaction:* Probenecid, valproic acid, ganciclovir, divalproex sodium, and estrogen contraceptives
- *Contraindications:* <3 months, lactation.
- *Cautions:* Penicillin, cephalosporin or other allergy, colitis, concomitant use with valproic acid, CNS disorders, renal impairment, meningitis, brain abscess, granulocytopenia, prolonged use, and pregnancy.

ANTINONTUBERCULOUS MYCOBACTERIAL DRUGS

Azithromycin

It is a macrolide with very long half-life, thereby imparting it the uniqueness of once daily dosing.

Brand names: Aziwok, Azithral, and Rowezy

- *Available as:* Tablet/capsule 250 and 500 mg; Suspension 100 and 200 mg/5 mL.
- *Indications:* Nontuberculous/atypical mycobacteria in combination with ATT comprising rifampicin and ethambutol; also, infections with *Staphylococcus aureus, Streptococcus, H. influenzae, Mycoplasma, Legionella;* typhoid, *Chlamydia trachomatis*, etc.
- *Dose:* 5 mg/kg/day (PO) OD on empty stomach for about 1 year. This dose is half of the usual short-term dose in acute infections.
- *Adverse drug reactions:* Hypersensitivity reactions, mild GIT upset including taste/smell perversion or loss, elevation of liver enzymes (reversible), pseudomembranous colitis (PMC), hearing loss (reversible), arthralgia, photosensitivity, seizures, Stevens–Johnson syndrome; acute renal failure; neutropenia; and prolongation of QT interval.
- *Drug interactions:* Antacids, digoxin, carbamazepine, phenytoin, theophylline, fluconazole, cyclosporine, and anticoagulants.
- *Contraindications:* Severe liver dysfunction and lactation.
- *Cautions:* Renal and hepatic dysfunction; it needs to be taken on empty stomach (1 hour before/2 hours after food).

Clarithromycin

It is a methoxy derivative of erythromycin.

Brand name: Claribid

- *Available as:* Tablet 250 and 500 mg; Suspension 75 mg/5 mL.
- *Indications:* Prophylaxis and treatment of *M. avium complex* disease, *Mycobacterium fortuitum, M. marinum,* and *Mycobacterium* abscesses in combination with ATT comprising rifampicin and ethambutol. Also, for upper

and lower respiratory infections (mild to moderate) and skin infections due to susceptible bacteria, say *H. influenzae, M. catarrhalis, M. pneumoniae, S. aureus, S. pneumoniae, C. trachomatis, and Legionella* spp.

- *Dose:* 7.5 mg/kg/day in two divided doses for about 1 year. This dose is around half of the dose for acute infections.
- *Drug interactions:* Theophylline, digoxin, rifampicin, carbamazepine, phenobarbital, phenytoin, midazolam, sodium valproate, oral anticoagulants, cisapride, primazole, ergot derivatives, drugs metabolized by P450, statins, warfarin, colchicines, quinidine, cyclosporine, bromocriptine, and zidovudine.
- *Contraindications:* Concomitant use of cisapride, pimozide, hypersensitivity to erythromycin, azithromycin, or clarithromycin.
- *Cautions:* Renal or hepatic impairment, arrhythmias, QT interval prolongation, pregnancy, and lactation.

Sulfamethoxazole with Trimethoprim (Cotrimoxazole)

A synergistic combination, in the fixed ratio of one part of trimethoprim (TMP) and five parts of sulfamethoxazole (SMZ). SMZ, a sulfa, inhibits synthesis of dihydrofolic acid by competitively inhibiting PABA. TMP blocks production of tetrahydrofolic acid and downstream biosynthesis of nucleic acids and protein by reversely binding to dihydrofolate reductase.

Brand names: Bactrim and Septran
- *Available as:*
  - Adult tablet 80 mg TMP and 400 mg SMZ.
  - 160 mg TMP and 800 mg SMZ
  - Pediatric tablet   20 mg TMP
                              100 mg SMZ, and

- Suspension (5 mL)   40 mg TMP
  200 mg SMZ
- Injection (5 mL)   80 mg TMP
  400 mg SMZ

- *Indications:* Nontuberculous mycobacteria in combination with ATT; also respiratory, GIT, urinary tract, ear, nose, and throat (ENT), skin/soft tissue infections; typhoid and paratyphoid fevers.
- *Dose:* Usual dose is 4–10 mg (up to 20 mg)/kg/day (O and IV), in terms of TMP, in two to three divided doses. In NTM, half of the conventional dose suffices. Duration is usually 1 year.
- *Adverse drug reactions:* Gastric upset, nausea, vomiting, glossitis, anorexia, malaise, skin rash, and rarely blood dyscrasias.
- *Contraindications:* Sulfonamide allergy and neonatal period; also any individual with G6PD deficiency; premature infants for first 3 months.
- *Cautions:* The injectable cotrimoxazole should never be given directly. The drug should be diluted in normal saline or 5% dextrose in a proportion of its 5 mL (1 ampule) to 125 mL of infusion. The rate of infusion should be about 2–6 mL/min. Infusion solution must be used within 6 hours of preparation G6PD deficiency.

Routine laboratory monitoring comprising complete blood count (CBC), periodic electrolytes, and creatine for renal function.

ANTILEPROSY DRUGS

Leprosy is caused by the *Mycobacterium leprae*. Once dubbed as an incurable disease, leprosy is now very much curable thanks to the availability of effective antileprosy drugs and favorable changes in therapeutic approach toward multidrug therapy (MDT) rather than a solitary drug therapy.

Clofazimine

A synthetic phendimetrazine tartrate derivative, acting by binding to mycobacterial DNA at guanine sites.

Brand name: Hansepran
- *Available as:* Capsule 50 and 100 mg.
- *Indications:* As a part of combination therapy for *M. leprae*.
- *Dose:* 1 mg/kg/day (PO) as a single dose with a maximum of 100 mg/day in combination with dapsone and rifampicin for 2 years. Thereafter, it is continued as a single agent for up to 1 year.
- *Adverse drug reactions:* Reversible skin and conjunctival discoloration (pink to tan-brown), dry itchy skin, rash, headache, dizziness, abdominal pain, diarrhea, vomiting, peripheral neuropathy, and elevation of liver transaminases.
- *Contraindications:* Hypersensitivity, G6PD deficiency, severe anemia (hemoglobin < 7 g%).
- *Caution:* It needs to be taken with food to enhance absorption. Routine laboratory monitoring for liver function is advisable.

Dapsone (Diaminodiphenyl Sulfone)

It is a sulfone antimicrobial resembling sulfonamides with same mechanism of action, acting as a competitive antagonist of PABA that is essential for bacterial synthesis of folic acid.

Brand name: Available under generic name only.
- *Available as:* Tablets 5, 10, 25, 50, and 100 mg.

- *Indication:* Leprosy in combination with other antileprosy drugs, say clofazimine, rifampicin, ethionamide; other uses: certain skin disorders including acne, chloroquine-resistant malaria (in combination with pyrimethamine). Topical use in dermatitis herpetiformis.
- *Dose:* 1–2 mg/kg/day (PO) as a single dose with a maximum of 100 mg/day for 3–10 years.
- *Adverse drug reactions*: Hemolytic anemia (especially in G6PD deficient subjects), pancreatitis, acute tubular necrosis, acute renal failure, albuminuria, increased liver enzymes, psychosis, tinnitus, peripheral neuropathy, photosensitivity, hypersensitivity syndrome characterized by fever, rash, malaise, and hepatic dysfunction; lepra reaction: a Jarisch–Herxheimer type of reaction (a sort of Arthus phenomenon) as a consequence of release of antigens from the killed *M. leprae* and consists of enlargement of existing skin lesions that may also become red, swollen, and painful, appearance of new lesions, fever, malaise, and other constitutional symptoms; sulfone syndrome: it develops 4–6 weeks following institution of therapy with dapsone usually in malnourished subjects, and consists of fever, desquamation of skin, enlargement of lymph nodes, icterus, and anemia.
- *Drug interaction:* Rifampin lowers dapsone levels seven- to 10-fold by accelerating plasma clearance in leprosy. This reduction does necessitate a change in dosage. Folic acid antagonists such as pyrimethamine may increase the likelihood of hematologic reactions. There is a mutual interaction between dapsone and TMP in which each raises the level of the other about 1.5 times.
- *Contraindication:* Hypersensitivity, G6PD deficiency, and severe anemia (hemoglobin < 7 g%).

- *Caution:* Exercise caution in subjects with G6PD deficiency and those on folic acid antagonists' therapy; periodic renal and hepatic function; CBC weekly during 1st month of therapy, weekly through 6 months of therapy, then every 6 months.
- *Special remarks:* Diaminodiphenyl sulfone (DDS) is the most commonly employed, the best and the most economical of all the antileprosy drugs. On account of increasing drug resistance, it is employed as a component of MDT.

Rifampicin

Brand names: R-cin, Rifamycin, and Siticox
- *Available as:* Capsule 150, 300, 450, and 600 mg; Syrup 100 mg/5 mL.
- *Indications:* Leprosy in combination with either dapsone or clofazimine (two-drug combination) or both (three-drug combination); tuberculosis; carriers of *N. meningitidis* resistant to penicillin and sulfas.
- *Dose:* 10–20 mg/kg/day (PO) as a single daily dose before food.
- *Adverse drug reactions:* Nausea, hypersensitivity reactions, hepatic dysfunction, orange-red staining of saliva, sputum, sweat, urine and stool, GIT upset, heartburn, rash, drowsiness, headache, confusion, numbness, cramps, visual disturbances, eosinophilia, and thrombocytopenia.
- *Contraindications:* Optic neuritis and jaundice.
- *Drug interactions:* Phenytoin, steroids, narcotics, alcohol, digoxin, hypoglycemic, oral contraceptives, and disulfiram.
- *Contraindications:* Hypersensitivity and liver dysfunction.
- *Caution:* Impaired liver and renal function. Alert the attendant regarding high-colored urine.

46
Chapter

Antiviral Drugs

INTRODUCTION

Antiviral drugs are a class of medication that are specifically for treating or preventing viral infections such as influenza, herpes virus infections, viral hepatitis, and human immunodeficiency virus (HIV).

Most viral diseases with the exception of those caused by HIV are self-limited illnesses that do not require specific antiviral therapy except when the infection is very severe.

The currently available antiviral drugs target the herpes, hepatitis, influenza, and HIV group of viruses.

ANTIHERPES AND ALLIED VIRUS DRUGS

Acyclovir

A synthetic purine nucleoside acts by inhibiting viral deoxyribonucleic acid (DNA) polymerase against human herpes viruses, including herpes simplex virus (HSV), types 1 and 2, varicella zoster virus (VZV), Epstein–Barr virus (EBV), and cytomegalovirus (CMV). In case of the last two microbes, its efficacy and, hence, utility is quite limited.

Brand name: Zovirax
- *Available as:* Tablet 200 mg; IV injection 250 mg/vial.
- *Indications:* Herpes simplex virus infections—particularly involving genitalia; herpes simplex encephalitis; neonatal

herpes simplex infection; primary HSV gingivostomatitis; long-term suppressive therapy in HSV infections; VZV infections; immunocompromised states.
- *Dose:*
  - *Neonates:* 30 mg/kg/day (IV) q 8 h
  - *Children:* 200 mg/m^2/day (IV) q 8 h
  - *Prophylaxis:* 200 mg (PO) five times a day for 5–10 days
- *Adverse drug reactions (ADRs):* Usually safe; transient skin rashes; occasionally gastrointestinal (GI) disturbances (nausea, vomiting, diarrhea, and abdominal pain); reversible neurologic reactions (dizziness, confusional states, hallucinations, and somnolence); hair loss, headache, and fatigue; rarely slight transient rise in serum bilirubin and liver-related enzymes, rise in blood urea and creatinine, and fall in hematologic indices.
- *Drug interactions:* Probenecid, other drugs affecting renal physiology could influence its pharmacokinetics.
- *Contraindication:* Hypersensitivity to acyclovir.
- *Cautions:*
  - Avoid rapid infusion which may cause reversible obstructive uropathy by crystallization of the drug in renal tubules.
  - Avoid prolonged use which can cause neutropenia.
  - Avoid high doses which can cause neurotoxicity.
  - Anti-influenza virus drugs.
  - Miscellaneous (nonselective) antiviral.

Adenine Arabinoside

Brand names: Vdarabine and Vra A
- *Available as:* Injection 200 mg/mL; topical; skin cream 5%, and ophthalmic ointment 3%.

- *Indications:* Herpes viruses, poxviruses, rhabdoviruses, hepadnaviruses and some ribonucleic acid (RNA) tumor viruses. Ophthalmic ointment is used in the treatment of acute keratoconjunctivitis and recurrent superficial keratitis caused by HSV-1 and HSV-2.
- *Dose*: 15–30 mg/kg OD (IV) for 10–21 days.
- *Adverse drug reactions:* Rarely, nausea, vomiting, *leukopenia, and thrombocytopenia.*
- *Caution:* The patient should be hospitalized for administration of the drug intravenously.
- *Special remarks:* On account of IV administration problem, its use is largely taken over by acyclovir that can be taken orally.

Cidofovir

An injectable *antiviral* agent primarily used to treat *cytomegalovirus* (CMV) *retinitis* in acquired immunodeficiency syndrome (AIDS) subjects. It inhibits viral replication by selectively inhibiting viral DNA *polymerases*.
- *Indications:* CMV, HSV, and VZV not responding to first-line agents, CMV retinitis, and respiratory papilloma (recurrent).
- *Dose*: 5 mg/kg/OD IV infusion.
- *Caution*: Appropriate hydration; make sure to administer oral probenecid before and after IV infusion.

Famciclovir

Brand name: Famtrex
- *Available as:* Tablets 125, 250, and 500 mg
- *Indications:* HSV and HZV infection

- *Dose:* Recurrent herpes labialis 1.5 g as a single dose once only.
  - Genital herpes simplex 250 mg TID for 5 days
  - Recurrent genital herpes 250 mg BID for 1 year
- *Adverse drug reactions:* Nausea, GI upset, diarrhea, headache, tired feeling, dizziness, mild itching, skin rash, and numbness.
- *Caution:* Avoid in acute renal failure.

Foscarnet

Brand name: Foscavir
- *Available as*: Injection 500 mg, 1 g vial.
- *Indications:* CMV, HSV, and HZV
- *Dose:* CMV in HIV/AIDS 180 mg/kg/day in three divided doses as slow IV infusion in 45–60 minutes for 3 weeks.
  - Acyclovir-resistant HSV and HZV in the immunocompromised 120 mg/kg/day (IV) in three divided doses for 3 weeks or until infects gets controlled whichever is later.
- *Adverse drug reactions:* Dizziness, dyselectrolytema, hypertension, and seizures.
- *Caution:* Ensure adequate hydration of the patient before administering this drug. Avoid in renal insufficiency.

Ganciclovir

A nucleoside analog structurally resembling acyclovir; inhibits viral DNA polymerase; effective against all herpes viruses (herpes simplex, herpes zoster, and Epstein–Barr virus, cytomegalovirus—CMV). Against CMV, it shows higher activity.

Brand names: Ganguard and Ganvir
- *Available as:* Tablet 250 mg; capsule 500 mg.
- *Indications:* Congenital CMV pneumonia and acquired CMV retinitis in HIV/AIDS.

- *Dose:* 10–15 mg/kg/day q 8 to 12 h for 14–21 days followed by long-term suppression therapy in a dose of 5–10 mg/kg/day thrice a week for 3 months.
- *Adverse drug reactions:* Reversible myelosuppression; risk of carcinogenicity and gonadal toxicity.
- *Caution:* Reduce dose in renal impairment/insufficiency, monitored according to creatinine clearance reduction.

Idoxuridine

Brand name: Rdinox
- *Available as*: Ophthalmic ointment (0.5%) and drops (0.1%).
- *Indication*: Herpetic keratitis.
- *Dose:* To be instilled in the eye several (4–6) times daily.

Isoprinosine

Brand name: Inosiplex
- *Available as:* Tablet 500 mg.
- *Indications:* Viral encephalitis, subacute sclerosing panencephalitis
- *Dose:* 25–50 mg/kg (PO) BD
- *Adverse drug reactions:* Feeling or being unwell, abdominal discomfort, *itching, rash,* and headache.
- *Caution*: Avoid in gout, renal disease, and during digitalization.

Trifluridine

Brand name: Viroptic
- *Available as:* Ophthalmic drops.
- *Indications:* Herpes simplex conjunctivitis/keratitis.
- *Dose:* One drop in each eye every 2 hours, not exceeding a total of nine drops/day. Once epithelialization has developed, dose may be reduced to one drop every 4 hours, not exceeding a total of five drops.

- *Adverse drug reactions:* Transient burning, stinging, local irritation, and *edema* of the eyelids.
- *Caution:* Avoid in pregnancy on account of its possible teratogenicity.

Valganciclovir

It is a product of ganciclovir.

Brand names: Valcept and Valgan
- *Indications:* CMV
- *Dose:*
  - Post-transplant (CMV prophylaxis) 15–20 mg/kg/dose (PO) 6 h for 100 days.
  - CMV retinitis for induction 900 mg/dose 12 h for 21 days followed by 900 mg/dose 6 h for maintenance.
  - CMV hepatitis/biliary atresia 250 mg/m^2/day for 3 weeks followed by 125 mg/m^2/day for additional 3 weeks.
- *Adverse drug reactions:* Fever, nausea, vomiting, diarrhea, headache, tremors, loss of balance or coordination, stuffy nose, sneezing, sore throat; neutropenia and thrombocytopenia.
- *Caution*: Avoid in kidney disease and pregnancy.

ANTIRETROVIRAL DRUGS

Abacavir

Brand names: ABC, Abamune, Abavir, Vrol, Ziagen
- *Available as:* Tablet 300 mg; suspension 20 mg/mL
- *Indication:* A second-line antiretroviral therapy in HIV/AIDS.
- *Dose:* 3 months to 12 years 8 mg/kg twice daily with a maximum of 600 mg/day.

- *Adverse drug reactions:* Gastrointestinal (GI) upset, diarrhea, anorexia, lethargy, fever, lipodystrophy, lactic acidosis, gross enlargement of liver with steatosis, myocardial infarction, hypersensitivity in the form of influenza-like illness (manifesting with cough, breathlessness, pharyngitis, fever, rash, abdominal pain, severe fatigue, myalgia, and arthralgia).
- *Drug interactions:* Retinoids (theoretical); may antagonize methadone; and may be potentiated by ethanol.
- *Contraindications:* Hepatic and renal dysfunction.
- *Caution:* Close monitoring for first every 2 weeks, 2 months for influenza-like symptoms due to hypersensitivity.

Didanosine

Brand name: Dinex
- *Available as:* Chewable tablet 100 mg.
- *Indication:* HIV infection, along with other ART.
- *Dose:* >2 weeks 240 mg/m^2 in one to two doses. Alternatively, 180 mg/m^2 daily in combination with zidovudine [ZDV, also known as azidothymidine (AZT)].
- *Adverse drug reactions:* GI upset, abdominal pain, rash, chills, fever, headache; pancreatitis; elevation of liver enzymes, amylase, and lipase; peripheral neuropathy, optic neuritis, hepatic dysfunction; and lipodystrophy.
- *Drug interactions:* Antagonistic for quinolones and tetracyclines. Potentiated by allopurinol, tenofovir, ganciclovir, ribavirin; and drugs causing pancreatitis.
- *Contraindications:* Pancreatitis; concurrent administration of allopurinol or ribavirin.
- *Caution:* Monitor serum amylase, retinal, and optic nerve changes, signs of mitochondrial dysfunction; pregnancy and lactation.

Efavirenz

Brand names: Efavir, Efcure, Eferven, Efrenz, and Sustiva
- *Available as:* Tablet/Capsule 50, 100, 200, and 600 mg; suspension 30 mg/mL.
- *Indication:* HIV infection with other antiretroviral therapy (ART).
- *Dose:* >3 years
  - 10–15 kg 200 mg OD
  - 15–20 kg 250 mg OD
  - 20–25 kg 300 mg OD
  - 25–32.5 kg 350 mg OD
  - 32.5–40 kg 400 mg OD
  - >40 kg/17 years 600 mg OD
- *Adverse drug reactions:* GI upset, drowsiness, headache, fatigue, fever, cough, dyspnea, skin rash, neuropathy, psychiatric reactions, and raised liver enzymes and amylase; lipodystrophy, gynecomastia, Stevens-Johnson syndrome, erythema multiforme; postural disturbances.
- *Drug interaction:* Cisapride, midazolam, ketoconazole, inducers of substrates of CYP344; alcohol, and grapefruit juice.
- *Cautions:* Monitor liver enzymes, serum amylase, lipids, and blood glucose. Monitor for psychiatric and CNS symptoms which may be precipitated by this therapy.

Lamivudine

Brand names: Hepavud, Heptec Ladiwin, and Lamnidac 100
- *Available as:* Tablet 150 mg
- *Indications:* Employed as an adjuvant to other antivirals in progressive HIV disease.
- *Dose:* >3 months 4 mg/kg BID with a maximum of 300 mg/day

- *Adverse drug reactions:* Neutropenia, anemia, thrombocytopenia, pure red cell aplasia, raised liver enzymes, raised serum amylase; headache, malaise, fatigue, GI upset, abdominal pain, insomnia, cough, nasal congestion, rhinorrhea, and throat discomfort. Fever, rash, alopecia, dizziness, depression, breathing problems, muscle pains, hepatitis, pancreatitis, peripheral neuropathy, lactic acidosis, lipodystrophy, paresthesia, and gross hepatomegaly with steatosis.
- *Drug interactions:* Intravenous ganciclovir, zalcitabine, foscarnet, cotrimoxazole, ZDV, ciprofloxacin, and pentamidine.
- *Contraindication:* Simultaneous use of zalcitabine.
- *Caution:* Monitor liver and kidney function, and signs of mitochondrial dysfunction.

Lopinavir

It is a second-line drug acting through protease inhibition.

Brand name: Ritomax-L Forte

- *Available as:* Capsule 200 mg in combination with ritonavir 50 mg.
- *Indication:* HIV in combination with other ART.
- *Dose:* 3–10 mg/kg/day in two divided doses with food to enhance bioavailability.
- *Adverse drug reactions:* Hyperglycemia, GI upset, abdominal pain, diarrhea, rash, insomnia, cough, headache, fat redistribution, pancreatitis, increased serum cholesterol and other lipids, hepatitis, myasthenia, extrapyramidal syndrome, skin striae, impotence, and QT prolongation.

- *Drug interactions:* Drugs metabolized by CYP3A or CYP2D6 including midazolam, cisapride, rifampicin; other retrovirals, warfarin, antiarrhythmics; anticonvulsants; steroids; and clarithromycin.
- *Contraindications:* Low neutrophil count <0.75 × 10^9/L, low hemoglobin level <7.5 g/dL; lactation.
- *Caution:* Monitor serum lipids, blood glucose renal and hepatic function.

Nelfinavir

Brand name: Nelvir

- *Available as:* Tablet 250 mg
- *Indication:* HIV infection (in combination with other ART).
- *Dose:* 3–13 years 50–55 mg/kg BD or 25–30 mg/kg TID.
- *Adverse drug reactions:* GI upset, nausea, diarrhea, flatulence, abdominal pain, rash; increased creatinine kinase, decreased nutrophils, increased transaminases, hepatitis, lipodystrophy, insulin resistance, diabetes, and hyperlipidemia.
- *Drug interaction:* Midazolam, triazolam, rifabutin, rifampicin, ergot derivatives, cisapride, carbamazepine, phenytoin, primozide, phenobarbital, amiodarone, quinidine, calcium antagonists, oral contraceptives, ritonavir, indinavir, saquinavir, azole, antifungals, erythromycin, azithromycin, clarithromycin, sildenafil, methadone, statins, fluticasone, and proton pump inhibitors (PPIs).
- *Contraindications:* Concurrent use of cisapride, pimozide, triazolam, midazolam, ergot derivatives, amiodarone, quinidine, lovastatin, simvastatin, sildenafil, moderate-to-severe liver disease, and lactation.

- *Caution:* Renal or hepatic impairment, hemophilia, diabetes, and monitoring for hyperglycemia or fat redistribution advisable.

Nevirapine

It is a nonnucleoside reverse transcriptase inhibitor specific for HIV-I transcriptase or human polymerase.

Brand name: Nevimune
- *Available as:* Tablet 200 mg
- *Indication:* HIV with advanced or progressive immunodeficiency in combination with other ARTs.
- *Dose:* Newborn 2 mg/kg OD in mother-to-child transmitted (MTCT) HIV. Later 150–200 mg/m^2/dose in two divided doses.
- *Adverse drug reactions:* Rash, nausea, vomiting, abdominal pain, fatigue, fever, headache, somnolence, myalgia, hepatitis, fat redistribution, Stevens-Johnson syndrome, toxic epidermal necrolysis, agranulocytosis, granulocytopenia, and anemia.
- *Drug interactions:* Ketoconazole, protease inhibitors, cimetidine, macrolides, rifampicin, rifabutin, warfarin, contraceptives, and saquinavir
- *Contraindications:* Renal failure, moderate-to-severe hepatic impairment, and lactation
- *Caution:* Monitoring of liver and renal function, hematologic status, and signs of severe dermatologic lesions, oral lesions, fever, and muscle and joint pains.

Stavudine

Brand name: Stavir
- *Available as:* Capsules 30 and 40 mg

- *Indications:* HIV with progressive or advanced immunodeficiency in combination with other agents.
- *Dose:*
  - >3 months
  - <30 kg 1 mg/kg BID
  - >30 kg 30 mg BID
- *Adverse drug reactions:* Peripheral neuropathy, pancreatitis, raised serum amylase, ALT, AST, lactic acidosis, hepatitis, liver failure, headache, pain, malaise, GI and CNS disturbances, fever, skin irritation; neoplasia, lipodystrophy, lymphadenopathy, macrocytosis, anorexia, myalgia, rash, diabetes, and gross hepatomegaly with steatosis.
- *Drug interactions:* Zidovudine, trimethoprim, doxorubicin, ribavirin, antihepatitis B or C therapy; enhanced risk of toxicity with neurotoxic, hepatotoxic, and pancreatotoxic (hydroxyurea and didanosine) drugs.
- *Contraindication:* Lactation <3 months.
- *Caution:* Monitor renal/liver function, mitochondrial dysfunction, lactic acidosis, serum lipids and blood glucose and physical signs of lipodystrophy and fat redistribution.

Tenofovir

It is a first-line ART for adolescents (just like adults) with HIV/AIDS.

Brand names: Teevir, Tenof, Tentide, Qvr, and Ricovir
- *Available as*: Tablet 100, 150, and 200 mg
- *Indications:* HIV/AIDS and chronic hepatitis B
- *Dose:* 300 mg single daily dose for 28 days
- *Adverse drug reactions:* Mild GT upset, depression, headache, dizziness, mild weakness; mild itching, and rash.

Zalcitabine (2′-3′-dideoxycytidine, DDC)

Brand name: Hivid
- *Available as:* Tablets 0.375 and 0.750 mg.
- *Dose*: 0.01 mg/kg TID.
- *Adverse drug reactions:* Peripheral neuropathy and pancreatitis.

Zidovudine

It is an antiviral agent that interferes with replication of HIV by inhibiting HIV RNA-dependent DNA polymerases.

Brand names: Retrovir and Zidovir
- *Available as:* Capsules/Tablets 100 and 300 mg; syrup 50 mg/5 mL.
- *Indication:* HIV infection both symptomatic and asymptomatic.
- *Dose:*
  - >3 months 180 mg/m^2 with a maximum of 200 mg every 6 hourly
  - 12 mg/kg/day in four divided doses (IV), or continuous IV infusion
- *Adverse drug reactions:* Headache, seizures, diarrhea, lactic acidosis, cholestasis, bone marrow suppression, rash, hepatotoxicity with hepatomegaly, and myopathy.
- *Drug interaction:* Rifampicin increases its metabolism whereas cimetidine, fluconazole, and valproic acid decrease it.
- *Contraindication:* Low neutrophil cell count <0.75 × 10^9/L or low hemoglobin (<7.5 g/dL); lactation.
- *Caution:* Monitor with blood tests at least every 2 weeks during first 3 months and then every month.

ANTI-INFLUENZA VIRUS DRUGS

Amantadine

It is an M2-inhibitor antiviral, a tricyclic amine, acting by blocking M2 protein ion channel. It changes pH of lysozymes.

Brand name: Amantrel

- *Available as:* Capsule 100 mg; syrup 50 mg/5 mL.
- *Indications:* Influenza A (both prevention and treatment); also herpes zoster, parkinsonism, drug-induced extrapyramidal reactions.
- *Dose:* 4–8 mg/kg/day (PO) q 8–12 h with a maximum of 150 mg/day and 200 mg/day before and after 10 years of age, respectively, for 2–7 days.
- *Adverse drug reactions:* Transient insomnia, nervousness, light-headedness, drowsiness, pedal edema, and livedo reticularis due to vasoconstriction.
- *Contraindications:* Gastric ulceration, epilepsy, nursing and pregnant mothers, and hypersensitivity to amantadine.
- *Caution:* Avoid its administration when the child is on quinine or quinidine.
- *Special remarks:* In view of widespread resistance, its use is no longer recommended by the World Health Organization (WHO) and the Centers for Disease Control and Prevention (CDC).

Oseltamivir

This antiviral agent is a neuraminidase inhibitor. Oseltamivir is not a substitute for early vaccination on an annual basis.

Brand names: Antiflu, Fluvir, and Tamiflu

- *Available as:* Capsule 75 mg. Powder for oral suspension to be constituted with water (12 mg/mL; available in glass bottles containing 25 mL of suspension)

- *Indications:* Treatment of uncomplicated acute illness due to influenza infection in patients aged 1 year and beyond who have been symptomatic for up to 48 hours.

    Prophylaxis of influenza in patients older than 1 year.
- *Dosage:*

Treatment: Optimal dose for adolescents and adults 75 mg BID for 5 days. Pediatric patients who cannot swallow, should receive the oral suspension.

- *1 to 12 years:*
  - <15 kg 30 mg
  - 15–23 kg 45 mg
  - 23–49 kg 60 mg
  - >40 kg 75 mg

All twice daily for 5 days.

It should preferably be administered within 48 hours after the onset of symptoms; most effective if initiated as soon as possible (<24 hours). The drug is generally well-tolerated.

Prophylaxis: Optimal dose for adolescents and adults 75 mg once daily for 10 days or up to 6 weeks during an epidemic. Pediatric patients who cannot swallow, should receive the oral suspension.

- *1–12 years:*
  - <15 kg 30 mg
- *15 to 23 years:*
  - 45 mg
  - 23–49 kg 60 mg
  - >40 kg 75 mg

All once daily for 10 days or up to 6 weeks during an epidemic.

Special dosage: Patients with a serum creatinine clearance between 10 and 30 mL/min are treated with 75 mg once daily for 5 days; the prophylactic dose is 75 mg every other day or 30 mg oral suspension everyday. No recommended dosing regimens are available for patients undergoing routine hemodialysis and continuous peritoneal dialysis treatment with end-stage renal disease.

- *Adverse drug reactions:* Nausea and vomiting which are generally mild-to-moderate in degree and usually occur on the first 2 days of treatment; GI bleeding, hemorrhagic colitis, respiratory infection, dizziness, fatigue, headache, insomnia, seizures, vertigo, delirium, confusion, abnormal behavior, delusions, hallucinations, agitation, anxiety, and nightmares.
- *Drug interactions:* Chlorpromazine, methotrexate, phenylbutazone; do not administer live-attenuated influenza vaccine (LAIV) within 2 weeks prior or 48 hours after treatment.
- *Contraindication:* Children <1 year age.
- *Caution:* Patients should be instructed to begin treatment with oseltamivir as soon as possible after the first appearance of flu symptoms. Similarly, prevention should begin as soon as possible following exposure:
  - Renal and hepatic impairment, hemodialysis, chronic cardiorespiratory disease, repeat courses, pregnancy, and lactation.
  - Transient gastrointestinal disturbance may be reduced by taking oseltamivir after a light snack.
  - Coadministration with food has no significant effect on the peak plasma concentration and the AUC.
  - Oseltamivir is not a substitute for an influenza vaccine. Patients should continue receiving an annual/seasonal vaccine according to the relevant national or local recommendations.

Rimantadine

It is an M2 inhibitor.

Brand name: Flumadine

- *Available as:* Capsule/Tablet 100 mg; syrup 50 mg 5 mL.
- *Indications:* Prophylaxis and treatment of influenza A infection. Treatment must be initiated within 48 hours after the onset of symptoms.
- *Dose:*
  - 100 mg BID. A dose reduction to 100 mg daily is recommended in patients with severe hepatic dysfunction, renal failure (CrCl ≤10 mL/min) and in elderly nursing home patients.
  - Children <10 years of age should receive 5 mg/kg but not exceeding 150 mg.
  - Children 10 years of age or older should receive the adult dose.
- *Drug interactions:* No significant interactions
- *Adverse drug reactions:* Gastrointestinal symptoms such as nausea, vomiting, diarrhea, dyspepsia; CNS disturbances such as insomnia, dizziness, tinnitus, ataxia; and skin rash.
- *Caution:* A dose reduction to 100 mg daily is recommended in patients with severe hepatic dysfunction, renal failure (CrCl ≤10 mL/min) and in old age.
- *Special remarks:* In view of widespread resistance, its use is no longer recommended by the WHO and the CDC.

Zanamivir

It is a neuraminidase inhibitor. Neuraminidase glycoprotein is essential in the infective cycle of influenza viruses. It simulates sialic acid, the natural substrate of neuraminidase.

Brand names: Relenza and Vlenza
- *Available as:* Powder along with inhalation device.
- *Indication:* Treatment of uncomplicated influenza (A and B) symptomatic over up to 2 days.
- *Dosage:*
  - *Treatment:* Inhalation of 10 mg twice daily for 2–5 consecutive days.
  - *Prophylaxis:* Not yet approved.
- *Adverse drug reactions:* A good safety profile and the overall risk for any respiratory event is low. Adverse events include bronchospasm especially in the setting of underlying airways disease, severe allergic reactions including oropharyngeal angioedema, dizziness, behavioral problems, arrhythmias, syncope, and seizures.
- *Drug interactions:* No clinically significant pharmacokinetic drug interactions are predicted based on data from in vitro studies.
- *Caution:* Avoid under 7 years and in patients with underlying airways disease (such as asthma or chronic obstructive pulmonary disease) in which risk of bronchospasm is significant.

MISCELLANEOUS (NONSELECTIVE) ANTIVIRAL DRUGS

Adefovir Dipivoxil

It is an endogenous immunomodulatory protein (precisely, a low molecular weight glycoprotein cytokine) exerting antiviral activity through induction of multiple effector proteins in virus-infected cells. This particular interferon has emerged as an effective antiviral agent.

Brand name: Roferon-A
- *Available as:* Injection (SC and IM) 3 million IU/dose.
- *Indications:* Hepatitis B, hepatitis C, and human papillomavirus (HPV) infection; anogenital warts caused by HPV; laryngeal and respiratory papillomatosis; and chronic myeloid leukemia and multiple myeloma.
- *Dose:* 2.5–10 million units/day (SC and IM) × 1 week followed by thrice a week for a total of 1–6 months.
- *Adverse drug reactions:* GIT upset, flu-like symptoms (fever, chills, myalgias, fatigue, and malaise), neuropathy (numbness, tremors, sleepiness, and seizures) bone marrow suppression (neutropenia and thrombocytopenia), thyroid dysfunction (hypo- as well as hyperthyroidism), alopecia, hepatic insufficiency, hypotension, and arrhythmias (transient).
- *Drug interactions:* Barbiturates, cancer chemotherapy, and theophyllines.
- *Contraindications:* Hypersensitivity, autoimmune hepatitis, and hepatic decompensation.
- *Cautions:* It should be used in combination with lamivudine and not as adefovir dipivoxil monotherapy to safeguard against prevention of drug resistance.

Ribavirin

It is a semisynthetic nucleoside antiviral drug.

Brand names: Rebetol, Ribavin, and Virazide
- *Available as:* Aerosol capsules 100 and 200 mg; syrup 50 mg/5 mL.
- *Indications:* Particularly useful in respiratory syncytial virus (RSV), hepatitis influenza virus, chronic hepatitis C, and HSV. In practice, primarily used for treatment of acute

bronchiolitis from RSV when the infant is critically ill or has underlying high-risk condition such as prematurity, chronic lung disease (cystic fibrosis) or congenital heart disease (CHD).

- *Dose:* Aerosol—6 g in 100 L sterile water, continuous aerosolization for 12-18 hours daily for 3-7 days.

  Or,

  2 g in 30-40 mL sterilized water for 2-3 h thrice daily for 3-7 days.

  Oral—10-15 mg/kg/day (PO) in three to four divided doses for 3-7 days.

- *Adverse drug reactions:* Hemolysis, anemia, flu-like symptoms, dizziness, weight loss, alopecia, rash, diabetes, pancreatitis, hyperuricemia, thrombotic thrombocytopenic purpura, thyroid disorders, dental and periodontal disorders, vision disorders, optic disk changes including papilledema and retinal detachment, psychiatric problems, cardiac arrest, and hypotension.

- *Drug interactions:* Alcohol, nucleoside reverse transcriptase inhibitors (NRTIs), stavudine, ZDV, didanosine, peginterferon α-2a.

- *Contraindications:* Pregnancy since it is a teratogenic drug; hypersensitivity to ribavirin or any component of the product, underlying hemoglobinopathies and autoimmune hepatitis.

- *Caution:* Avoid in asthma; closely monitor renal, cardiac, hematologic, and biochemical parameters before and at 2-4 weeks' intervals during therapy.

- *Special remarks*: It is very expensive.

Chapter 47

Antifungal Drugs

INTRODUCTION

Antifungal drugs (antimycotic drugs) are a pharmaceutical fungicide or fungistatic agents used to treat and prevent mycoses such as thrush (candidiasis), ringworm, athlete's foot, serious systemic infections such as cryptococcal meningitis. Oral antifungal drugs currently in use include fluconazole, ketoconazole, itraconazole, and terbinafine. These agents are reserved for extensive or severe infection for which topical antifungal agents are inappropriate or ineffective. The drugs may be fungicidal or fungistatic. The drugs target fungal cell membrane and the fungal cell wall that are supposed to be protective parts of the cell that can cause the cell to leak and die when damaged.

Four major types of antifungal drugs are:
1. Polyenes
2. Azoles
3. Allylamines
4. Echinocandins

POLYENES

Amphotericin B

Brand name: Fungizone
- *Available as:* Injection 50 mg vial.

Chapter 47: Antifungal Drugs

- *Indications:* Progressive and potentially fatal fungal infections; also leishmaniasis.
- *Dose:* 250 µg/kg/day. Increase gradually to 1 mg/kg/day (IV infusion).
- *Adverse drug reactions (ADRs):* Nausea, vomiting, diarrhea, anorexia, epigastric pain, headache, muscle and joint pains, anemia, impaired renal/hepatic function, fever, rash, anaphylaxis; arrhythmias; blood dyscrasia, neuropathy, dyselectrolytemia, and dyspnea.
- *Drug interactions:* Steroids, aminoglycosides, cardiac glycosides, polymyxins, other antifungals, diuretics, vancomycin, cyclosporine, pentamidine, anticancer drugs, and leukocyte transfusions.
- *Contraindications:* Renal and hepatic dysfunction.
- *Caution:* Exercise caution in its concomitant use with aminoglycosides, vancomycin, cyclosporine, and other nephrotoxic drugs which enhance the renal impairment of amphotericin B (AMB). Monitor hepatic and renal functions, blood counts, electrolytes. Avoid rapid infusion.

Fluconazole

Brand name: Forcan

- *Available as:* Capsule 50, 150, and 200 mg; injection 2 mg/mL, 100 mL infusion bottle.
- *Indications:* Mucosal candidiasis, systemic candidiasis, cryptococcosis (meningitis)—prophylaxis against fungal infections after cytotoxic chemotherapy/radiotherapy and in immunocompromised hosts.
- *Dose:* 3–6 mg/kg/day once a day (PO) in children >1 year age.
- *Adverse drug reactions:* Nausea, abdominal pain, taste perversion, headache, dizziness, rash, exfoliative dermatitis, and hepatotoxicity.

- *Drug interaction:* Rifampicin, anticoagulants, theophylline, cyclosporine, cisapride, phenytoin, short-acting benzodiazepines, zidovudine, cimetidine, and thiazide.
- *Contraindications:* Pregnancy and lactation.
- *Caution:* Impaired renal function.

AZOLES

Itraconazole

It is a first generation triazole.
Brand name: Candistat
- *Available as:* Capsule 100 mg.
- *Indications:* Vulvovaginal, oropharyngeal candidiasis, pityriasis versicolor, dermatophytosis, onychomycosis, histoplasmosis, coccidioidomycosis (including meningeal involvement), paracoccidioidomycosis, sporotrichosis, systemic mycosis; also, for prevention of relapse in subjects with AIDS and disseminated histoplasmosis.
- *Dose:* 3–5 mg/kg/day OD
  - Fungal infection with chronic granulomatous disease—5–10 mg/kg/day once or in two divided doses
  - Disseminated histoplasmosis—6–8 mg/kg/day
- *Adverse drug reactions:* Nausea, vomiting, hypokalemia (with excess dose), headache, neuropathy, allergic reactions, hair loss, cholestatic jaundice, hepatitis, and congestive heart failure (CHF).
- *Drug interactions:* Such drugs as H_2 blockers and gastric proton-pump inhibitors that cut down the gastric acidity reduce its blood levels by 50%. Rifampicin, isoniazid, phenytoin, phenobarbital, carbamazepine, and cisapride also decrease its blood levels to some extent.
- *Contraindications:* Pregnancy and lactation.

- *Cautions:* Avoid prolonged use, and in decreased gastric acidity and hepatic and renal impairments. Monitor liver and renal status.

Ketoconazole

Brand name: Funazole
- *Available as:* Tablet 200 mg
- *Indications:* Superficial and systemic fungal infections
- *Dose:* 3.3–6.6 mg/kg/day OD
- *Adverse drug reactions:* Hepatotoxicity
- *Contraindications:* Liver dysfunction and children <2 years
- *Caution:* Avoid in liver disease. Monitor liver function test (LFT) during therapy.

Miconazole

Brand names: Daktarin and Micogel
- *Available as:* Topical gel and powder.
- *Indications*: Fungal and gram-positive bacterial infections of the skin, nails, and vagina.
- *Dose:* Apply to lesions twice daily and continue 10 days beyond the healing of the lesions. Nail disease needs at least 3 months' therapy.
- *Drug interaction:* Warfarin.
- *Caution*: Avoid contact with eyes and during lactation, pregnancy, and superinfections.

Voriconazole

It is a second generation triazole with enhanced antifungal spectrum.

Brand names: Fungiver, Verkab, Veritek, Veritop, Verz, and Vorage
- *Available as:* Tablet 50 and 200 mg

- *Indications:* Invasive aspergillosis, candidemia in nonneutropenic subjects, fluconazole-resistant serious invasive *Candida* infections.
- *Dose:* Recommended for >2 years age.
  - <25 kg 6–10 mg/kg/day in two divided doses
  - 25–40 kg 200 mg every 12 h for two doses (loading dose) followed by 100 mg every 12 h
  - 40 kg 400 mg every 12 h for two doses followed by 200 mg every 12 h
- *Adverse drug reactions:* Elevated LFT, rash, visual disturbances, including transient photophobia and blurred vision.
- *Drug interactions:* Rifampicin, phenobarbital, and carbamazepine lower its concentrations. It raises the levels of cisapride, cyclosporine, omeprazole, quinidine, tacrolimus, and warfarin.
- *Contraindications:* Pregnancy and lactation.
- *Cautions:* Monitor liver and renal function.

ALLYLAMINES

Terbinafine

Brand name: Exifine

- *Indications:* Dermatophyte infections of skin and nails
- *Available as:* Tablet 125 and 250 mg. Topical 1% cream.
- *Dose:*
  - 125–250 mg OD for 4–12 weeks, higher dose is for fingernail infections. In case of big toenail infection, 3–6 months therapy is recommended.
  - For topical application, 1% cream is required to be massaged into affected area once or twice daily for 1–2 weeks, avoiding the eyes and mucous membrane.
- *Adverse drug reactions:* Gastrointestinal (GI) upset, taste disturbance, headache, fatigue, malaise, hypo- or

Chapter 47: Antifungal Drugs

paresthesia, rash, arthralgia, myalgia; liver dysfunction; hematologic dysfunction in the form of pancytopenia, thrombocytopenia, agranulocytosis, Stevens–Johnson syndrome, psoriasis, and systemic lupus erythematosus (SLE)-like skin lesions.
- *Drug interactions:* Hepatic enzyme inhibitors-like cimetidine, inducers like rifampicin, drugs affecting cytochrome P450; antidepressants, β-blockers, monoamine oxidase inhibitors (MAOIs) type B; and cyclosporine.
- *Contraindications:* Liver disease (active or chronic) and lactation.
- *Caution:* Monitor LFT.

MISCELLANEOUS ANTIFUNGALS

Griseofulvin

Brand names: Grisactin Forte and Walavin-250
- *Available as:* Tablet 250 mg
- *Indications:* Fungal infections of skin, hair, and nails.
- *Dose:* 10–20 mg/kg/day (PO) in four divided doses.
- *Adverse drug reactions:* Gastrointestinal tract (GIT) upset, drowsiness, headache, urticaria, photosensitivity, and SLE precipitation.
- *Drug interaction:* Alcohol, barbiturates, coumarin anticoagulants, and oral contraceptives.
- *Contraindications:* Porphyria, hepatocellular failure, hypersensitivity, monilial infection, pregnancy, and SLE.
- *Caution:* Lactation and long-term use.

Nystatin

Brand name: Mycostatin
- *Available as:* Tablet 5 lakh units; Suspension 1 lakh units/mL.

- *Indications:* Fungal infections, especially *Candida albicans* affecting intestines.
- *Dose:*
  - *Newborn:* 4 lakh units/day (PO) in divided doses
  - *Later period:* 1-2 million units/day in four divided doses
- *Adverse drug reactions:* GIT upset in the form of nausea, vomiting, and diarrhea, especially in high doses; hypersensitivity reactions.
- *Drug interactions:* None
- *Contraindication:* Allergy
- *Caution:* Avoid giving feed for some time after the medication; continue therapy for a few days after the lesions have disappeared.

Antiparasitic (Intestinal) Drugs

Chapter 48

INTRODUCTION

Antiparasitic drugs are a class of drugs that are employed for the treatment of parasitic diseases such as harboring the gastrointestinal tract (GIT) (helminths like nematodes, trematodes and cestodes, and protozoa such as amebas and giardia), and extraintestinal infestations such as malarial parasite, mites, ticks, and flees. This chapter deals with intestinal parasitic infestations only.

ANTIPROTOZOAL DRUGS

Albendazole

It is a broad-spectrum agent belonging to the benzimidazole group of drugs. It mainly acts by inhibiting the tubular polymerization that results in loss of cytoplasmic microtubules and also by decreasing glucose uptake.

Brand names: Albezole, Emanthal, Nemozole, and Zentel

- *Available as:* Tablet 400 mg; syrup 200 mg/5 *actions:* Giardiasis. Also employed for the treatment of infestation with nematodes and cestodes including hydatid disease.
- *Dose:* Under 2 years—200 mg; later 400 mg (PO) for 5 successive days in giardiasis.

- *Adverse drug reactions (ADRs):* Abdominal discomfort, diarrhea/constipation, dizziness, rash, fever, reversible alopecia, hematological and liver enzyme changes; convulsions and meningism in cerebral disease; acute renal failure, aplastic anemia, agranulocytosis, and rash.
- *Drug interactions:* Theophylline, oral contraceptives, oral hypoglycemic, anticonvulsants, anticoagulants, potentiated by dexamethasone, praziquantel (PZQ), cimetidine, etc.
- *Contraindication:* Pregnancy.
- *Cautions:* Avoid in liver disease, lactation, and hyperactive onchodermatitis; make sure the tablet is properly chewed before it is swallowed.

Diloxanide Furoate

It is a purely luminal amebicide.

Brand names: Amicline and Furamide

- *Available as:* Tablet 500 mg.
- *Indications:* Intestinal amebiasis—prevention, symptom-free cyst passers, and acute/chronic intestinal. It is effective as an intraluminal amebicidal with no role in hepatic amebiasis.
- *Dose:* 20 mg/kg/day in three divided doses for 7–10 days.
- *Adverse drug reactions:* Very safe. Occasionally, nausea, flatulence, and abdominal discomfort; rash, urticaria, and pruritus.
- *Drug interactions:* None.
- *Contraindications:* Hypersensitivity to diloxanide furoate.
- *Caution:* Avoid in lactation and pregnancy.

Chapter 48: Antiparasitic (Intestinal) Drugs

Furazolidone

Brand name: Furoxone
- *Available as:* Tablet 100 mg; suspension 25 mg/5 mL.
- *Indications:* Giardiasis; also nonspecific diarrhea, bacterial diarrhea, cholera, and typhoid fever.
- *Dose:* 6–10 mg/kg/day in three to four divided doses for 7–10 days.
- *Adverse drug reactions:* High-colored urine, nausea, vomiting, arthralgia, rash, hemolytic anemia in G6PD deficiency, hypotension, and headache.
- *Drug interactions:* Alcohol, tyramine-containing foods; monoamine oxidase inhibitors (MAOIs), and sympathomimetic amines.
- *Contraindication:* G6PD deficiency and neonates.
- *Caution:* Tell the parents/child about development of high-colored urine during therapy. This is harmless.

Metronidazole

Brand names: Emigyl, Flagyl, Giardyl, Monizole, Metrogyl, and Unimezole
- *Available as:* Tablets 200, 400, and 800 mg; suspension 100 and 200 mg/5 mL; injection 2 mg/mL.
- *Indications:* Giardiasis. Also, in amebiasis; trichomoniasis; anaerobic infections; antibiotic-associated diarrhea; acute ulcerative gingivitis; and dracunculiasis.
- *Dose:*
  - 10–20 mg/kg/day (PO) for 5–7 days in divided doses for giardiasis
  - 20–50 mg/kg/day (PO) for 10 days in divided doses for amebiasis
  - 21 mg/kg/day (IV) in three divided infusions for severe amebiasis and anerobic infections

- *Adverse drug reactions:* Metallic taste lasting for some days, nausea, vomiting, headache, diarrhea, dizziness, rash, itching, furred tongue, incoordination, leukopenia, hypotension, and poor tolerance with alcohol.
- *Drug interactions:* Phenobarbital, phenytoin, hepatic enzyme inducers, alcohol, oral anticoagulants, cimetidine, and disulfiram.
- *Contraindications:* Active central nervous system (CNS) disease, blood dyscrasias, first trimester of pregnancy, and lactation.
- *Caution:* May avoid in children weighing <15 kg.

Nitazoxanide

Brand names: Nitarid and Netazox

- *Available as:* Syrup 100 mg/5 mL; tablets 200 and 500 mg.
- *Indications:* Giardiasis, amebiasis, cryptosporidiosis, fascioliasis, *C. parvum*. Also in ascariasis, trichuriasis, *Hymenolepis nana (H. nana)*, and *H. pylori*.
- *Doses:*
  - 7–10 mg/kg/dose BD × 3 days
  - 1–4 years 100 mg BD
  - 4–11 years 200 mg BD
  - >11 years 500 mg BD

  It should be administered with food.
- *Adverse drug reactions:* GIT upset including abdominal pain, anorexia, headache, dizziness, eye or urine discoloration, increased creatinine/serum glutamic pyruvic transaminase (SGPT).
- *Drug interaction:* Highly protein-bound drugs.
- *Contraindication:* Diabetes mellitus.

- *Cautions:* Avoid giving on empty stomach; avoid in children <1 year, in hepatic/biliary impairment, immunocompromised state, diabetes, pregnancy, and lactation.

Ornidazole

Brand names: Zil and Ornid
- *Available as:* Tablet 500 mg.
- *Indications:* Giardiasis, amebiasis, trichomoniasis, and anaerobic infections.
- *Dose:*
  - *L. giardia:* 40 mg/kg/day for 2 days.
  - *E. histolytica:* 40 mg/kg/day for 3 days.
  - *Anaerobes:* 40 mg/kg/day in two divided doses for 5–7 days.
- *Adverse drug reactions:* GI upset (nausea, vomiting, and anorexia), furrowed tongue, unpleasant taste, urticaria, angioedema, dark urine, leukopenia, and neuropathy and epileptiform seizures on chronic therapy.
- *Drug interactions:* Alcohol and anticoagulants.
- *Contraindications:* First trimester of pregnancy, lactation; hypersensitivity; neurologic disorders and blood dyscrasias.
- *Caution:* Avoid in subjects suffering from CNS disorders.

Paromomycin

It is an aminoglycoside antibiotic.
Brand name: Humatin
- *Available as:* Capsule 250 mg.
- *Indications:* Giardiasis and amebiasis. Though relatively less effective, this drug is permitted for use even in pregnancy. Additional indications include tapeworms, visceral leishmaniasis, cryptosporidiosis, etc.

- *Dose:*
  - *L. giardia:* 30 mg/kg/day in three divided doses for 10 days.
  - *E. histolytica* (*eradication of cysts*): 30 mg/kg/day in three divided doses for 10–15 days.
- *Adverse drug reactions:* GI upset, rash, pruritus, dizziness, vertigo, hematuria, and myalgia.
- *Drug interaction:* Atracurium.
- *Contraindication:* Hypersensitivity.
- *Caution:* Avoid driving during treatment.
- *Special remarks:* Permitted even in pregnancy and lactation.

Secnidazole

Brand name: Secnil forte

- *Available as:* Tablet 2 g.
- *Indications: E. histolytica, L. giardia,* and *T. vaginalis.*
- *Dose:* 30 mg/kg with a maximum of 2 g as a single dose once only.
- *Adverse drug reactions:* Mild GI upset (nausea, vomiting, diarrhea, epigastric pain, and anorexia), fatigue, headache, rash, urticaria, seizures, peripheral neuropathy; and leukopenia.
- *Drug interaction:* Alcohol, disulfiram, and warfarin.
- *Contraindication:* Lactation and pregnancy.

Tinidazole

Brand names: Fasigyn, Tiniba, and *ALIDAC*

- *Available as:* Tablets 150, 300, 500, 600, and 1,000 mg.
- *Indications:* Giardiasis and amebiasis. Also urogenital trichomoniasis, ulcerative gingivitis, and anaerobic infections.

- *Doses:*
  - 50–60 mg/kg as a single dose for giardiasis and trichomoniasis.

  Or
  - 10–15 mg/kg/day for 5–7 days
  - 50–60 mg/kg/days on 3 successive days for amebiasis. In severe intestinal amebiasis and/or amebic liver abscess, a 5-day course is preferred.
- *Adverse drug reactions:* GIT upset, metallic taste, furred tongue, urticaria, angioedema, neuropathy, dark urine, and leukopenia.
- *Drug interaction:* Alcohol.
- *Contraindications*: Neurologic disorders, blood dyscrasias, lactating mothers, and first trimester of pregnancy.
- *Cautions:*
  - Avoid concomitant use of alcohol.
  - Discontinue in case of neurologic adverse reactions.
  - Avoid in liver disease, lactation, and hyperactive onchodermatitis.

ANTHELMINTICS

Albendazole

Brand names: Albezole, Emanthal, Nemozole, and Zentel
- *Indications:* Ascariasis, enterobiasis, ancylostomiasis, trichuriasis, strongyloidiasis, and teniasis; neurocysticercosis; filariasis (in combination with ivermectin). Also effective in giardiasis as already detailed.
- *Dose:* Most helminths 200–400 mg as single dose every 6 months in National Program of India. Neurocysticercosis 15 mg/kg/day for 28 days.

For details, see under "Antiprotozoal Drugs" in this very chapter.

Ivermectin

It is a broad-spectrum antiparasitic and antimite drug.

Brand name: Ascapil
- Available as: Tablet 6 mg/
- *Indications:* Strongyloidiasis, ascariasis, cutaneous larva migrans; also scabies, lice, filariasis, and onchocerciasis.
- *Dose:*
  - *Ascariasis:* 150–200 µg/kg once
  - *Strongyloidiasis:* 200 µg/kg once only
  - *Trichuriasis:* 200 µg/kg OD for 3 days
  - *Filariasis:* 150 µg/kg once; to be repeated every 6–12 months until the patient becomes symptom free
  - *Cutaneous larva migrans:* 200 µg/kg OD for 1–2 days
  - *Onchocerciasis (River blindness):* 150 µg/kg once only
  - *Loaiasis:* 150 µg/kg once only
  - *Lice:* 200 µg/kg OD × 3 days (day 1, 2, and 10)
  - *Scabies:* 200 µg/kg once only
- *Adverse drug reactions:* GI upset, worsening of asthma, rash, fever, headache, dizziness, giddiness, chest pain, pruritus, and seizures; abnormal liver function test (LFT); rarely ataxia, mydriasis and respiratory paralysis may occur when given in high doses. Disease-specific ADRs are known.
- *Drug interaction:* Warfarin.
- *Contraindication:* Pregnancy.
- *Caution:* Avoid <5 years of age and <15 kg weight. Do not exceed 12 mg total dose.

Levamisole

Brand names: Vermisol and Vizole
- *Available as:* Tablets 50 and 159 mg; syrup 50 mg/5 mL.

- *Indications:* Ascariasis, ancylostomiasis; also for immunopotentiation.
- *Doses:*
  - *Ascariasis:* 2.5 mg/kg (PO) as a single dose
  - *Ancylostomiasis:* 2.5–5 mg/kg/dose every 6 hours till four doses are given.
  - *Immunopotentiation:* 2 mg/kg/day on alternate days for 4–6 weeks.

  It is advisable to give a repeat course after a month to prevent/treat reinfestation/recurrence.
- *Adverse drug reactions:* GI upset, insomnia, altered taste, bodily pains, dermatitis, and flu-like symptoms depression.
- *Drug interaction:* Warfarin.
- *Contraindications:* Liver and kidney insufficiency.
- *Cautions:* Avoid in pregnancy, lactation, and rheumatoid arthritis.

Mebendazole

Brand names: Pantelmin, Mebex, and Wormi

- *Available as:* Tablet 100 mg; syrup 100 mg/5 mL; granules 200 mg/5 g sachet.
- *Indications:* Ascariasis, enterobiasis, ancylostomiasis, trichuriasis, strongyloidiasis, *T. solium,* and *T. saginata.*
- *Dose:*
  - Threadworm 1 tablet/5 mL (single dose once only)
  - Roundworm 1 tablet/5 mL (single dose once only)
  - Hookworm 1 tablet/5 mL (single dose once only)
  - *Trichuris trichiura* 1 tablet/5 mL twice daily for 3 successive days
  - *T. solium* 2 tablets/5 mL twice daily for 3 successive days

- *T. saginata* 2 tablets/5 mL twice daily for 3 successive days
- *Strongyloides stercoralis* 2 tablets/5 mL twice daily for 3 successive days
- *Adverse drug reactions:* Slight GIT upset, abdominal pain, diarrhea, exanthema, urticaria, and angioedema.
- *Drug interactions:* Cimetidine and metronidazole.
- *Contraindications:* Pregnancy and lactation.

Mepacrine

Brand names: Quinacrine and Atabrine

- *Available as:* Tablet 100 mg.
- *Indications:* Giardiasis and *H. nana* infestation.
- *Dose:*
  - *L. giardia:* 5 mg/kg/day in three divided doses for 5–7 days.
  - *H. nana:* 15 mg/kg (maximum 8 g) as a single dose preferably through Ryle's tube followed by a mild purgative.
- *Adverse drug reactions:* Very bitter. GI upset, jaundice-like skin and mucous membrane discoloration, rash, seizures, and psychosis.
- *Drug interaction:* None.
- *Contraindications:* Advanced liver disease, psychosis, blood disorders, and hypersensitivity.
- *Cautions:* When a large dose is to be given as in case of tapeworms, it is advisable to give it through a Ryle's tube preceded by an antiemetic. Secondly, in order to flush out the worms, it is important to give a mild purgative after the administration of the drug through the tube.

Pyrantel Pamoate

Brand name: Nemocid

- *Available as:* Tablets 125 and 250 mg; suspension 100 mg, 250 mg/5 mL.
- *Indications:* Ascariasis, enterobiasis, ancylostomiasis, trichuriasis, and strongyloidiasis.
- *Dose:* 10 mg/kg with a maximum of 500 mg as a single administration. A repeat dose may be given after a fortnight. Whereas, as low a dose as 5 mg/kg may suffice for ascariasis, heavy infestation with hookworm needs either an extended course of 3 days or 20 mg/kg/day dose for 2 days.
- *Adverse drug reactions:* Rash, pruritus, gastrointestinal upset, disturbed taste, rise in body temperature, hepatotoxicity, myasthenia-like symptoms; leukopenia, thrombocytopenia, and albuminuria.
- *Precaution:* Hepatic insufficiency.

Niclosamide

Brand name: Niclosan

- *Available as:* Chewable tablet 500 mg.
- *Indications:* Tapeworm infestations.
- *Dose:*
  - 40 mg/kg (PO) as a single dose with a maximum of 2 g for *T. solium*, *T. saginata,* and *Diphyllobothrium latum* (fish tapeworm).
  - For *H. nana*, the same dose needs to be given for 5–7 successive days.
- *Adverse drug reactions:* GIT upset (nausea, vomiting, diarrhea, stomatitis, and pain in abdomen), rarely cysticercosis in *T. solium* infestation, ataxia, headache, rash, sleep disturbances, and paresthesia.

- *Precautions:* Tablets must be chewed thoroughly before being swallowed or finely ground and mixed with some liquid before these are ingested. The child must receive a purgative 1–2 hours after drug administration to clear the bowel of the dead segments before these are digested. This is important to safeguard against risk of cysticercosis from the liberated ova.

Nitazoxanide

Brand names: Nitarid and Nitazox

Indications: Ascariasis, trichuriasis, and *H. nana*. Also giardiasis, amebiasis cryptosporidiosis, fascioliasis, *C. parvum*, and *H. pylori*.

For details, see under "Antiprotozoal Drugs" in this very chapter.

Paromomycin

It is an aminoglycoside antibiotic.

Brand name: Humatin
- *Available as:* Capsule 250 mg.
- *Indications:* Tapeworms; also *L. giardia* and *E. histolytica*.
- *Additional:* Visceral leishmaniasis and cryptosporidiosis.
- *Dose:*
  - *Tapeworms:* 40–50 mg/kg/day in four divided doses every 15 minutes (in *H. nana*, it is given once a day for 7 days).

For details, see under "Antiprotozoal Drugs" in this very chapter.

Piperazine

Brand name: Antepar
- *Available as:* Tablet 500 mg; syrup 750 mg/5 mL.
- *Indications:* Ascariasis (first-line drug for ascariasis with intestinal or biliary obstruction) and oxyuriasis (enterobiasis).
- *Dose:*
  - *Ascariasis:* 100–150 mg/kg as a single administration

    Or

    50–75 mg/kg OD for 2 days
  - *Oxyuriasis (enterobiasis):* 50–75 mg/mg/kg/day
- *Adverse drug reactions:* Rash, vomiting, blurring of vision, and muscle weakness may precipitate/aggravate seizures.
- *Contraindication:* Seizure disorder.
- *Caution:* Avoid in epileptic children. It is advantageous to repeat the course after a month for preventing recurrence/relapse.
- *Special remarks:* The drug is no longer in routine use.

Praziquantel

A pyrazinoisoquinoline derivative, readily absorbed from the gut, metabolized in liver, and crosses the blood-brain barrier (BBB).

Brand name: Biltricide
- *Available as:* Tablet 500 mg.
- *Indications:* Tapeworm infestation; cysticercosis (now second-line choice to albendazole), *D. latum, E. granulosus,* and *schistosomes liver flukes.*

- *Dose:*
  - 50–100 mg/kg/day (PO) in three divided doses for 7–28 days for neurocysticercosis in which case dexamethasone therapy to counter high intracranial tension and inflammatory flare-up is also indicated.
  - 5–10 mg/kg (PO) single dose once only for tapeworms and liver fluke. In case of a poor response, 15–25 mg/kg single dose may be given.
  - 40 mg/kg as a single dose in schistosomiasis in which it should be considered the drug of choice.
- *Adverse drug reactions:* Headache, malaise, dizziness, nausea, vomiting, and abdominal pain; occasionally, urticaria, pruritus, and low-grade fever; and localized edematous reaction due to its parasiticidal effect on cysts in cerebrum.
- *Contraindications:* Hypersensitivity, intraocular cysticercosis, and rifampicin (a strong CYP-450 inducer).
- *Caution:* Breastfeeding needs to be interrupted for 3 days after the dose for nursing mothers.

Chapter 49

Antiparasitic (Extraintestinal) Drugs

INTRODUCTION

Extraintestinal parasitic infections/infestations include malarial parasite, mites, ticks, and flees.

Antimalarial drugs are employed for the treatment and prevention of malaria infection. Most such drugs target the erythrocytic stage of malaria infection, which is the phase of infection that is responsible for symptomatic illness in the form of high fever with chills and rigors. Four major drug classes currently in use for treating malaria include artemisinin derivatives, quinoline-related compounds, antifolates, and antimicrobials. So far, no single drug that can eradicate all forms of the malarial parasite's lifecycle is available. Understandably, one or more classes of drugs are frequently given at the same time to synergistic effect. Moreover, treatment regimens are dependent on the geographical location of infection, the likely *Plasmodium* species, and the severity of disease.

Notwithstanding availability of quite a number of antimalarial drugs, the World Health Organization (WHO) and the Indian Academy of Pediatrics (IAP) strongly recommend artemisinin-based combination therapy (ACT) in falciparum malaria that shows a very high level of resistance to the time-honored chloroquine.

ANTIMALARIAL DRUGS

Amodiaquine Hydrochloride

Brand name: Camoquin

- *Available as:* Tablet 200 mg.
- *Indications:* Malaria, both treatment and prophylaxis.
- *Dose:* 10 mg/kg day with a maximum dose of 600 mg (PO) as single dose. If maintenance dose required (as in case of unimmunized children), give 5 mg/kg/day for 2 more days.
- *Adverse drug reactions (ADRs):* Diarrhea, vomiting, and vertigo are the most commonly encountered; agranulocytosis, hepatitis, peripheral neuropathy, corneal deposits, visual disturbances, and skin and nail pigmentation (with frequent use).
- *Contraindication:* Concurrent administration of other antimalarials.
- *Caution:* Monitor regularly with blood, liver, and ophthalmic tests.
- *Remarks:* Also available as plain amodiaquine (Basoquin-Pfizer) providing 150 mg base/5 mL.

Artemether

A derivative of artemisinin, the active principle of *Artemisia annua* employed in Chinese traditional medicine, as "Qinghaosu". It is lipid soluble and given either orally or intramuscularly (never intravenously).

Brand names: Arte plus and Lumerax

- *Available as:*
  - Tablet artemether 20 mg and lumefantrine 120 mg
  - Intramuscular (IM) injection 80 mg/mL

- *Indication:* Acute falciparum malaria. Oral for uncomplicated chloroquine/multidrug-resistant (MDR) and injectable for complicated malaria.
- *Dose:*
  - 5–15 kg one tablet, 15–25 kg two tablets, and 25–35 kg three tablets
  - *Adolescents:* Four tablets. This dose is to be administered stat and then at 8, 24, 36, 48, and 60 hours.
  - *IM dose:* Day 1—3.2 mg/kg. Then, 1.6 mg/kg OD for 4 days (total dose 9.6 mg/kg).
- *Adverse drug reactions:* Headache, dizziness, sleep disorders, gastrointestinal tract (GIT) upset, palpitation, anorexia, pruritus, rash, arthralgia, myalgia, asthma, fatigue, QT prolongation, paresthesia, gait disturbances, and liver dysfunction.
- *Contraindications:* G6PD deficiency and immunocompromised states.
- *Drug interactions:* Inhibitors of CY344, drugs prolonging QT interval, neuroepileptics, antifungals, antidepressants, macrolides, quinolones, cisapride, and other antimalarials.
- *Caution:* Severe cardiac, renal, and hepatic impairment. Monitor electrocardiograph (ECG) and potassium.

Artesunate

This too is a derivative of artemisinin. It is water-soluble and given orally, intramuscularly, or intravenously.

Brand names: Arnate and Falcigo
- *Available as:* Tablet 50 mg; injection 60 mg/vial.
- *Indication:* Acute falciparum malaria. Oral for uncomplicated chloroquine/MDR and injectable for complicated malaria.

- *Doses:*
  - 4 mg/kg (PO) followed by 2 mg/kg on day 2 and 3 and 1 mg/kg on day 4–7.
  - Injection 2–4 mg/kg/dose (IM and IV) stat. Then, 1.2 mg/kg/dose (IM and IV) after 12–24 hours.
  - Thereafter 1.2 mg/kg/dose (IM and IV) OD × 6 days.
- *Adverse drug reactions:* Headache, dizziness, sleep disorders, GIT upset, palpitation, anorexia, pruritus, rash, arthralgia, myalgia, asthma, fatigue, QT prolongation, paresthesia, gait disturbances, and liver dysfunction.
- *Contraindications:* G6PD deficiency, immunocompromised states.
- *Drug interaction:* Inhibitors of CY344, drugs prolonging QT interval, neuroepileptics, antifungals, antidepressants, macrolides, quinolones, cisapride, and other antimalarials.
- *Caution:* Severe cardiac, renal, and hepatic impairment. Monitor ECG and potassium.

Chloroquine Sulfate

Brand names: Nivaquine, Lariago, and Resochin

- *Available as:* Tablet 200 mg (150 mg base); syrup 50 mg/5 mL (base); and injection 40 mg/mL (base).
- *Indications:* Malaria, reactional states in leprosy; at times rheumatoid arthritis, discoid lupus erythematosus; and extraintestinal amebiasis.
- *Dose:* For *Plasmodium vivax*—In terms of base, starting dose 10 mg/kg, then repeat 5 mg/kg at 6, 24, and 48 hours intervals (total of 25 mg/kg). For *P. falciparum*—10 mg/kg stat followed by 10 mg/kg at 24 hours and 5 mg/kg at 48 hours. Total dose remains 25 mg/kg.
  - *Prophylactic dose:* 5 mg/kg once a week.

- For cerebral malaria, dose is 5–10 mg/kg (maximum of 300–400 mg base) which should be given intramuscularly. If intravenous administration is considered essential, 1/10th of the calculated dose may be given intravenously and the remaining intramuscularly. Parenteral overdose may cause fatal convulsions and cardiovascular collapse.
- Parenteral administration may also be indicated in malaria in an unconscious child or in the presence of persistent vomiting.

- *Adverse drug reactions:* Nausea, vomiting, headache, visual disturbances, hepatic dysfunction, blood dyscrasias, pruritus, rash, neurologic changes, dystonic reactions, susceptibility to phenothiazine toxicity, rarely retinopathy may occur with its long-term use.

    In the event of gross overdosage, vomiting should be induced or gastric lavage done promptly. This should be followed by appropriate resuscitative measures. Tracheal intubation with artificial respiration, use of vasopressor agents and cardiac massage are indicated. Intravenous molar lactate (1/6) is of value to counter the quinidine-like action of chloroquine on the myocardium. To enhance excretion of chloroquine.

- *Contraindications:* Retinal or visual field changes; injectable form must not be given to children <5 years.
- *Drug interactions:* Antacids, cimetidine, digoxin, mefloquine, cyclosporine, rabies vaccine, anticoagulants, neostigmine, physostigmine, amiodarone, hepatotoxic agents, and ampicillin.
- *Caution:* Avoid administration during dehydration. Else, dystonic reaction may occur.

Doxycycline

Brand names: Biodoxi and Doxypal

- *Available as:* Tablet 100 mg.
- *Indications:* Malaria prophylaxis, treatment of complicated malaria in conjunction with other antimalarials. Also several bacterial, protozoal, and rickettsial infections.
- *Dose:* 2–5 mg/kg/day (maximum 200 mg) as a single dose or in two divided doses.
- *Adverse drug reactions:* Nausea, vomiting, abdominal pain, dryness of mouth, *Clostridium difficile*-associated diarrhea (CDAD); photosensitivity, Stevens–Johnson syndrome; hemolytic anemia; superimposed infections, e.g., vaginitis; pseudotumor cerebri (on withdrawal); infrequently, esophagitis; in young children (<8 years), tooth discoloration (permanent staining), enamel hypoplasia, and retarded growth of fibula.
- *Contraindications:* Known hypersensitivity; children <8 years.
- *Drug interactions:* Antacids, laxatives, oral iron, oral anticoagulants; carbamazepine, phenytoin, and barbiturates reduce its half-life.
- *Cautions:* Monitor hepatic and renal parameters. Avoid exposure to sunlight/ultraviolet rays during therapy. Avoid in children < 8 years in the wake of risk of permanent staining of teeth and growth retardation.

Lumefantrine

It is an antimalarial agent, a blood schizonticide active against erythrocytic stages of *Plasmodium falciparum*, for treating acute uncomplicated malaria. It is available in combination with artemether for improved efficacy.

Brand names: Actizo, Anther, ARH-L, and Lumerax

- *Available as:* In combination with artemether. Lumefantrine 120 mg and artemether 20 mg/tablet/5 mL.
- *Indications:* Acute uncomplicated malaria caused by *Plasmodium falciparum* including malaria acquired in chloroquine-resistant areas.
- *Doses:*
  - <3 years   1 tablet BD for 3 days
  - 4–8 years   2 tablets BD for 3 days
  - 9–14 years   3 tablets BD for 3 days
  - 14 years   4 tablets BD for 3 days
- *Adverse drug reactions:* Cough, vomiting, anorexia, and headache. Rarely, serious adverse ADRs like QT prolongation, bullous eruption, urticaria, hypersensitivity reaction, and angioedema.
- *Contraindication:* Cardiac arrhythmias.
- *Drug interaction:* Methoxyamphetamine.
- *Cautions:* Avoid grapefruit since it predisposes to enhanced adverse effects. Always take it with food or milk.

Mefloquine

Brand name: Meflotas

- *Available as:* Tablet 250 mg.
- *Indications:* Resistant malaria; also for prophylaxis.
- *Doses:*
  - For prophylaxis, once a week.
  - 5–19 kg—¼ tablet
  - 20–30 kg—½ tablet
  - 31–45 kg—¾ tablet
  - Adolescents—1 tablet
  - *For treatment:* 15 mg/kg/day with a maximum of 1 g in one or two doses 6–8 hourly.

- *Contraindications:* Hypersensitivity to quinine, severe hepatic impairment, active depression, generalized anxiety disorder, and seizures.
- *Drug interactions:* Quinine, ketoconazole, rifampicin, drugs affecting cardiac conduction, β-blockers, calcium-channel blockers, antihistaminics, phenothiazines, anticonvulsants, tricyclic antidepressants, and oral typhoid vaccine.
- *Cautions:* Pregnancy, lactation, renal, and hepatic impairment, epilepsy, and cardiac conduction disorders, children <14 years.

Primaquine Phosphate

Brand names: Malirid and PMQ

- *Available as:* Tablets 2.5, 5, 7.5, and 15 mg
- *Indications:* Malaria for obtaining radical cure especially *P. vivax* and *P. ovale*.
- *Dose:* To be administered for 14 successive days in the dose varying with age preferably after excluding significant G6PD deficiency. In terms of body weight, dose is 0.25 mg/kg/day for 14 days. According to National Antimalaria Program (NAMP), a 5-day course is sufficient. In case of falciparum malaria, dose is 0.75 mg/kg but once only. Beyond 12 years, dose is 15.0 mg.
  Subjects with borderline G6PD deficiency should receive a dose of 0.7 mg/kg once only in case of falciparum infection and once a week for 3 weeks in case of vivax malaria.
- *Adverse drug reactions:* GIT upset, intravascular hemolysis, anemia, methemoglobinemia, and agranulocytosis.
  Primaquine needs to be given to subjects with *P. falciparum* infection as well for gametocytocidal action. However, it is

sufficient to give it once only but in two to three times the dose for vivax malaria. It is to be noted that primaquine therapy should not be started right from the 1st day when antimalarial treatment is initiated. This is likely to precipitate complications and may result in fatality. Also, remember that primaquine should not be given to malaria cases unless the hemoglobin level is 7 g% or above.

- *Contraindications:* G6PD deficiency, systemic lupus erythematosus (SLE), rheumatoid arthritis, bone marrow depression, when hemolysis-producing agents are being administered.
- *Drug interaction:* Quinacrine
- *Cautions:* Monitoring of CBC; severe anemia with Hb <7 g/dL, pregnancy, and lactation. Primaquine needs to be given to only MP-positive cases preferably after excluding G6PD deficiency if facility is available.

Pyrimethamine with Sulfamethoxypyrazine

Brand name: Metakelfin

- *Available as:* Tablet containing 500 mg sulfamethopyrazine (SMP) and 25 mg pyrimethamine.
- *Indication:* Malaria especially falciparum resistant to chloroquine.
- *Doses:*
  - 25 mg/kg, with reference to SMP, or 1 mg/kg with reference to pyrimethamine as a single dose
  - For prophylaxis, same dose at fortnightly intervals
- *Adverse drug reactions:* Rash (mild and transient), blood dyscrasia, acute hemolytic anemia in G6PD deficiency.
- *Contraindication:* Allergy to sulfas.

- *Caution:* Avoid its use in G6PD deficiency. It is a suppressive treatment and needs to be followed by primaquine therapy in positive cases.

Pyrimethamine with Sulfadoxine

Brand names: Laridox, Malocide, and Croydoxin FM
- *Available as:* Tablet containing 500 mg sulfadoxine (sulfadimethoxine) and 25 mg pyrimethamine.
- *Indications:* Malaria, especially falciparum, resistant to chloroquine.
- *Dose:* 25 mg/kg with reference to sulfadoxine or 1 mg/kg with reference to pyrimethamine as a single dose.
- For prophylaxis, same dose should be repeated at fortnightly intervals.
- *Adverse drug reactions:* Vomiting, pruritus, leukopenia, rash (mild and transient), blood dyscrasia and acute hemolytic anemia, especially in G6PD deficiency. Rarely, it may cause Stevens–Johnson syndrome, hepatitis, psychosis, vertigo, and renal complications.
- *Contraindication:* Allergy to sulfas.
- *Caution:* Avoid its use in individuals with G6PD deficiency. It is a suppressive treatment and needs to be followed by primaquine therapy in positive cases.

Quinine Sulfate

Brand names: Cinkona, Falciquin, Qininga, and Res-Q
- *Available as:*
  - Tablets 100 and 300 mg
  - Injections 150 and 300 mg/mL
- *Indication:* Malaria resistant to routine antimalarial drugs.

- *Dose:* 25 mg/kg/day in three divided doses (PO) for 7 days. 20 mg/kg/dose (IV) by slow infusion over 4 hours. Repeat 10 mg/kg at intervals of 8 hours till clinical response occurs and patient can swallow tablets.
- *Adverse drug reactions:* Acute hemolytic anemia, vertigo, thrombocytopenia, tinnitus, headache, dizziness, abdominal pain, nausea, vomiting, diarrhea, blurring of vision, flushing, confusion; rash lupus-like syndrome, Stevens–Johnson syndrome; blood dyscrasias, acute renal failure, hypoglycemia, chest pain, AV block; and cinchonism.
- *Contraindications:* Tinnitus, optic neuritis, myasthenia gravis, hemoglobinuria, prolonged QT interval, G6PD deficiency, hemolytic uremic syndrome, thrombocytopenia, blackwater fever-associated previous quinine administration, and hypersensitivity.
- *Drug interactions:* Antacids, muscle relaxants, theophylline, anticoagulants, erythromycin, drugs prolonging QT interval (quinidine, procainamide, and amiodarone).
- *Cautions:* Atrial fibrillation, cinchonism, renal/hepatic impairment, conduction defects, heart block, cardiac arrhythmias, hypoglycemia, hypokalemia, bradycardia; pregnancy, and lactation. Blood glucose monitoring needed.

ANTIFILARIAL DRUGS

Diethylcarbamazine

Brand names: Banocide and Hetrazan
- *Available as:* Tablets 50 and 100 mg. Syrup, 100 mg/ 5 mL.
- *Indications:* Filariasis, Loeffler's pneumonia, and ocular larva migrans.

- *Dose:*
  - Children with no demonstrable filarial in blood (say, tropical eosinophilia): 6 mg/kg/day in three divided doses for 14 days.
  - Children with demonstrable filarial in blood:
    - *Day 1:* 1 mg/kg as a single dose.
    - *Day 2:* 1 mg/kg TDS.
    - *Day 3:* 1-2 mg/kg TDS.
    - *Day 4-14:* 6 mg/kg/day in three divided doses.
  - *Loeffler's pneumonia (A. lumbricoides):* 15 mg/kg OD for 4 days.
  - *Ocular larva migrans:* 6 mg/kg/day in three divided doses.
- *Adverse drug reactions:* Dizziness, headache, nausea, arthralgia, and conjunctival congestion; rarely psychosis.
- *Caution:* Lactation and renal impairment.

ANTILEISHMANIA DRUGS

Amphotericin B

See Chapter 47 (Antifungal Drugs)

Pentamidine Isethionate

Brand names: Pentacarinat and Pentam

- *Available as:* Injection 300 mg.
- *Indications:* Leishmaniasis (antimony resistance/intolerance) and *Pneumocystis carinii* (*P. jirovecii*) pneumoniae.
- *Dose:*
  - *Localized leishmaniasis:* 2-3 mg/kg/dose (IM) on alternate days for 4-7 injections.
  - *Systemic leishmaniasis:* 2-4 mg/kg/dose (deep IM) on alternate days for 15-24 injections.

- *P. carinii:* 4 mg/kg/day (in IV dextrose over 1 hour) for 14 days.
- *Prophylaxis:* 4 mg/kg/dose (IM and IV) every 2–4 weeks.
- *Adverse drug reactions:* Hypotension, hypoglycemia, nephrotoxicity, and risk of diabetes.
- *Caution:* It is important to give IV dose slowly in dextrose over 1 hour period. When administered IM, injection should be deep enough.

Sodium Stibogluconate

Brand name: Pentavalent antimony

- *Available as:* Injection 100 mg/mL in 100 mL bottle.
- *Indication:* Visceral and localized leishmaniasis.
- *Doses:*
  - *Localized cutaneous:* 10 mg/kg/day (IV and IM) for 10 days.
  - *Diffuse cutaneous:* 20 mg/kg/day for 20 days.
  - *Mucosal and visceral leishmaniasis:* 20 mg/kg/day for an extended period varying from 28 to 40 days.
  - *Relapse:* Therapy may be given for 60 days.
- *Adverse drug reactions:* Nausea, myalgia, arthralgia; fall in hemoglobin, total leukocyte count (TLC) and platelet counts; raised liver transaminases, and ECG changes (nonspecific flattening/inversion of T wave).
- *Caution:* Slow IV injection which should be discontinued in case of substernal pain or cough.

ANTI-TOXOPLASMOSIS DRUGS

Pyrimethamine

Brand name: Daraprim

- Available as: Tablet 25 mg.

- *Indication:* Toxoplasmosis.
- *Doses:*
  - *Congenital:* 2 mg/kg/day (PO) in two divided doses for 2 days followed by 1 mg/kg/day (PO) OD for 2-6 months. Thereafter, 1 mg/kg/day for 3 alternate days in a week till completion of 12 months of course.
  - *Acquired:* 2 mg/kg/day (PO) in two divided doses for 2 days followed by 1 mg/kg/day in two divided doses for 4-6 weeks.

  Simultaneous administration of sulfadiazine (vide infra) is an essential part of therapy of toxoplasmosis.
- *Adverse drug reactions:* Bone marrow depression; photosensitivity, rash, glossitis, and convulsions.
- *Cautions:* Advisable to coadminister folinic acid (calcium leucovorin) to safeguard against inhibition of folic acid synthesis leading to bone marrow depression.

Sulfadiazine

Brand name: Zad-G

- *Available as:* Tablet 500 mg; injection 250 mg/mL; and cream 2.5% and 5%.
- *Indications:* Toxoplasmosis; urinary tract infection, meningococcal meningitis; bacterial skin infections; and alternative prophylaxis against acute rheumatic fever.
- *Doses:*
  - 100–150 mg/kg/day (PO) in divided doses; 100 mg/kg/day (IV) in divided doses.
  - 500 mg to 1 g daily for alternative prophylaxis (patients allergic to penicillin) in rheumatic fever.
- *Adverse drug reactions:* Allergic reactions including Stevens–Johnson syndrome, crystalluria, cyanosis, jaundice, purpura, and hemolytic anemia in G6PD deficiency.

Chapter 49: Antiparasitic (Extraintestinal) Drugs

- *Contraindication:* Hypersensitivity.
- *Caution:* Generous intake of water needed during therapy; avoid in G6PD deficiency subjects.

ANTISCABIES AND ANTIPEDICULOSIS DRUGS

Scabies is a skin infestation caused by a mite, *Sarcoptes scabiei*.

Benzyl Benzoate

Brand names: Babesol and Benzol

- *Available as:* Lotion 25%.
- *Indications:* Scabies and pediculosis.
- *Dose/Application:* For scabies, to be applied topically to the whole body from neck to toes, avoiding inflamed/raw areas of skin, eyes and face, and mucous membrane for 3 days. Each application should be followed by a thorough bath 12–24 (preferably 24 hours) hours later. 3 days therapy suffices.
- For pediculosis, application to the affected areas once (sometimes, a couple of repeat applications) is sufficient.
- *Adverse drug reactions:* Blister formation, crusting, itching, oozing, reddening, or scaling of skin, difficulty in urinating (dribbling), jerking movements, and sudden loss of consciousness.
- *Caution:* Avoid contact with eyes, face, urethral meatus, mucous membrane (inside of nostrils, lips), and inflamed/raw areas.

Crotamiton

Brand name: Crotorax

- *Available as:* Cream 10% and lotion 10%.
- *Indications:* Scabies and pediculosis.

- *Dose:* Topical application (nearly whole body for scabies and affected area for pediculosis).
- *Adverse drug reactions:* Allergic reaction and skin irritation.
- *Caution:* Avoid application over raw, broken skin, and eyes.

Gamma: Benzene Hexachloride

Brand names: Scaboma and Welscab
- *Available as:* Lotion 1%
- *Indications:* Scabies
- *Dose:* Topical application (lotion, shampoo, and cream).
- *Adverse drug reactions:* Allergic reaction and seizures.
- *Caution:* Avoid application over raw, broken skin, and in premature infants.

Ivermectin

See Chapter 48: Antiparasitic (Intestinal) Drugs.

Permethrin

It is a first-line drug for scabies and pediculosis.

Brand names: Clerkin, Permard, Permite, Permisol, and Scabitol-P
- *Available as:* Cream 5% and lotion 5%.
- *Indications:* Scabies and pediculosis.

ANTI-SCHISTOSOMIASIS DRUGS

See Praziquantel (PZQ) in Chapter 48: Antiparasitic (Intestinal) Drugs.

Section 4

Unclassified Drugs

50. Miscellaneous Drugs

Chapter 50: Miscellaneous Drugs

ATORVASTATIN

It is a synthetic lipid-lowering agent; acts by inhibiting the liver enzyme, *3-Hydroxy-3-methylglutaryl-coenzyme A (HMG-CoA) reductase*, that plays a key role in production of cholesterol in the body.

Brand names: Atocor, Atorlip, Atorva, Avas, Castor, Lipicure, Liponorm, and Lipitor

- *Available as:* Tablets 10, 20, and 40 mg.
- *Indications:* For lowering lipid levels in blood.
- *Dose:* 10–20 mg daily at unlike other statins that require administration at bedtime at any fixed time.
- *Adverse drug reactions:* Unexplained muscle pain, tenderness, or weakness; confusion and memory problems; fever, unusual tiredness, and dark-colored urine; swelling, weight gain, reduced/increased urine output, increased thirst, increased urination, hunger, dry mouth, and fruity breath odor.
- *Cautions:* Avoid <10 years of age and concurrently with another statin.

ATOVAQUONE

It may mention antimalarial drugs and in text of cotrimoxazole (*Pneumocystis carinii*)

Brand name: Mepron
- *Available as:* Suspension 750 mg/5 mL.
- *Indication:* Pneumocystis carinii (*Pneumocystis jiroveci*) pneumonia (PCP) as an alternative to cotrimoxazole (second choice), in *combination* with *proguanil* for the treatment and prevention of malaria.
- *Dose:*
  - <40 kg 30–40 mg/kg/day (PO) as a single dose
  - >40 kg 750 mg dose (PO) in three divided doses for 21 days
- *Adverse drug reactions:* Allergic reactions, depression, fever, cough, flu-like manifestations, stomatitis with white patches, and hepatotoxicity.
- *Caution:* Store in a dry place at room temperature; no freezing.

CHOLESTYRAMINE

Brand names: Prevalite and Questran
- *Available as:* Sachet 4 g
- *Indications:* Pruritus in liver disease (high bile salts), diarrhea from high fecal bile acids, and high blood cholesterol (as a statin).
- *Dose:* 200–250 mg/kg/day (PO) in three divided doses.
- *Adverse drug reactions:* Constipation, malabsorption (fat-soluble vitamins—A, D, and E), and hyperchloremic acidosis.
- *Caution:* Avoid in biliary atresia/obstruction. Do not swallow the content of the sachet as such. Instead dissolve it in water and then drink.

DEXTRAN-40

It is a sterile and nonpyrogenic preparation of low molecular weight dextran (40,000) in 5% dextrose. Injection or

0.9% sodium chloride injection, administered by intravenous infusion.

Brand name: Lomodex-40
- *Available as:* IV infusion of high molecular weight dextran-70 in 0.9% saline and 5% dextrose.
- *Indications:* Hypovolemic shock, cerebrovascular accident; prevention of deep vein thrombosis.
- *Dose:* Subject to child's condition.
- *Adverse drug reactions:* Most effective and yet safe. Rarely, allergic reactions, volume overload, *pulmonary edema, cerebral edema*, platelet dysfunction, and acute renal failure.
- *Contraindication:* Medical conditions with fluid overload.
- *Caution:* Avoid in chronic renal insufficiency and diabetes mellitus.

DEXTRAN-70

It is a sterile nonpyrogenic preparation of complex branched glucose polysaccharides of high-molecular weight (70,000). Dextran-70 is used as a plasma-volume expander for restoration of circulatory volume.

Brand name: Lomodex-70
- *Available as:* IV infusion of high molecular weight dextran-70 in 0.9% saline, 5% dextrose. Also, lubricant eye drops.
- *Indications:* For short-term expanding plasma volume during surgery, in hypovolemic shock due to trauma and dehydration, or specific cases of hemorrhage, and prevention of postoperative deep-vein thrombosis. Also, as a lubricant in eye drops.

- *Dose:* Subject to child's condition.
- *Adverse drug reactions:* Most effective and yet safe. Rarely, allergic reactions, volume overload, *pulmonary edema, cerebral edema,* platelet dysfunction, and acute renal failure.
- *Contraindication:* Thrombocytopenia causing bleeding.
- *Caution:* Avoid in chronic renal insufficiency and diabetes mellitus.

FLUNARIZINE

It is a weak calcium-channel plus sodium-channel blocker in brain.

Brand names: Flunarin, Nariz, Nomigrain, and Sibelium
- *Available as:* Capsule 5 and 10 mg
- *Indication:* Migraine
- *Dose:* 5 mg OD (PO)
- *Adverse drug reactions:* Vomiting, diarrhea/constipation, dizziness/light-headedness/headache, dryness of the mouth, flushing, increased appetite, weight gain, and unusual tiredness or weakness.
- *Caution:* It is a preventive agent and should be avoided in acute attack of migraine.

GLUCAGON

A *peptide hormone*, produced by α-*cells* of the *pancreas*, having action just opposite that of insulin, i.e., it raises the concentration of *glucose* and *fat* in the bloodstream. It is the main catabolic hormone in the body.

Brand names: Glucagon and Glucagon Novo
- *Available as:* Injection 1 mg vial and 10 mg vial

- *Indications:* Hypoglycemia (drug-induced or insulin-induced, intractable in large for gestational age neonates), as an antidote in β-blocker toxicity.
- *Dose:* Weight <25 kg 0.5 mg and >25 kg 1 mg (SC, M, and IV)
- *Adverse drug reactions:* Allergic reactions, nausea, and vomiting.
- *Caution:* Avoid in starvation, chronic hypoglycemia, and adrenal insufficiency.

MODAFINIL

It is a strong central nervous system (CNS) stimulant belonging to amphetamine class.

Brand names: Modafil, Modalert, Modfi, and Provake

- *Available as:* Tablets 100 and 200 mg.
- *Indications:* Narcolepsy.
- *Dose:* 100–300 mg OD (morning).
- *Adverse drug reactions:* Tachycardia, tremors, skin reactions, and psychiatric reactions.
- *Caution:* Avoid <12 years of age.

OMEGA-3 FATTY ACIDS

Brand names: Maxepa, Maxiguard, and Mega-3

- *Long-chain polyunsaturated fatty acids:* (1) Eicosapentaenoic (EPA), (2) docosahexaenoic acid (DHA), and (3) arachidonic acid (AA). These are health-friendly, especially for brain growth and development.
- *Available as:* Softgel capsule, drops, usually providing DHA and EPA in combination with vitamin E and micronutrients.
- *Indications:* Infants and children at risk of neurologic disorder or cardiovascular disease, pregnancy, and lactation.

ORAL REHYDRATION SALT (ORS)

Brand names: Electral, Electrobion, Punarjal, Prolyte, Speedral, and Walyte

- *Available as:* Sachet 6 and 30 g with the composition shown in **Table 1**.
- *Indications:* Prevention and therapy of dehydration, especially in diarrhea.
- *Dose:* For prevention of dehydration: 10 mL/kg of body weight after each loose bowel movement.
- *For treatment of dehydration:* 10 mL/kg of body weight until the lost fluids are replaced (usually 4–6 hours).

TABLE 1: Composition of low osmolarity Oral Rehydration Salt (ORS) in 1 L water.

Ingredients with amount	
Sodium chloride	2.6 g
Trisodium citrate	2.9 g
Potassium chloride	1.5 g
Glucose	13.5 g
Strength	
Sodium	75 mEq/L
Chloride	65 mEq/L
Potassium	20 mEq/L
Glucose	75 mOsm/L
Overall osmolarity	300 mOsm/L

Note: Adverse drug reactions and Caution appear above the ORS heading and refer to Omega-3 supplements.

- *Adverse drug reactions:* Omega-3 supplements (DHA/EPA) can make bleeding more likely, especially when simultaneously on nonsteroidal anti-inflammatory drugs (NSAIDs).
- *Caution:* Avoid in bleeding diathesis.

- *Adverse drug reactions:* Edema that was sometimes encountered in infants on standard WHO ORS is rare with low osmolarity ORS.
- *Caution:* Avoid ORS in renal insufficiency and allergy to any of its ingredients.

PANCURONIUM BROMIDE

Brand names: Pancuronium and Pavulon

- *Available as:* Injection 2 mg/mL, 1 mg/mL, and 2 and 10 mL vials.
- *Indications:* Adjunct to general anesthesia to facilitate tracheal intubation, and to provide skeletal muscle relaxation during surgery or mechanical ventilation.
- *Dose:* 0.0–0.1 mg (50–100 µg)/kg/dose (IV) every 30–60 minutes. Maintenance: 10–20 µg/kg/dose every 60–90 minutes.
- *Adverse drug reactions:* Increased saliva, skeletal muscle weakness, drooling, rash, bronchospasm, flushing, redness, tachycardia, low blood pressure, and high blood pressure.
- *Caution:* Monitor heart rate, BP, and assisted ventilation status.

PIRACETAM

It is a neuronal, vascular, and cognitive enhancer.

Brand names: Alcetam, Cetam, Neuropil, Nootropil, Normabrain, and Pretam

- *Available as:* Tablets 400 and 800 mg; Suspension 500 mg/5 mL.
- *Indications:* Learning disability, psychomotor retardation, and cortical myoclonus (as adjunct).
- *Dose:* 30–50 mg/kg which may be reduced to 15–25 mg/kg once the optimal effect is attained.

- *Adverse drug reactions:* Depression, general excitability, somnolence, and weight gain.
- *Special remarks:* Not approved by Food and Drug Administration (FDA).

PROBIOTICS

Friendly benign microorganisms employed for restoring the normal ecosystem of the gut and, thereby, displacing the pathogenic bacteria.

Brand names: Bifilac, Bnift, Darolac, Ecoflora, Econorm, Gnorm, Nutrolin-B, and Vizylac
- *Available as:* Sachet/capsule containing *Saccharomyces boulkdarii, Lactobacillus boulardii* or *Lactobacillus sporogenes* usually along with vitamins and/or zinc.
- *Indications:* Diarrheas (acute, persistent, antibiotic-associated, and pseudomembranous colitis), *H. pylori* infection, inflammatory bowel disease, irritable bowel syndrome, 3-month colic, infantile eczema; and necrotizing enterocolitis (prevention).
- *Dose:* One sachet/capsule BD.
- *Adverse drug reactions:* Usually safe. Common ADRs include abdominal detention bloating, gastroesophageal, mild diarrhea, constipation; occasionally flu-like symptoms; rarely, sepsis.
- *Caution:* Child needs to take extra fluids and cut down on sugar during the course of probiotic therapy.

PROSTAGLANDIN E1

Brand names: Alprostadil, Alprostin, and Prostin VR Pediatric
- *Available as:* Injection 500 µg/mL ampule.
- *Indications:* Ductus-dependent congenital heart disease (tetralogy of Fallot, pulmonary atresia with intact ventricle

septum, left heart syndrome, transposition of the great arteries (TGA) with intact ventricular septum, coarctation of aorta, aortic stenosis, pulmonary stenosis, etc.)

- *Dose:* Loading dose 0.05–0.4 µg/kg/min as continuous IV infusion through umbilical artery catheter, or a large vein at the level of ductus arteriosus.
- Maintenance dose after opening of ductus is 0.01 µg/kg/min.
- *Adverse drug reactions:* Short-term—flushing, apnea, hypotension, convulsions, and defective platelet aggregation.
- Long-term (after some weeks)—cortical hyperostosis, fat necrosis, and intimal mucosal insult.
- *Caution:* Avoid in neonates with respiratory distress.

PYRITINOL (PYRIDOXINE DISULFIDE AND PYRITHIOXINE)

It is a seminatural analog of water-soluble vitamin B6, and it is supposed to work by increasing the ability to deliver glucose into the brain to increase energy and stimulate brain function.

Brand name: Encephabol

- *Available as:* Tablets 100 and 200 mg; Suspension 100 mg/5 mL.
- *Indications:* Behavioral disorders. Also, in dementia.
- *Dose:* 50–100 mg (PO) OD.
- *Adverse drug reactions:* Nausea, headache, drowsiness, gastrointestinal (GI) upset, tingling, prickling, or burning sensations of the hands and feet, anorexia, and insomnia.
- *Special remarks:* Once a favorite prescription, at present this agent no longer finds a favorable recommendation from the academicians in view of doubtful evidence of beneficial outcome.

RITUXIMAB

Genetically engineered monoclonal antibodies used to treat diseases which are characterized by having too many B cells, overactive B cells, or dysfunctional B cells.

Brand names: Reditux and Mabtas
- *Available as:* 100 mg/10 mL vial, 500 mg/50 mL vial
- *Indications:* Autoimmune disorders [Juvenile idiopathic arthritis, systemic lupus erythematosus (SLE), autoimmune anemia], leukemias (CD20-positive *CLL*), lymphomas (both Hodgkin and non-Hodgkin), *multiple sclerosis*, and *chronic inflammatory demyelinating polyneuropathy.*
- *Dose:* 37.5 mg/m^2 (IV) once a week for 2 weeks.
- *Adverse drug reactions:* Allergy reaction (rash, itchiness, edema, breathlessness, and hypotension), reactivation of *hepatitis B* in those previously infected, *progressive multifocal leukoencephalopathy, and toxic epidermal necrolysis.*
- *Caution:* Avoid shaking and freezing the vial.

SIDENAFIL

Brand names: Alsigra, Aronix, Grandipam, Liberize, Slagra, Nipatra, and Viagra
- *Available as:* Tablets 25 and 50 mg
- *Indications:* Pulmonary arterial hypertension (PAH); also erectile dysfunction.
- *Dose:*
  - Newborn: 0.3–1 mg/kg/dose 8–12 hours.
  - Later age: 0.25–0.5 mg/kg/dose 8–12 hours.
- *Adverse drug reactions:* Nose bleeds, headache, upset stomach and heartburn, flushing of the skin, difficulty

in sleeping, worsening shortness of breath, and nasal congestion.
- *Caution:* Avoid in kidney disease, liver disease, sepsis, etc.

SURFACTANT

It is a surface tension-reducing agent.

Brand names: Bovine: Survanta, and Synthetic: Exosurf

- *Indications:*
  - Rescue therapy in respiratory distress syndrome (RDS) of moderate-to-severe intensity
  - *Prophylaxis of RDS:* When gestational age <29 weeks
  - Severe meconium aspiration syndrome (MAS)
  - Acute/adult respiratory distress syndrome (ARDS)
- *Available as:* Survanta: 4 and 8 mL vials. Curosurf: 1.5 and 3 mL vials. Infasurf: 3 and 6 mL vials. Exosurf: 10 mL vial.
- *Dose:* 100–200 mg/kg/dose of phospholipids I intratracheal (ITL).
- *Bovine:* 4 mL/kg/dose IT. A dose needs to be divided into four parts, each 1 mL/kg and administered in each of the four positions. Repeat every 6 hourly if required to a maximum of four doses.
- *Artificial:* 5 mL/kg/dose (IT). A dose needs to be divided into two parts, each administered in two positions. Repeat after 12 hours.

  Box 1 lists the dose of various brands of surfactant.
- *Adverse drug reactions:* Reflux of the administered dose, airway obstruction, apnea, pulmonary hemorrhage [usually in preterm neonates with patent ductus arteriosus

BOX 1: Dose of available surfactant brands.

- Survanta—2.5 mL/kg/dose in four aliquots
- Curosurf—2.5 mL/kg/dose (initially), 1.25 mL/kg (subsequent doses)
- Infasurf—3 mL/kg/dose
- Exosurf—5 mL/kg/dose

(PDA)], bradycardia, hypotension/hypertension, and hypoxemia.
- *Monitoring:*
  - *During administration:* Heart rate, oxygen saturation, ECG, and blood pressure.
  - *Posttherapy:* Arterial blood gases (ABG) for hyperoxia and hypocarbia.

TRIPLE DYE

- *Indication:* As an antiseptic for topical application.
- *Available as:* Acriflavin 1.14 g, gentian violet 2.29 g, brilliant green 2.29 g, and spirit/distilled water 1,000 mL.
- *Dose:* It may be employed to the umbilical stump only in the beginning.
- *Caution:* The old practice of frequent application to umbilical stump subsequently is no longer recommended.

URSODEOXYCHOLIC ACID/URSODIOL

Brand names: Urso, Ursocol, and Udihep
- *Available as:* Tablets/capsules 150, 250, and 300 mg.
- *Indications:* Neonatal cholestasis [especially total parenteral nutrition (TPN)-induced], sclerosing cholangitis, cystic fibrosis with liver disease, and gallstone (for dissolution).

- *Dose:*
  - *Neonates:* 10-15 mg/kg/day in one to three divided doses.
  - *Infants:* 30 mg/kg/day divided q 8-12 hours.
  - *Adolescents:* 300 mg at bedtime for 5-12 months.
- *Adverse drug reactions:* Diarrhea, dyspepsia, biliary pain, rhinitis, pruritus, and headache.
- *Contraindications:* Advanced liver disease/severe liver dysfunction and complete biliary tract obstruction.

Section 5

Drug Therapy in Neonates

51. Drug Dosage in Neonates
52. Emergency Drugs in Neonates

Chapter 51

Drug Dosage in Neonates

INTRODUCTION

Drug dosage in neonates is particularly a very sensitive matter since neonates have remarkable differences in physiology. This affects their drug absorption, distribution, metabolism, and elimination. Under-dosing may cause poor efficacy and therapeutic effect. Overdosing may result in adverse drug reactions.

GENERAL

Acetaminophen

10–15 mg/kg/dose (PO) q 4–6 hours.

Acetazolamide

25 mg/kg (PO) once a day to start; increase to bid, tid, and qid over 4–7 days.

Adenosine

0.05 mg/kg (IV) stat; every 2 minutes increase bolus dose by 0.05 mg/kg until a clinical response follows or a maximum dose of either 0.25 mg/kg or 12 mg is reached.

Albumin Human

0.5–1 g/kg/dose.

Albuterol

- 0.1–0.5 mg/kg/dose pm or q 2–6 hours (nebulizer solution).
- 0.1–0.3 mg/kg/dose q 6–8 hours (PO).

Alprostadil (Prostaglandin)

0.05–0.1 mg/kg/min as continuous IV infusion; may be slowly increased to a maximum of 0.4 mg/kg/min or wean as low as 0.005 µg/kg/min depending on response.

Aminophylline

6 mg/kg (IV and O) loading dose; maintenance dose 2.5–3.0 mg/kg/dose q 12 hours (IV and O).

Amrinone Lactate

- 0.75 mg/kg IV bolus over 2–3 minutes, follow with 3–5 mg/kg/min.
- Continuous IV infusion.

Antihemophilic Factor

Units required = weight (kg) × 0.5 × desired increase in factor VIII (% of normal).

Atropine Sulfate

0.2 mg/kg 30 minutes preoperative; follow same dose every 4–6 hours.

Bumetanide

0.01–0.05 mg/kg/dose every 24–48 hours.

Caffeine Citrate

10 mg/kg (O and IV) loading dose, then maintenance dose 5–10 mg/kg/day as one or two doses/day.

Calcitriol (Vitamin D Analog)

- 0.05 mg/kg/day (IV)
- 1.0 mg/day (PO).

Calcium Salts

2.4 mEq/kg/day in divided doses.

Captopril

- 0.01 mg/kg every 8–12 hours (premature).
- 0.05–0.1 mg/kg/dose every 8–24 hours; titrate upward to response, maximum dose 0.5 mg/kg/dose every 6–24 hours (full-term).

Carnitine

8–16 mg/kg/day (IV infusion).

Chloral Hydrate

25 mg/kg/dose (PO).

Chlorothiazide

- 20–40 mg/kg/day divided every 12 hours (PO).
- 2–8 mg/kg/day divided every 12 hours (IV).

Cimetidine

5–10 mg/kg/day (O, IM, and IV) divided every 8–12 hours.

Cisapride

0.15–0.3 mg/kg/dose 3–4 times daily.

Citrate Solutions

2–3 mEq/kg/day (PO) m three to four divided doses with water after meals.

Clonidine

1 µg/kg every 6–8 hours; then up to 2 mg/kg/dose every 4 hours.

Dexamethasone

- 0.25 mg/kg (IV) every 12 hours for three to four doses in airway edema or extubation starting over 4 hours before scheduled extubation.
- 0.25 mg/kg/dose (O andIV) every 12 hours for six doses; taper over 1–6 weeks in bronchopulmonary dysplasia.

Digoxin

10–30 µg/kg (IV), then 5–10 µg/kg/day maintenance dose.

Dihydrotachysterol

0.05–0.1 µg/day.

Dobutamine

2–20 µg/kg/min.

Dopamine

1–20 mg/kg/min (IV) at infusion rate (mL/h) = 6 × weight (kg) × desired dose (µg/kg/min)/mg/drug/100 mL IV fluid.

Dornase α (DNA Enzyme)

2.5 mL one to two times daily nebulized with Pulmo-Aide or Pari-Proneb compressor in cystic fibrosis.

Doxapram

2.5–3.0 mg/kg (IV), then follow with IV infusion of 1 mg/kg/h with maximum of 2.5 mg/kg/h.

Epinephrine (Adrenaline)

0.01–0.03 mg/kg (0.1–0.3 mL/kg of 1:1,000 solution) every 3–5 min (IV, 1 Tr).

Erythropoietin (Epoetin)

100–500 units/kg/dose every 1–2 days for 10–21 days.

Folic Acid

25–35 µg/day.

Glucagon

0.3 mg/kg/dose (IM, SC, and IV) with a maximum of 1 mg.

Granulocyte Colony-stimulating Factor

5 µg/kg/dose daily for three to six doses.

Hydralazine

- 0.25–1.0 mg/kg/dose (PO) every 6–8 hours.
- 0.1–0.5 mg/kg/dose (IV) every 6–8 hours.

Hydrochlorothiazide

2–4 mg/kg/day in two divided doses.

Hydrocortisone

Congenital adrenal hyperplasia 0.5–0.7 mg/kg/day (IV), follow with 0.3–0.4 mg/kg/day (¼ in morning, ¼ at noon, and ½ at night).

Adrenal Insufficiency

1–2 mg/kg (IV bolus) followed with 25–150 mg/day.

Shock

35–50 mg/kg (IV) followed with 50–150 mg/kg/day divided every 6 hours for 48–72 hours.

Indomethacin

0.10–0.25 mg/kg/dose every 12 hours for three to six doses for closure of patent ductus arteriosus (PDA).

Insulin

Regular insulin 0.01–0.10 units/kg/h continuous IV infusion or 0.1–0.2 units/kg every 6–12 hours.

Intravenous Immune Globulin (IVIG)

500–750 mg/kg (IV) once only.

Levothyroxine

8–10 µg/kg/day.

Lorazepam

0.05–0.20 mg/kg/dose (IV) over 2–5 minutes; may be repeated in 10–15 minutes in status epilepticus.

Magnesium Sulfate

25–50 mg/kg/dose (IV) every 8 hours for two to three doses.

Methadone

0.05–0.2 mg/kg/dose every 12 hours; thereafter, taper dose according to abstinence score.

Metoclopramide

0.033–0.100 mg/kg/dose (O and IM) every 8 hours for gastroesophageal Reflux (GER).

Midazolam

0.15–0.50 mg/kg/min (IV) continuous infusion; 0.05–0.15 mg/kg (IV) bolus every 2–4 hours.

Morphine

0.05–0.2 mg/kg/dose (IM, IV, and SC) every 2–4 hours; 0.025–0.05 mg/kg/h continuous IV infusion as analgesic.

Naloxone

0.1 mg/kg (IV) with a maximum of 2 mg; may repeat every 2–3 minutes until desired effect; continuous IV infusion may also be employed.

Phenobarbital

10–20 mg/kg (O and IV) loading dose followed by 3–4 mg/kg/24 hours (O and IV) q 12–24 hours as maintenance dose as an anticonvulsant.

Phenytoin

15–20 mg/kg (IV), not exceeding 0.5 mg/kg/min loading dose followed by 5 mg/kg/24 hours (O and IV) q 12–24 hours as maintenance dose as anticonvulsant.

Primidone

12–20 mg/kg/24 hours (PO) q 8–12 hours.

Propranolol

- 0.25 g/kg/dose (PO) q 6–8 hours. Gradually build up the dose for desired response to a maximum 5 mg/kg/24 hours.
- 0.01 mg/kg (IV) over 10–15 minutes. Gradually build up the dose for desired effect to a maximum/mg/kg/24 hours.

Ranitidine

1.5–2 mg/kg/24 hours (O and IV) q 12 hours. For continuous 24 hours IV infusion 0.04 mg/kg/h with a maximum 1 mg/kg/24 hours.

Spironolactone

1–3 mg/kg/day (PO) divided q 12–24 hours.

Theophylline

6–10 mg/kg loading dose then 2–4 mg/kg/dose every 12 hours.

Tolazoline

1–2 mg/kg (IV) loading dose followed by 1–2 mg/kg/h continuous IV infusion.

Tromethamine (Tham)

0.3 M solution (mL) = weight (kg) × base deficit (mEq/L).

Ursodeoxycholic Acid (Ursodiol)

10–15 mg/kg/day (PO) qd.

Valproic Acid

20 mg/kg (PO) loading dose followed by 10 mg/kg/dose every 12 hours.

Vitamin E

25–50 units/day (PO).

ANTIMICROBIAL DRUGS

Antibiotics

Amikacin

≤7 *days:*
1,200–2,000 g: 7.5 g/kg q 12–18 hours
>2,000 g: 10 mg/kg q 12 hours

>7 *days:*
>1,200–2,000 g: 7.5 mg/kg q 8–12 hours
>2,000 g: 10 mg/kg q 8 hours

Administer IM or IV over 30–60 minutes.

Amoxicillin

50 mg/kg/day (PO, IM, and IV) in divided doses q 12 hours under 1 week, q 8 hours at 1–3 weeks, q 6 hours at >3 weeks.

Amoxicillin-clavulanate (Coamoxiclav)

30 mg/kg/day (PO and IV) divided q 12 hours, increasing to q 8 hours after the perinatal period.

Ampicillin

≤7 days:

≤2,000 g:
- 50 mg/kg/day (IM and IV) q 12 hours for septicemia.
- 100 mg/kg/day divided q 8 hours for meningitis.

>2,000 g:
- 75 mg/kg/day divided q 8 hours for septicemia
- 150 mg/kg/day divided q 8 hours for meningitis.

>7 days:

<1,200 g:
- 50 mg/kg/day (IM and IV) q 12 hours for septicemia.
- 100 mg/kg/day divided q 12 hours for meningitis.

<1,200–2,000 g:
- 75 mg/kg/day (IM and IV) divided q 8 hours for septicemia.
- 150 mg/kg/day divided q 8 hours for meningitis.

>2,000 g:
- 100 mg/kg/day (IM and IV) divided q 6 hours for septicemia.
- 200 mg/kg/day divided q 6 hours for meningitis.

Azithromycin

- 10 mg/kg/day (PO) for 3 days.
- 10 mg/kg/(PO) on first day, then 5 mg/kg/day for 4 days.

Aztreonam

≤7 days:
- ≤2,000 g: 60 g/kg/day (IM and IV) divided q 12 hours.
- >2,000 g: 90 mg/kg/day divided q 8 hours.

>7 days:
- <1,200 g: 90 mg/kg/day divided q 8 hours.
- >2,000 g: 120 mg/kg/day divided q 6-8 hours.

Carbenicillin

≤7 days:
- ≤2,000 g: 225 mg/kg/day (IM and IV) divided q 8 hours.
- >2,000 g: 300 mg/kg/day divided q 6 hours.
- *>7 days* 300-400 mg/kg/day divided q 6 hours.

Cefaclor

20-40 mg/kg/day (PO) divided q 8-12 hours.

Cefadroxil

20-30 mg/kg/day (PO) divided q 12 hours.

Cefoperazone

100 mg/kg/day (IM and IV) divided q 12 hours.

Cefotaxime

- ≤7 days: 100 mg/kg/day (IM and IV) divided q 12 hours.

>7 days:
- <1,200 g: 100 mg/kg/day divided q 12 hours.
- >1,200 g: 150 mg/kg/day divided q 8 hours.

Cefazolin

≤7 days:	40 mg/kg/day (IM and IV) divided q 12 hours.
>7 days:	40–60 mg/kg/day (IM and IV) divided q 8 hours.
<1,200 g:	10 mg/kg/day (IM and IV) divided q 12 hours.
1,200–2,000 g:	15 mg/kg/day divided q 8 hours.
>2,000 g:	20 mg/kg/day divided q 8 hours.

Ceftazidime

≤7 days:	100 mg/kg/day (IM and IV) divided q 12 hours.
>7 days:	
<1,200 g:	100 mg/kg/day (IM and IV) divided q 12 hours.
≥1,200 g:	150 mg/kg/day (IM and IV) divided q 8 hours.

Ceftriaxone

50–75 mg (IM and IV) q 24 hours.

Cefuroxime

40–100 mg/kg/day (IM and IV) divided q 12 hours.

Cephalexin

25–100 mg/kg/day (PO) divided q 6–8 hours.

Chloramphenicol

20 mg/kg (IV) loading dose, then 12 hours later by:

≤7 days:	25 mg/kg/day (IV) q 24 hours.
>7 days:	
≤2,000 g:	25 mg/kg/day (IV) q 24 hours.
>2,000 g:	50 mg/kg/day (IV) divided q 12 hours.

Clindamycin

≤7 days: ≤2,000 g: 10 mg/kg/day (IM and IV) divided q 12 hours.

Erythromycin

≤7 days:	20 mg/kg/day (PO) divided q 12 hours.
>7 days:	
<1,200 g:	20 mg/kg/day divided q 12 hours.
≥1,200 g:	30 mg/kg/day divided q 8 hours.

Gentamicin

≤7 days:	
1,200–2,000 g:	2.5 mg/kg/ q 12–18 hours.
>2,000 g:	2.5 mg/kg/ q 12 hours.
>7 days:	
1,200–2,000 g:	2.5 mg/kg q 8–12 hours.
>2,000 g:	2.5 mg/kg q 8 hours.

Administer IM and IV over 30–60 minutes.

Imipenem-cilastatin

≤7 days:	
<1,200 g:	20 mg/kg (IM, IV) q 18–24 hours.
>1,200 g:	40 mg/kg divided q 12 hours.
>7 days:	
1,200–2,000 g:	40 mg/kg q 12 hours.
>2,000 g:	60 mg/kg q 8 hours.

Methicillin

≤7 days:

- 1,200–2,000 g:
  - 50 mg/kg/day (IV) q 12 hours for sepsis.
  - 100 mg/kg/day divided q 12 hours for meningitis.
- >2,000 g:
  - 75 mg/kg/day divided q 8 hours for sepsis.
  - 150 mg/kg/day divided q 8 hours for meningitis.

>7 days:

1,200–2,000 g:	75 mg/kg q 8 hours for sepsis 150 mg/kg/day divided q 8 hours.
>2,000 g:	- 100 mg/kg divided q 6–8 hours for sepsis. - 200 mg/kg/day divided q 6 hours.

Metronidazole

0–4 weeks:

<1,200 g:	7.5 mg/kg (O and IV) q 48 hours.

<7 days:

1,200–2,000 g:	7.5 mg/kg/day (PO and IV) q 24 hours.
>2,000 g:	15 mg/kg/day (PO and IV) divided q 12 hours.

>7 days:

1,200–2,000 g:	15 mg/kg/day (PO and IV) divided q 12 hours.
>2,000 g:	30 mg/kg/day (PO and IV) divided q 12 hours.

Mezlocillin

≤7 days:	150 mg/kg/day (IV) divided q 12 hours.
>7 days:	225 mg/kg divided q 8 hours.

Nafcillin

≤7 days:

1,200–2,000 g:	50 mg/kg/day q 12 hours.
>2,000 g:	75 mg/kg/day divided q 8 hours.

>7 days:

1,200–2,000 g:	75 mg/kg q 8 hours.
>2,000 g:	- 100 mg/kg divided q 6–8 hours for sepsis. - 200 mg/kg/day divided q 6 hours for meningitis.

Oxacillin

≤7 days:
1,200–2,000 g: 50 mg/kg/day q 12 hours.
>200 g: 75 mg/kg/day divided q 8 hours.

<7 days:
≤1,200 g: 50 mg/kg/day divided q 12 hours.
1,200–2,000 g: 75 mg/kg/day q 8 hours.
>2,000 g: 100 mg/kg/day divided q 6 hours.

Penicillin G

≤7 days:
1,200–2,000 g:
>2,000 g:
- 50,000 units/kg/day q 12 hours.
- 75,000 units/kg/day divided q 8 hours for sepsis.
- 150,000 units/kg/day divided q 8 hours for meningitis.

<7 days:
≤1,200 g:
- 50,000 units/kg/day divided q 12 hours for sepsis.
- 100,000 units/kg/day divided q 12 hours for meningitis.

1,200–2,000 g:
- 75,000 units/kg/day divided q 8 hours for sepsis.
- 225,000 units/kg/day divided q 6 hours for meningitis.

>2,000 g:
- 100,000 units/kg/day divided q 6 hours for sepsis.
- 200,000 units/kg/day divided q 6 hours for meningitis.

Penicillin G (Benzathine)

>1,200 g: 50,000 units/kg once (IM).

Penicillin G (Procaine)

>1,200 g: 50,000 units/kg (IM) qd.

Piperacillin

≤7 days: 150 mg/kg/day (IV) divided q 8–12 hours.
>7 days: 200 mg/kg (V) divided q 6–8 hours.

Sulfadiazine

100 mg/kg/day (PO) divided q 12 hours with pyrimethamine 2 mg/kg/day (PO) qd (with folinic acid) for toxoplasmosis.

Ticarcillin

≤7 days:
<2,000 g: 150 mg/kg/day (IV) divided q 8–12 hours.

>7 days:
>2,000 g: 225 mg/kg/day divided q 8 hours.

>7 days:
<1,200 g: 150 mg/kg/day divided q 12 hours.
1,200–2,000 g: 225 mg/kg/day divided q 8 hours.
>2,000 g: 300 mg/kg/day divided q 6–8 hours.

Tobramycin

≤7 days:
1,200–2,000 g: 2.5 mg/kg q 12–18 hours.
>2,000 g: 2.5 mg/kg q 12 hours.

>7 days:
1,200–2,000 g: 2.5 mg/kg q 8 to 12 hours.
>2,000 g: 2.5 mg/kg q 8 hours.

Administer IM and IV over 30–60 minutes.

Vancomycin

≤7 days:

<1,200 g:	15 mg/kg/day (IV) divided q 24 hours.
1,200–2,000 g:	15 mg/kg/day divided q 12–18 hours.
>2,000 g:	30 mg/kg/day divided q 12 hours.

>7 days:

<1,200 g:	15 mg/kg/day divided q 24 hours.
1,200–2,000 g:	15 mg/kg/day divided q 8–12 hours.
>2,000 g:	45 mg/kg/day divided q 8 hours.

Antiviral Drugs

Acyclovir: 30–45 mg/kg/day (IV) divided q 8 hours for HSV encephalitis.

Vidarabine (Ara-A): 15–30 mg/kg/day (IV) infusion over 18–24 hours for HSV infection.

Lamivudine: 4 mg/kg/day (PO) divided q 12 hours used in combination with zidovudine in HIV.

Nelfinavir: 30 mg/kg/day (PO) divided q 8 hours.

Nevirapine: 5 mg/kg (PO) qd for 14 days followed by 240 mg/m^2/day (PO) divided q 12 hours for 14 days and thereafter 400 mg/m^2/day divided q 12 hours.

Zidovudine:
- 8 mg/kg/day (PO) divided q 6 hours.
- 6 mg/kg/day (IV) divided q 6 hours.

Antifungal Drugs

Fluconazole: 6 mg/kg (PO and IV) qd first day qd for 14–21 days.

Miconazole: 5–15 mg/kg/day (IV) divided q 8–24 hours.

Nystatin: 100,000 units (topical) 4 times a day.

Emergency Drugs in Neonates

INTRODUCTION

Most common emergency situations warranting drug therapy in neonates are resuscitation, sepsis, apnea, cardiac conditions, seizures, hypoxia, etc. It is important that Neonatal Intensive Care Units (NICUs) remain preparted with the drugs and their administration in these situations.

Box 1 lists commonly employed emergency drugs in neonates.

BOX 1: Emergency drugs in neonates.

Adrenaline: 1:10,000 (0.1 mg/mL)
- *Dose*:
  - 0.1–0.3 mL/kg IV (preferred)
  - 0.3–1 mL/kg endotracheal tube (ETT)

For bradycardia:
- Repeat q 3–5 minutes as needed
- Never give via artery

Sodium bicarbonate: 4.2% (0.5 mEq/mL)
- *Dose*: 2 mEq/kg IV

For metabolic acidosis:
- Give IV over at least 2 minutes
- Assure adequate ventilation before administration

Contd...

Contd...

Volume expanders:
- *Dose:* 10 mL/kg IV
- Normal saline (preferred)
- Ringer lactate and O-negative whole blood
- Give IV over 5–10 minutes

Atropine: 1 mg/10 mL (0.1 mg/mL)
- *Dose:* 0.02 mg/kg IV, ETT
- May repeat in 5 minutes for bradycardia

Defibrillation:
- *Dose:* 2 joules/kg

Naloxone: 0.4 mg/mL
- *Dose:* 0.1 mg/kg IV (preferred) or IM
- May repeat dose × 3 as needed

For narcotic-induced respiratory depression:
Avoid use if suspected maternal narcotic addiction or methadone use.

Calcium gluconate: 100 mg/mL
- *Dose:* 100 mg/kg IV. Give over 5–10 minutes
- May repeat in 10 minutes, if needed

Calcium chloride: 10% 1 g/10 mL (100 mg/mL)
- *Dose:* 20 mg/kg IV
- Infuse over 1 minute. May repeat in 10 minutes, if needed

Adenosine: 3,000 µg/mL (6 mg/2 mL)
- Mix 1 mL of adenosine in 9 mL NS = 300 µg/mL
- *Dose:* 50 µg/kg rapid IV push (1–2 seconds) closest to IV insertion site, follow immediately with rapid saline flush. May repeat q 1–2 minutes as needed. May increase by 50 µg/kg/dose to a maximum dose of 300 µg/kg for supraventricular tachycardia

Section 6

Pharmacotherapy in Pediatric Emergencies

53. Important Emergency Drugs
54. Pharmacotherapy of Common Pediatric Emergencies

53
Chapter

Important Emergency Drugs

INTRODUCTION

Common emergency situations needing pharmacotherapy include respiratory, gastrointestinal, neurological and cardiac conditions, dehydration and dyselectrolytemia, resuscitation, poisoning and envenomations. The Pediatric Intensive Care units (PICUs) need to remain ready with the pharmacotherapy of such emergencies.

- *Adenosine:* 0.05–0.3 mg/kg/dose with a maximum of 6 mg/dose IV in 1–2 seconds. Then, 0.2 mg/kg dose with a maximum of 12 mg/dose every 2–5 minutes until supraventricular tachycardia (SVT) is controlled.
- *Adrenaline (Epinephrine):*
  - 1 in 1,000, 0.01 mL/kg/dose with a maximum of 0.5 mL/dose (IM). Same dose may be repeated after a gap of 15–20 minutes.
  - 1 in 10,000; 0.1 mL intravenous or endotracheal for cardiac arrest; same dose through nebulizer.
- *Aminophylline:* A loading dose of 5–7 mg/kg (IV), diluted in saline (25 mL). Then, 0.5–0.9 mg/kg/h IV infusion in acute severe asthma.
- *Atropine:* 0.02 mg/kg/dose (IV and SC)

- *Calcium gluconate:* Glucose, 10%, 1–2 mL/kg/dose, diluted with equal volume of distilled water, in 10 minutes until heart rate falls <100 minutes.
- *Dexamethasone:* 0.5 mg/kg/dose (V) every 6 hours.
- *Diazepam:* 0.3 mg/kg/dose (IV) in 1–2 minutes. If seizures fail to respond, repeat doses may be given after 15 minutes and 45 minutes of the initial dose.
- *Dobutamine:* A continuous IV infusion of 5–20 µg/kg/min
- *Dopamine:* A continuous IV infusion of 5–20 µg/kg/min
- *Fentanyl:* A continuous IV infusion of 1–5 µg/kg/dose every 1–4 hours. Rate 1–5 µg/kg/h.
- *Furosemide:* 1–2 mg/kg/dose (PO and IV) with maximum daily dose of 6 mg/kg.
- *Hydrocortisone:*
  - *Acute severe asthma/status asthmaticus:* 25–50 mg/kg/dose (IV) 4–6 hours.
  - *Endotoxic shock:* 50 mg/kg to begin with followed by 50–150 mg/kg/day in four divided doses as for 2–3 days.
  - Acute adrenal insufficiency 50 mg/m^2/day
  - *Congenital adrenal hyperplasia:* 10–15 mg/m^2/day (one-fourth at noon and half at night). Maintenance dose: 0.3–0.4 mg/kg/day (divided).
- *Ketamine:*
  - *Intramuscular:* 2.5–5 mg/kg/dose
  - *Intravenous:* 0.5–2 mg/kg/dose
- *Lignocaine:* IV bolus 1 mg/kg/dose every 5 minutes, the total dose not exceeding 5 mg/kg. Then, 10–50 µg/kg/min IV infusion. Total daily dose must not exceed 5 mg/kg/day.
- *Lorazepam:* 0.05–0.1 mg/kg/dose with maximum of 4 mg/dose (IV and IM). If response in controlling seizure attack is unsatisfactory, repeat the dose.

Chapter 53: Important Emergency Drugs

- *Methylprednisolone:*
  - IV bolus 30 mg/kg in 10-15 minutes once a day × Spray (intranasal) 0.2
- *Midazolam:* IV bolus 0.2 mg/kg. Then, continuous IV infusion 0.75-10 µg/min.
- *Morphine:* 0.1-0.2 mg/kg/dose (SC and IV)
- *Naloxone:* 0.1 mg/kg (IV) every 2-3 min × 3 doses. Total dose must not exceed 2 mg.
- *Nifedipine:* 0.3-0.5 mg/dose (sublingual)
- *Paraldehyde:*
  - 0.1-0.2 mg/kg dose (deep IM), using a glass syringe
  - 0.3 mL/kg/dose (per rectum)
- *Phenobarbital:* Loading dose of 15-20 mg/kg/dose (IV) in 15-20 minutes. Subsequently, 5-8 mg/kg/day in two divided doses.
- *Phenytoin:* Loading dose of 15-20 mg/kg/dose (IV) in 15-20 minutes. Subsequently, 5-8 mg/kg/day in two divided doses.
- *Salbutamol:*
  - *Injection (IM/SC/IV):* 4-6 µg/kg/dose every 6-8 hours.
  - *Nebulization:* 0.1-0.15 mg/kg/dose in 1.5 mL saline every 2-6 hours.
- *Sodium bicarbonate:*
  - 7.5% solution of $NaCO_3$ (mEq or mL) = Base deficit × weight (kg) × 0.6
  - Roughly, $NaCO_3$ may be given in the dose of 1-2 mEq/kg/dose (IV). Rather than injection the neat solution, dilute it with equal volume of distilled water or double volume of glucose (5%).
- *Terbutaline sulfate:*
  - *Injection (IM/SC/IV):* 3-5 µg/kg/dose every 6-8 hours.
  - *Nebulization:* 0.08-0.13 µg/kg/dose in 1.5 mL saline every 2-6 hours.

54 Chapter
Pharmacotherapy of Common Pediatric Emergencies

ACUTE BRONCHIOLITIS
Pharmacotherapy
- Humidified oxygen
- Nebulization, employing hypertonic saline, or racemic epinephrine, 2.5%, diluted with water, for 5 minutes. Bronchodilators and steroids are usually not needed.
- Antiviral agent, ribavirin aerosol, in case of severe bronchiolitis causing significant respiratory distress in a child suffering from immunodeficiency or lung disease such as asthma, cystic fibrosis (CF), etc.

Supportive Measures
- Attention to Airway, Breathing, and Circulation (ABC)
- Fluid and nutrition
- Ventilatory care for respiratory failure.

ACUTE DIARRHEA WITH DEHYDRATION
Pharmacotherapy
- *Rehydration:*
  - Low osmolarity (245 mmol) oral rehydration solution (ORS) in mild-to-moderate dehydration

Chapter 54: Pharmacotherapy of Common Pediatric Emergencies

- IV fluids in severe dehydration or child not responding to ORS or not accepting it
- *Zinc supplements:*
  - *<6 months:* 10 mg/day (PO) for 2 weeks
  - *>6 months:* 20 mg/day (PO) for 2 weeks

Probiotics (optional): Saccharomyces boulardii, Lactobacillus acidophilus, Lactobacillus sporogenes, etc.

- *Antibiotic therapy in bacterial diarrhea:* Cotrimoxazole (8–10 mg/kg/day in terms of trimethoprim, in two to three divided doses), nalidixic acid (50 mg/kg/day in four divided doses), etc.
- *Vitamin A supplements (optional):*
  - *<6 months:* 50,000 units/day
  - *6 months–1 year:* 100,000 units/day
  - *>1 year:* 200,000 units/day
- *Antisecretory drug:* Racecadotril 1.5 mg/kg/dose thrice daily (optional).

Supportive Measures

- Maintain good nutrition.
- Avoid antimotility drugs (e.g., *diphenoxylate HCl or loperamide*) especially in under-5s.

ACUTE EPIGLOTTITIS

Pharmacotherapy

- Humidified oxygen
- *Intravenous antibiotic therapy:*
  - *Ampicillin:* 50–100 mg/kg/day in four divided doses
  - *Chloramphenicol:* 50 mg/kg/day in four divided doses

Third generation cephalosporins, e.g. ceftriaxone 20–80 mg/kg/day (IV) in 1 or 2 doses
- *Antipyretics:* Paracetamol (acetaminophen) 15 mg/kg/dose every 6–8 hours, or 50 mg/kg/day in three to four divided doses.

Supportive Measures
- Airway, breathing, and circulation monitoring
- Intravenous fluid drip
- Severe respiratory distress may warrant.
  - Nasotracheal intubation
  - Needle cricothyrotomy
  - Tracheostomy.

ACUTE GLOMERULONEPHRITIS

Pharmacotherapy
- Injection penicillin (procaine), 4 lakh (IM) OD for 1–2 weeks (if acute tonsillitis present, i.e., poststreptococcal glomerulonephritis) or a macrolide like azithromycin.
- Antihypertensive drug, say nifedipine.
- For congestive cardiac failure (CCF), furosemide, adequate digitalization, or dopamine infusion.
- Anticonvulsant drug other than phenobarbital in case of seizures.

Supportive Measures
During oliguric phase:
- Bed rest
- Restriction of salt and protein
- For renal failure, dialysis.

ACUTE KIDNEY INJURY (ACUTE RENAL FAILURE)

Pharmacotherapy

- Normal saline, 20 mL/kg for 1 hour followed by IV mannitol, 0.5 g/kg
- *No response:* Repeat normal saline, 20 mL/kg for 1 hour.
- No/poor response (urine output <1 mL/kg/hour) IV furosemide, 1 mg/kg at rate of 4 mg/min
- *No diuresis after 2 hours:* IV furosemide, 10 mg/kg at same rate.
- *Poor response:* Low-dose dopamine, 2.5 mg/kg/min.

Supportive Measures

- Salt restriction
- Monitoring of BP, electrolytes, input-output, renal function test (RFT), etc.

ACUTE OTITIS MEDIA

Pharmacotherapy

- Amoxicillin or coamoxiclav, 50 mg/kg/day in two to three divided doses for 10–14 days.
  Or,
- A single dose therapy using ceftriaxone may give equally good results.
- Paracetamol, 10–15 mg/kg/dose every 6–8 hours until fever and pain are over (about 3 days).

Supportive Measures

- Upper airway decongestant therapy
- *Failure of conservative treatment:* Incision of the drum under anesthesia.
- *Drum already burst:* Swabbing and cleansing of the ear canal repeatedly.

ACUTE SEVERE ASTHMA (STATUS ASTHMATICUS)

Pharmacotherapy

- Warm humidified oxygen
- Nebulization employing salbutamol respiratory solution, 0.5 mL in 2 mL of normal saline, over 5 minutes. It is first given every 20 minutes for four times followed by every 2 hours.
- Injection adrenaline, 1:1,000 solution, 0.01 mL/kg (SC)
- IV fluid drip, 150% (one-and-a-half time) of normal maintenance requirement
- Injection hydrocortisone, 10 mg/kg (IV) stat followed by 4 mg/kg every 6 hours. If readily available, methylprednisolone, 2–3 mg/kg should be preferred.
- *Response poor:* Nebulization with ipratropium bromide respiratory solution, 0.5 mL in 2 mL normal saline plus salbutamol. The two are supposed to provide synergistic effect.
- *Response still poor:* IV aminophylline, 6 mg/kg/bolus in 5% dextrose with equal dilution, over 20 minutes. Follow with IV aminophylline infusion, 1 mg/kg/h.
- *Response continues to be poor:* Magnesium sulfate (50%) infusion, 0.1–0.2 mL/kg in 30 mL saline over 30 minutes.
- *Last resort:* Intubation plus ventilator support.

Supportive Measures

- Airway, breathing, and circulation
- Oxygen
- Hydration
- Nutrition.

ACUTE TONSILLITIS

Pharmacotherapy

- Amoxicillin, 30–40 mg/kg/day in three divided doses for 5–7 days
  Or,
  Azithromycin, 10 mg/kg OD for 3–5 days
- *Nonsteroidal anti-inflammatory drug (NSAID):* Paracetamol, 10–15 mg/kg/dose 6–8 hourly, or ibuprofen, 10 mg/kg/dose, 6–8 hourly for 3–5 days.

Supportive Measures

- Saline gargles
- Good nutrition.

ANAPHYLAXIS

Pharmacotherapy

- Humidified oxygen
- Injection adrenaline (epinephrine) 1:1,000 solution, 0.01 mL/kg IM (preferred choice) or SC. Repeat every 15 minutes, if required.
- Injection hydrocortisone (Efcorlin), 10 mg/kg (IV). Repeat 3 mg/kg every 4 hours, if required.
  Or,
- Methylprednisolone, 2 mg/kg/dose IV. Follow with 1 mg/kg/dose every 6 hours.
- Injection diphenhydramine (Benadryl), 1 mg/kg (IV and IM) over 5 minutes. This assists to counter the systemic effects of histamine.
- Dopamine IV infusion, 5–15 mg/kg/min by continuous IV infusion in case of presence of peripheral circulatory failure (PCF).

- Salbutamol nebulization or IV aminophylline for bronchospasm.
- *Postreaction:* Prednisolone (Wysolone), 1 mg/kg/day q 8 hours plus antihistaminic (cetirizine or loratadine) for 3 days.

Supportive Measures

- *Airway, breathing, and circulation:* Maintain airway patency, breathing, and circulation. At times, even intubation, tracheostomy or cricothyroidotomy may be warranted.
- Maintain fluid and electrolyte balance.
- Maintain appropriate nutrition.

ANTIBIOTIC-ASSOCIATED DIARRHEA (SEVERE)

Pharmacotherapy

- Metronidazole (high dose), 20–40 mg/kg/day in two to three divided doses (PO), and 21 mg/kg/day (IV infusion)
- If poor response, vancomycin, 40–50 mg/kg/day (IV)
- If poor response, vancomycin + metronidazole
- *Refractory case:* Fidoxomicin, 4–6 mg/kg/day (PO and IV) in two divided doses.

Supportive Measures

- Withdraw the offending antibiotics.
- Probiotics
- Maintenance of hydration and nutrition.

BLOODY DIARRHEA/ACUTE BACILLARY DYSENTERY (SHIGELLOSIS)

Pharmacotherapy

- Ampicillin (50–100 mg/kg/day in four divided doses), cotrimoxazole (8–10 mg/kg/day in terms of trimethoprim,

in two to three divided doses), nalidixic acid (50 mg/kg/day in four divided doses), or tetracycline (only >8-year-old), etc.
- *Zinc supplements:*
  - *<6 months:* 10 mg/day (PO) for 2 weeks
  - *>6 months:* 20 mg/day (PO) for 2 weeks
    Probiotics (optional): Saccharomyces boulardii, Lactobacillus acidophilus, Lactobacillus sporogenes, etc.; 10 billion organisms/dose twice daily.
- *Vitamin A supplements (optional):*
  - *<6 months:* 50,000 units/day
  - *6 months–1 year:* 100,000 units/day
  - *>1 year:* 200,000 units/day.

Supportive Measures
- Correction of dehydration/dyselectrolytemia
- Correction of malnutrition
- Avoidance of antimotility drugs like loperamide and diphenoxylate.

BACTERIAL MENINGITIS

Pharmacotherapy

Antibiotic Therapy

- *Age birth to 3 months:* In view of gram-negative pathogens, start ampicillin + aminoglycoside/cefotaxime. Subsequent therapy depends on culture and sensitivity report and/or clinical response.
- *Age 3 months to 12 years:* In the wake of *H. influenzae, S. pneumoniae,* and *N. meningitidis* being the dominant pathogens, initial therapy should be ceftriaxone/

cefotaxime or ampicillin + chloramphenicol. Subsequent therapy depends on culture and sensitivity report and/or clinical response.
- IV mannitol
- Corticosteroids over a brief period
- Anticonvulsant therapy.

Supportive Measures
- Maintenance of hydration and nutrition
- Good nursing care.

CONGESTIVE CARDIAC FAILURE

Pharmacotherapy

- *Loop diuretic:* Furosemide, 1 mg/kg/dose remains the diuretic of first choice to relieve pulmonary edema. When higher doses are required, add spironolactone—a potassium-sparing weak diuretic. Diuretic therapy promotes water and sodium excretion via kidneys, thereby diminishing ventricular preload and pulmonary edema.
- Digoxin, employed at its lower dose ranges **(Table 1)**, should be considered the second-line agent after furosemide, and is best restricted to subjects with supraventricular arrhythmias.
- Vasodilators for decreasing afterload, especially in CCF associated with left-right shunt, cardiomyopathy, severe aortic or mitral insufficiency.
- Angiotensin-converting enzyme (ACE)-inhibitors, such as captopril and enalapril, decrease afterload and to some extent preload, water and sodium retention by reducing production of aldosterone.

TABLE 1: Recommended dosage for digitalization in congestive cardiac failure/supraventricular arrhythmias.

Age	Digitalizing dose (oral)*	Digitalizing dose (IV/IM)*	Maintenance dose (oral)**	Maintenance dose (IV/IM)**
Preterm	30 mg/kg	25 mg/kg	8–10 mg/kg/day (two divided doses)	6–8 µg/kg/day
Term–2 years	65–75 mg/kg	50 mg/kg	8–10 mg/kg/day (two divided doses)	12–15 mg/kg/day
2–10 years	30–40 mg/kg	25 mg/kg	8–10 mg/kg/day (two divided doses)	6–8 mg/kg/day
>10 years	1–1.5 mg	0.5–1 mg	125–250 mg/kg/day	100–400 mg/day

Digitalizing dose: Half of the calculated dose is given initially with one-fourth the dose given q 8 h twice.
**Maintenance dose*: It is given twice a day in young children and once a day in older children and adolescents.

- *Inotropic agents:*
  - Dopamine
  - Dobutamine
- Beta-blockers.

Supportive and Other Measures
- Complete rest
- Cautious treatment of anemia.

DIABETIC KETOACIDOSIS
Pharmacotherapy
- *First hour:* Normal saline/Ringer lactate 10–20 mL (IV bolus) plus
- Insulin infusion (drip) 0.1 unit/kg/hour

- *Second hour and afterward:* Saline (0.45%) drip + insulin 0.1 unit/kg/hour + KCl, 40 mEq/L
- During the next 23 hours, 85 mL/kg deficit + maintenance – bolus is administered.
- Once blood sugar has come down to 250–300 mg/dL, 0.45% saline is replaced by 0.5 saline in 5% dextrose. While KCl is continued at the rate of 40 mEq/L, insulin may be reduced to 0.05 unit/kg/hour.
- In case pH >7.30, total CO_2 >15 mEq/L, electrolytes are within normal range, subcutaneous insulin may be initiated. However, it should be ensured that the insulin infusion continues for 1 hour after giving SC insulin injection.
- In case this is a known case of diabetes, old insulin regimen should be resumed.
- In case this is a fresh diabetic child, insulin should be started in the dose of 0.1–0.25 unit/kg divided 6–8 hourly subcutaneously. This establishes the daily insulin requirement of the child. Subsequently, child should be put on combination insulin regimen.

Supportive Measures
- Close monitoring of potassium status (through ECG), hemodynamic status, urinary output, and evidence of raised intracranial pressure (RICP)
- Finding out precipitating factor (say, an infection or another stress factor) and treating it
- Clinical and biochemical monitoring for best outcome.

HEAT STROKE
Pharmacotherapy
- Oxygen 100%

Chapter 54: Pharmacotherapy of Common Pediatric Emergencies

- *Rapid cooling:*
  - Stripping
  - Cold sponging
  - Cool environment
- *IV fluids:* 20 mL/kg normal saline over 20 minutes. If IV route not accessible, employ intraosseous (IO) route. After 20 minutes, if pulse still not felt, repeat normal saline in same dose.
- Dopamine IV infusion, 10 mg/kg/min if pulse continues to be not felt and hypotension persists.
- Anticonvulsant therapy. Injection diazepam, 0.3 mg/kg followed by phenobarbital or phenytoin.
- IV mannitol 20%, 7 mL/kg to control cerebral edema causing RIP.
- Attention to disseminated intravascular coagulation (DIC) manifestations:
  - Gastrointestinal wash with cold fluid
  - Injection vitamin K
  - Fresh frozen plasma, 10 mL/kg.

HEMATEMESIS (VARICEAL BLEED)

Pharmacotherapy

- Octreotide bolus, 1 mg/kg bolus, followed by 1 mg/kg/hour infusion
- IV antibiotics (say, ampicillin 50 mg/kg/day in four divided doses) to prevent such complication as spontaneous bacterial peritonitis.

Supportive Measures

- Initial resuscitation/stabilization of vitals
- Blood transfusion

Interventional Therapy

- Endoscopic variceal band ligation, sclerotherapy, and glue injection
- In case endoscopic therapeutic options fail, transjugular intrahepatic portosystemic shunt (TIPS).

HYPERCYANOTIC SPELL

Pharmacotherapy

- After comforting and placing the child in knee-chest position, administer humidified oxygen by face mask.
- Morphine 0.1–0.2 mg/kg (IV)
- IV fluid replacement and volume expansion; blood transfusion if child is anemic.
- Sodium bicarbonate for combating metabolic acidosis
- Propranolol, 0.1–0.2 mg/kg (IV)
- Increase systemic vascular resistance by IV vasopressin like methoxamine or phenylephrine, titrating the dose to increase systemic systolic blood pressure by 20%.
- Surgical repair of the defect or systemic-to-pulmonary artery anastomosis.

Supportive Measures

Place the child in knee-chest position.

HYPERTENSIVE CRISIS

Background

Aim is to lower high BP promptly (though not suddenly) to prevent occurrence of end organ damage. The stepwise phased reduction of BP should be as follows:

- One-third of the target reduction in first 6 hours

Chapter 54: Pharmacotherapy of Common Pediatric Emergencies

- One-third of the target reduction in next 24 hours
- Remaining one-third reduction in 48–72 hours.

Pharmacotherapy

- Sublingual nifedipine, 0.25–0.5 mg/kg/dose, or IV nitroprusside, 0.5 mg/kg/min, or labetalol, 0.2 mg/kg (IV) in 2 minutes, is the current choice.
- After control of severe hypertension in the first 6–12 hours, oral antihypertensive therapy should gradually replace the parenteral one.

Supportive Therapy

Bed rest.

IDIOPATHIC APNEA OF PREMATURITY

Pharmacotherapy

- IV theophylline, 6 mg/kg/dose as loading dose
- *Maintenance dose:* 6 mg/kg/day divided Q6H/Q8H/Q12H (IV/PO)
- Infuse slowly over a minimum of 20 minutes. Else, the neonate may develop arrhythmias.

Supportive Measures

- Tactile stimulation
- Continuous positive airway pressure (CPAP)
- Mechanical ventilation.

KEROSENE OIL POISONING

Pharmacotherapy

- Antacid (Mucaine gel, diovol, and gelusil) for countering gastric irritation

- Antibiotics for safeguarding from superimposed bacterial infection (pneumonia) though of doubtful value.

Supportive Measures
- Oxygen/respiratory support
- Decontamination of skin
- Avoidance of gastric lavage and induced vomiting.

MALARIA

A. *P. Vivax* and Chloroquine-sensitive *P. Falciparum* Malaria

Chloroquine 10 mg base/kg stat followed by 5 mg/kg at 6, 24, and 48 hours (a total of 25 mg/kg)

In vivax infection, primaquine should be given in a dose of 0.25 mg/kg/day for 14 days for preventing a relapse.

In falciparum infection, a single dose of primaquine, 0.75 mg/kg, should be given for gametocytocidal action.

B. Chloroquine-resistant *P. Falciparum* Malaria

Artesunate, 4 mg/kg once daily for 7 days. Next day, 25 mg/kg of sulfadoxine and 1.25 mg/kg of pyrimethamine should be given as a single dose.

Or,

Artemisinin-based combination therapy (ACT)—artemether plus lumefantrine—for 3 days.

For gametocidal action, a single dose of primaquine, 0.75 mg/kg, should be given.

Supportive Treatment
- Antipyretics for fever and tepid sponging for hyperpyrexia

- Fluid and electrolytes
- Attention to nutrition.

MENINGOENCEPHALITIS
Pharmacotherapy
- Antibiotics cover to combat any etiologic or superadded bacterial infection.
- Anticonvulsant such as phenobarbital, phenytoin, lorazepam, etc.
- Antipyretic like paracetamol
- Mannitol for reduction of RICP
- Corticosteroids (doubtful value).

Supportive Measures
- Maintenance of fluid and electrolyte balance and nutrition
- Tepid sponging for controlling high temperature
- Careful repeated withdrawal of cerebrospinal fluid for reduction of RICP.

NEONATAL SEIZURES
Pharmacotherapy
- Phenobarbital (the gold standard), 20 mg/kg (IV) slowly over 10 minutes followed by, in case of no response, two doses, each 10 mg/kg, at 5 minutes interval. Total dose should not exceed 40 mg/kg. Maintenance dose is 5 mg/kg once a day.
- If no response, phenytoin, 20 mg/kg (IV) slowly over 20 minutes as loading dose. Maintenance dose is 5 mg/kg once a day.
- *Intractable seizures:* Lorazepam, 0.05 mg/kg/dose (IV) or midazolam, 0.05–0.15 mg/kg (IV) q 2–4 hours.

If the cause is not traceable and response to anticonvulsant therapy and/or correction of biochemical and metabolic abnormalities is unsatisfactory, it is advisable to give a therapeutic trial with pyridoxine (vitamin B_6), 25–50 mg, calcium gluconate, 5–10 mL of 10% solution, by slow IV injection, and 1–2 mL/kg of 50% glucose diluted with distilled water.

Unless there is an indication for a long-term therapy, an anticonvulsant (say, oral phenobarbital) is continued for only 4–12 weeks following control of convulsions and then gradually withdrawn.

Supportive Measures

- Stabilization of vitals (ABC)
- Stabilization of metabolic/biochemical abnormalities such as hypoglycemia and hypocalcemia.

NONVARICEAL BLEED

Pharmacotherapy

- Proton pump inhibitor (PPI) such as pantoprazole as an initial IV bolus followed by continuous infusion **(Box 1)**.
  As soon as the subject is stabilized and accepting oral feeds, route of pantoprazole may be changed over to oral but in a dose that is double the IV dose.
- Treatment for *H. pylori,* if infection is present.

BOX 1: Intravenous dose of pantoprazole in nonvariceal hematemesis.

- *Under 40 kg weight:* 0.2 mg/kg followed by 0.2 mg/kg/h for 72 hours.
- *Over 40 kg weight:* 80 mg followed by 8 mg/h.

- Surgical options in case of rebleeding following endoscopic therapy.

Supportive Measures
- Initial resuscitation/stabilization of vitals
- Endoscopic administration of sclerosant, thermal coagulation or placement of hemoclips.

ORGANOPHOSPHATE POISONING

Pharmacotherapy
- Injection atropine 0.04 mg/kg every 5 minutes until signs of atropinization appear. Do not exceed a total of 10 mg/kg/day.
- Pralidoxime chloride (PAM), 25–50 mg/kg (IV) in normal saline with 12 hours of ingestion. PAM reactivates cholinesterase enzyme and acts by substrate competition mechanism at the neuromuscular junction.
- Anticonvulsant therapy, e.g., diazepam 0.3 mg/kg/dose (IV).

Supportive Measures
- Shift the patient away from the source and place of the poison.
- Wash whole body with soap and water.
- Irrigate eyes with distilled water.
- Airway, breathing, and circulation. Intubation may be required for the comatose child.
- Oxygen
- Gastric lavage with $KMnO_4$
- Milk of magnesia through Ryle's tube
- IV drip. Observe extra caution to protect against pulmonary edema.

PNEUMONIA

Pharmacotherapy

Antibiotics based on clinical judgment about the likely organisms **(Box 2)**.

Supportive Measures

- Antipyretics for fever; tepid sponging for hyperpyrexia
- Suctioning of excessive secretions/mucus
- Oxygen therapy for hypoxia
- Fluid management for adequate hydration
- Nutrition management
- Close monitoring.

BOX 2: Antibiotic therapy in pneumonia.

- *Community acquired*
- *Mild illness:*
  - Initiate with cotrimoxazole (8–10 mg/kg/day q 12 h, in terms of trimethoprim) or amoxicillin (40–50 mg/kg/day q 8 h) orally
  - If response unsatisfactory, coamoxiclav, cefuroxime axetil, or cefpodoxime
- *Severe illness:*
  - Cefuroxime, ceftriaxone, or cefotaxime (IV) plus aminoglycoside (IV)
  - Suspected *Staphylococcus aureus*: Penicillin, ampicillin, or amoxicillin plus cloxacillin
- *Suspected methicillin-resistant Staphylococcus aureus:* Vancomycin, linezolid or teicoplanin
- *MDRS:* Vancomycin or linezolid
- *Klebsiella:* Cefotaxime or ceftriaxone (IV)
- *Nosocomial:* Antibiotics to cover *E. coli, Klebsiella, Proteus, S. aureus, Pseudomonas,* and anaerobes along with metronidazole

(IV: intravenous)

RESPIRATORY DISTRESS SYNDROME/HYALINE MEMBRANE DISEASE

Pharmacotherapy

- Exogenous surfactant (preferably bovine), administered intratracheally (IT) as preventive as well as rescue therapy. *See* Chapter 50 (Miscellaneous Drugs) for precise details.
- Antibiotics cover
- Indomethacin, ibuprofen, or mefenamic acid for accompanying patent ductus arteriosus (PDA).

Supportive Measures

- Humidified incubator care
- *Oxygen:* Initially 70-90 mm Hg but cut down as soon as possible.
- Continuous positive airway pressure/assisted ventilation
- IV fluids with sodium bicarbonate
- Exchange transfusion.

SCORPION STING

Most of the manifestations of scorpion sting are due to autonomic storm.

Pharmacotherapy

- For pain relief, give a NSAID (say paracetamol), local ice packs, 2% xylocaine or dehydroemetine locally.
- Diazepam to quieten the restless child, allay anxiety and prevent myocardial stress.
- For autonomic storm - Prazosin, 30 mg/kg/dose. Repeat after 3 hours and then every 6 hours till improvement.
- For pulmonary edema – Diuretic

- For hypotension – IV dobutamine, 5–15 mg/kg/min
  Or,
  Sodium nitroprusside
  Or,
  Nitroglycerine, IV infusion, 0.5 mg/kg/min.

Supportive Measures

- Airway, breathing, and circulation (vitals) monitoring
- Application of tourniquet proximal to the location of sting to cut down absorption of toxin
- Oral and IV fluids to prevent development of hypovolemia
- Monitoring is essential to safeguard from pulmonary edema.
- Poor response to supportive and pharmacotherapy: Mechanical ventilation.

SNAKEBITE

Pharmacotherapy

- Tetanus prophylaxis
- Dopamine drip, 5–15 mg/kg/min if the child is hypotensive.
- Antivenom serum (AVS), preferably within 4 hours of the bite. However, no patient should be deprived of its possible benefit even if he arrives late and has indication for its use. In our experience of treating a large number of snakebite cases, it continues to be of value even after 24 hours of bite.
  - Mild envenomation (only local swelling without any systemic manifestations): 20 mL
  - Moderate envenomation (Local swelling with mild systemic manifestations): 50–90 mL
  - Severe envenomation (Severe systemic manifestations): 100–150 mL and even more

BOX 3: Steps of antivenom serum desensitization.

- *Step 1:* Scratch test
- *Step 2:* Intradermal injection
- *Step 3:* Subcutaneous injection
- *Step 4:* Intravenous administration

- Injection dexamethasone shield should be employed against hypersensitivity reactions even if AVS sensitivity testing turns out to be negative.
- AVS sensitivity test should always be done beforehand by instilling a drop of AVS into eye. Positive test is indicated by conjunctival congestion. Desensitization is attained in steps **(Box 3)**.
   Any evidence of hypersensitivity reaction is an indication for adrenaline, 0.1 mL (SC).

Supportive Measures

- Immobilization of the affected part which should be kept at a lower level to reduce travel of the venom to upper body.
- Application of a bandage above the bite site, provided that it occludes the lymphatics only and not the blood flow.
- Airway, breathing, and circulation
- Oxygen
- IV drip
- Ventilatory care in case of respiratory failure.

STATUS EPILEPTICUS/ACUTE SEIZURES
Pharmacotherapy

- Injection diazepam, 0.1–0.3 mg/kg (IV) slowly, rate not exceeding 2 mg/min for a maximum of three doses
   Per rectum diazepam, 0.2–0.5 mg/kg

Or,
Injection lorazepam, 0.05–0.1 mg/kg (IV) slowly
Per rectum lorazepam, 0.05–0.1 mg/kg
Sublingual lorazepam, 0.05–0.1 mg/kg
Or,
Injection midazolam, 0.15–0.3 mg/kg (IV)
Buccal or nasal midazolam, 0.5 mg/kg

- *Response poor:* Phenytoin or fesophenytoin, 15–30 mg/kg (IV) at the rate of 1 mg/kg/min followed 12–18 hours later by maintenance dose of 3–9 mg/kg/24 hours in two divided doses.
  Or,
  Phenobarbital, 15–20 mg/kg (loading dose) IV followed 12–18 hours later by maintenance dose of 3–5 mg/kg/24 hours in two divided doses.
- *Response poor:* Diazepam infusion
  Or,
  Midazolam infusion, 0.2 mg/kg/h
  Or,
  Propofol infusion, 1–2 mg/kg, 2–10 mg/kg/h
  Or,
  Valproic acid, 10–15 mg/kg (loading dose) IV
  Or,
  Paraldehyde (5%), 150–200 mg/kg IV slowly for 15–20 minutes followed by infusion of 20 mg/kg/h (in glass and not plastic syringe)
- *Response poor:* Barbiturate-induced coma by thiopental, 2–4 mg/kg for 24 hours.
  Or,
  General anesthesia, using halothane or isoflurane by a well-trained personnel with anesthetic gas scavenging equipment for prolonged periods.

Chapter 54: Pharmacotherapy of Common Pediatric Emergencies

Supportive Measures

- Airway, breathing, and circulation
- Start IV/IO line
- Do blood sugar, serum calcium, and magnesium levels
- If blood sugar <40 mg%, give IV 10% dextrose, 5 mL/kg
- *Seizures controlled:* Maintain dextrose drip 8 mg/kg/min
- *No response:* Give IV 10% calcium gluconate 1 mL/kg diluted 1:1 with 5% dextrose
- *Seizures controlled:* Evaluate for the cause and put the child on oral maintenance calcium 100 mg/kg/day
- *No response:* Anticonvulsant therapy as outlined in pharmacotherapy.

Section 7

Immunization and Vaccines

55. Conventional and New Vaccines for Routine Use
56. Combination Vaccines
57. Immunization Schedules in India
58. Adverse Events Following Immunization

Chapter 55: Conventional and New Vaccines for Routine Use

INTRODUCTION

Immunization is crucial for providing the child a protection against several infectious diseases that otherwise are known to cause much morbidity and mortality. In India, National Immunization Schedule is the most widely practiced schedule that provides free vaccines against priority infectious diseases. In collaboration with the international agencies such as the World Health Organization (WHO) and the United Nations Children's Fund (UNICEF), efforts remain in progress to develop and constantly improve India's National Immunization Schedule and to expand its reach to all parts of the country. For instance, pneumococcal conjugate vaccine (PCV) and *Haemophilus influenzae* type B (Hib) vaccines stand incorporated in the Universal Program for Immunization (UPI) in recent years in some parts of the country with a promise to extend their reach in rest of the country.

The Indian Academy of Pediatrics schedule includes additional vaccines for covering yet more diseases and is widely followed in office practice. The schedule keeps undergoing changes from time to time in keeping with the changing concepts.

BACILLUS CALMETTE–GUÉRIN VACCINE

Brand name: Tubervac

- *Available as:* 10 and 20 dose vials/long-necked ampoules plus diluents 0.5 mL and 1 mL, respectively
- *Indication:* Prophylaxis against severe forms of tuberculosis, e.g., tuberculous meningitis, miliary tuberculosis (efficacy 50–80%; protective efficacy for pulmonary tuberculosis 50%).
- *Dose:* 0.1 mL (0.05 mL if specifically indicated by the manufacturer), regardless of the age and weight, intradermally with a special tuberculin syringe and a 26G/27G needle. The best site is top (convex aspect) of left shoulder at the level of deltoid insertion for easy visualization of the scar and optimum lymphatic drainage. Sterile saline (not an antiseptic) should be employed for cleaning the surface.
- *Response:* Normally, after 2–3 weeks, a a tiny papule develops, growing up to 5 mm by the end of 5–6 weeks. It heals with a slight ulceration, ending up in a scar after 6–12 weeks. Moreover, slight cervical/axillary lymphadenitis may also develop. It is self-limiting and resolves spontaneously in a few months.
- *Adverse events following immunization (AEFI):* Accelerated reaction, deep ulceration with superimposed sepsis, significant ipsilateral cervical and/or axillary lymphadenitis with suppuration (BCGosis) which is managed by antibiotic therapy and/or surgical excision. Earlier practice of isoniazid (INH) therapy for 3–6 months needs to be discouraged. A chest X-ray should always be done in such cases to exclude evidence of tuberculosis. Rarely, osteitis, osteomyelitis, keloid formation, and

Chapter 55: Conventional and New Vaccines for Routine Use

disseminated tuberculosis in immunocompromised infants.
- *Contraindication:* None whatsoever.
- *Cautions:*
  - Avoid in immunocompromised states, especially cellular immunodeficiency.
  - Keep a gap of 4 weeks between catch-up Bacillus Calmette-Guerin (BCG) and measles or measles, mumps, and rubella (MMR) vaccine.
- *Storage:* 2–8°C (upper shelf of refrigerator); and must be used within 4–6 hours after reconstitution. Protect from light.
- *Special remarks:* BCG vaccine was supposed to provide protection against serious forms of tuberculosis (say miliary and meningeal tuberculosis) to the magnitude of 50–80% and pulmonary tuberculosis around 50%. In view of the South India's famous Chengalpattu (previously known as Chingleput) study observations, protective value.

DIPHTHERIA, TETANUS, AND WHOLE CELL PERTUSSIS

It is a combination of diphtheria toxoid, tetanus toxoid, and killed whole cell pertussis bacilli on adjuvants in the form of insoluble aluminum salts.

Brand names: DTwP and Triple
- *Indication:* Combined protection against diphtheria, tetanus, and pertussis (whooping cough).
- *Available as:* 0.5 mL, providing diphtheria toxoid 20–30 limit of flocculation (LF), tetanus toxoid 5–25 LF, and pertussis 20,000 million.

- *Dose:* 0.5 mL (IM), preferably at anterolateral aspect of thigh at 6, 10, and 14 weeks with boosters at 16–18 months and 4–6 years.

  Now both Universal Immunization Program (UIP) and Indian Academy of Pediatrics (IAP) schedule recommend DTP (not DT) as such for the second (4–6 years) booster too.
- *Adverse event following immunization:* Local induration and even abscess at injection site, febrile reaction, seizures, excessive crying, pseudotumor cerebri; occasionally, 1–3 hours after injection, collapse (pallor, sweating, and slow pulse), allergic skin reactions, encephalitis, provocation/activation of poliomyelitis during an epidemic of disease.
- *Contraindications:*
  - History of anaphylaxis or development of encephalopathy within 7 days following previous DTwP/DTaP vaccination is the only absolute contraindication.
  - Progressive/evolving neurological disease is a relative contraindication.
  - DTP should be temporarily deferred in acute febrile illness. Moreover, DTwP should not be given in children >7 years.
- *Storage:* 2–8°C/35–46°F (lower shelf of refrigerator).
- *Caution:* Be prepared to handle anaphylactic reactions. Avoid administering immunoglobulin concurrently.

DIPHTHERIA-TETANUS TOXOID

It is an alum-precipitated dual antigen, diphtheria and tetanus, and toxoid.

Brand name: Dual antigen
- *Available as:* Injection single dose ampule. Injection multidose (10 mL) vial.

- *Indications*: Active protection against diphtheria and tetanus in infants and children who cannot be given pertussis for one or the other reason until 7 years of age.
- *Dose*: 0.5 mL (IM) over anterolateral aspect of thigh (not buttocks).
- *AEFI:* Mild local reaction with painful swelling at the injection site.
- *Contraindication:* Children >7 years of age. In older children, risk of AEFIs from high dose of diphtheria toxoid can be high.
- *Caution:* Avoid administration in buttocks in the wake of risk of injury to sciatic nerve and poor absorption due to excessive fat.

DIPHTHERIA, TETANUS, AND PERTUSSIS (ACELLULAR TRIPLE VACCINE)

Brand names: Infanrix and Tripacel

- It is a combination of diphtheria toxoid, tetanus toxoid, and acellular pertussis bacilli on adjuvants in the form of insoluble aluminum salts.
- *Available as:* 0.5 mL providing diphtheria toxoid 20–30 Lf, tetanus toxoid 5–25 Lf, and pertussis vaccine 20,000 million.
- *Special remarks:* Only advantage of DTaP (which is expensive) over DTwP is reduction in the incidence of adverse drug reactions (ADRs). Else, its efficacy is similar to DTaP.

HAEMOPHILUS INFLUENZAE TYPE B CONJUGATE VACCINE

Brand names: Hiberix, ActHiB, and Hibpro

- *Available as:* Single or in combination with DTP, Hepatitis B, inactivated polio vaccine (IPV), etc.

- *Indications:* Active immunization of infants above 2 months against diseases caused by Hib; all children with hyposplenia (functional or anatomical).
- *Dose*: 0.5 mL IM
  - *2–6 months:* Three doses at intervals of 1–2 months; booster at 18 months.
  - *6–12 months:* Two doses at intervals of 1 month; one dose between 12 and 15 months; booster at 18 months
  - *1–5 years:* Only one dose.
- *AEFI:* Mild erythema and tender swelling at the injection site, pyrexia, excessive crying, irritability, restlessness, anorexia, vomiting, and diarrhea.
- *Contraindications:* Known hypersensitivity, acute severe febrile illness, age >6 years.
- *Caution:* Be prepared for an inadequate response in subjects on immunosuppressive therapy or with immunodeficiency.
- *Storage:* 2–8°C/35–46°F (preferably in middle shelf of refrigerator).

HEPATITIS A VACCINE

Brand names: Inactivated—Havrix and Avaxim. Live attenuated—Biovac

- IAP recommends it at 12 months of age followed by a booster at 18–24 months.
- *Available as:* Though most of the vaccines are inactivated (killed), a live-attenuated Chinese vaccine (Biovac and Wockhardt) is also available.
  - Havrix 720 Junior providing 720 enzyme-linked immunosorbent assay (ELISA) units/0.5 mL
  - Havrix 1,440 providing 1,440 ELISA units/0.5 mL

BOX 1: High-risk situations needing hepatitis A vaccine on priority.

- Chronic liver disease
- Hepatitis B and C carriers
- Immunodeficiency (both congenital and acquired)
- Transplant recipients
- Adolescents seronegative for HAV who are leaving home for residential school.
- Travelers to countries with high endemicity for hepatitis A

(HAV: hepatitis A virus)

- *Indication:* Active immunization against hepatitis A virus (HAV) infection, especially in healthy children who are less likely to have developed natural immunity because of sophisticated lifestyle, provided that the parents can afford it. It is also indicated in high-risk groups **(Box 1)**.
- *Dose:* Havrix—age 12 months to 18 years 10.5 mL [(720 ELISA units) IM], 19 years and above—1 mL (1,440 ELISA units) IM
  - *Avaxim:* Cut-off age for 1 mL dose is 15 years.
  - The recommended site of injection is anterolateral part of thigh in infants and deltoid muscle in children and adolescents. In subjects with bleeding diathesis, say thrombocytopenia, it should be administered subcutaneously.
  - Two doses at 6 months interval are recommended.
  - In case of live-attenuated vaccine (Biovac), single dose is considered enough though two doses give yet better seroconversion and higher antibody titer.
- *AEFIs:* Transient erythema and tender swelling over injection site, nausea, vomiting, anorexia, malaise, headache, fatigue, and pyrexia.

- *Contraindications:* Acute severe febrile illness, known hypersensitivity.
- *Storage:* 2–8°C/35–46°F (preferably, middle shelf of refrigerator).

HEPATITIS B VACCINE

Brand names: Engerix B, Genevac B, Revac B, and Shanvac

- *Available as:* 20 µg/mL; 0.5 mL, 1 mL, and multidose vials.
- *Indications:* Prophylaxis of HBV infection. This, the first anti-cancer vaccine, should be considered a universal vaccine as recommended by the WHO.
- *Dose:*
  - <18 years 0.5 mL (10 µg) IM in the deltoid region (children) and anterolateral aspect of thigh (infants and neonates)
  - >19 years 1.0 mL (20 µg) IM in the deltoid region
  - National: At 6, 10, and 14 weeks (a total of three doses).
  - IAP: At birth (zero dose) and then at 6, 10, and 14 weeks (a total of four doses).
- *Protective efficacy:* >90%
- *AEFIs:* Only minor, say soreness, erythema and induration at the injection site; infrequently fatigue, flu-like symptoms, malaise, dizziness, headache, paresthesia, abnormal liver function tests, nausea, vomiting, diarrhea, abdominal pain, arthralgia, myalgia, rash, pruritus, urticaria, syncope, hypotension, anaphylaxis, and serum sickness.
- *Contraindications:* Hypersensitivity and severe acute febrile illness.
- *Storage:* 2–8°C/35–46°F (preferably in lower shelf of refrigerator); should never be allowed to freeze.

Chapter 55: Conventional and New Vaccines for Routine Use

- *Special remarks:* All brands are equally good. Hepatitis B immunoglobulin (HBIG) must be given along with Hepatitis B vaccine in case of exposure to hepatitis B (perinatal, sexual, and occupational) in susceptible individuals.

HUMAN PAPILLOMA VIRUS VACCINES

Brand names: Cervarix and Gardasil

- *Indication:* Protection against cervical cancer, the most important cause of common cancer-related mortality in Indian women. IAP recommends this vaccine to all females who can afford it.
- *Dose:* 0.5 mL (IM) in deltoid, preferably at 10–12 years of age. The catchup vaccine is permitted up to the age of 26 years. Three doses at 0, 2, and 6 months are recommended in case of Gardasil and at 0, 1, and 6 months in case of cervarix.
- *AEFI:* Syncope
- *Cautions*:
  - To guard against syncope, the vaccine should be administered in a sitting/lying down position and the vaccine should be observed for 15 minutes postvaccination.
  - Avoid in pregnancy.
  - Efficacy and immunogenicity in immunocompromised children are relatively low.
- *Contraindications:* History of previous hypersensitivity to any vaccine component.
- *Storage:* 2–8°C/35–46°F
- *Special remarks*: Following reports of deaths allegedly from this vaccine, two Indian Council of Medical Research

(ICMR)—sponsored research studies in India were suspended pending outcome of an enquiry. The vaccine was, however, neither withdrawn nor its administration suspended.

MEASLES VACCINE

Brand name: M-vac

- A live-attenuated vaccine, usually including Schwartz, Edmonston–Zagreb, Moraten, and Edmonston-B strains. The vaccines manufactured in India are formulated from Edmonston–Zagreb strain grown on human diploid cells or purified chick embryo cells.
- *Available as*: Single and multidose vials, providing at least 1,000 TCID-50/0.5 mL.
- *Indications:* Active immunization against measles.
- *Dose 0.5 mL (SC and IM)*
  - *National:* At 9–12 months. Then at 15–18 months as MMR.
  - In high-risk situations, it may well be administered earlier. In that event, it is best repeated after an interval of 6 months or so.
  - *IAP:* At 9 months, 15 months, and 4–6 years as MMR.
- *Adverse drug reactions:* Febrile reactions for a day or two from 5th to 12th postvaccination day, febrile seizures, local erythema and soreness over the injection site, malaise, headache, slight gastrointestinal upset, rhinopharyngitis; toxic shock syndrome; very infrequently, encephalitis and thrombocytopenic purpura.
- *Contraindications:* Acute febrile illness, hypersensitivity to neomycin, severe immune deficiency (both primary and secondary), immunosuppressive therapy, recent

γ-globulin administration, active untreated tuberculosis, and history of severe allergic reactions to constituents.
- *Caution:* Never administer by IV route. Observe special precaution in subjects with seizure disorder.
- *Storage:* 2–8°C/35–46°F.

MEASLES, MUMPS, AND RUBELLA VACCINE

Brand names: Tresivac and Priorix
- *Indications:* Active combined immunization against MMR
- *Dose and schedule*
  - *National:* A single injection (SC and IM) at 16–24 months of age (at least 3 months following measles vaccine).
  - *IAP:* At 9 months, 15 months, and 4–6 years.
- *AEFI:* Fever, febrile seizures, parotitis, and lymphadenitis. There is no causal relationship of MMR vaccine with autism. Same applies to the preservative for inactivated vaccines, i.e., thimerosal, which had also been incriminated for causing neurodevelopmental disorders, including autism.
- *Contraindications:* Allergy to egg protein, recent administration of immunoglobulins, congenital, or acquired immune deficiency.
- *Storage:* 2–8°C/35–46°F (preferably, top shelf of refrigerator).

INACTIVATED POLIO VACCINE

Salk strain type, killed (inactivated) vaccine, providing 95–100 protective efficacy.

Brand names: Polprotec and Imovax
- *Available as:* As such and in combination with other vaccines.

- *Indications:* Now that eradication of polio is round the corner, over and above the oral polio vaccine (OPV), the enhanced IPV has been introduced in the IAP immunization schedule. In addition to routine immunization against polio, it is especially indicated in immunocompromised children and for boosting the eradication endeavors.
- *Dosage:* 0.5 mL (SC and IM) at 6, 10, and 14 weeks followed by IPV at 16–18 months and 4–6 years.
- *Adverse drug reactions:* No significant side-effects recorded so far.
- *Contraindication:* Severe hypersensitivity.
- *Storage:* 2–8°C/35–46°F.

ORAL POLIO VACCINE

Sabin strain type and live-attenuated vaccine that also indices humoral immunity, providing per dose efficacy of 30% worldwide and 10–15% in India. A highly heat-sensitive vaccine, having shelf-life of 6 months at 2–8°C. At –20°C, it zooms to 2 years. It is just 1–3 days at room temperature.

Brand names: Bromide and Biopolio
- *Indication:* Protection against poliomyelitis
- *Dose and schedule:* Two to three drops directly into child's mouth

  National: At birth (zero dose), 6, 10, and 14 weeks. Along with the 14 weeks dose of OPV, an IPV dose is also given. Following these four primary doses, booster doses are administered at 15–18 months and 5th year. Thus, a total of six doses are recommended. Pulse polio doses are in addition to these basic doses.

  IAP: At birth OPV (zero dose). Booster at 6 months, 9 months, 15–18 months, and 5th year. In between, at 6th, 10th, and 14th week, IPV is given.

- *AEFIs:* Practically no side effects are seen; rarely vaccine-associated paralytic poliomyelitis (VAPP).
- *Contraindications:* Severe vomiting and diarrhea; immunodeficiency.
- *Storage:* Vaccine carrier for transport to outreach center: 2–8°C/35–46°F.
- *Clinical level:* Freezer (–5 to –15°C). State and district levels: –20°C. protected from light.

PNEUMOCOCCAL POLYSACCHARIDE VACCINE

Brand names: Pneumo-23 and Pneumovax-23

- Unlike PCV-7, PCV-10, and PCV-13, this is an unconjugated vaccine, containing 23 serotypes that must not be administered <2 years of age on account of its immunogenicity. Furthermore, it is T-cell independent, has low immunologic memory, and fails to reduce nasopharyngeal carriage, and provides herd immunity.
- *Indications:* In children >2 years with high risk of serious pneumococcal infections (nephrotic syndrome, asplenia, splenectomy, and immunocompromised states), sickle-cell anemia, chronic renal failure, and cerebrospinal fluid (CSF) rhinorrhea. **Box 2** lists the detailed high-risk situations.
- *Dose:* 0.5 mL (SC and IM) as a single dose. Maximum two lifetime doses. Immunologic hypersensitivity may occur following repeated doses.
- *AEFIs:* Quite safe except for local injection site reactions, low-grade fever, irritability, drowsiness, relapse of stabilized idiopathic thrombocytopenic purpura (ITP), purpura; rarely skin rash, arthralgia, myalgia, headache, fatigue; Guillain-Barré syndrome (GBS); arthus-like reactions on revaccination.

BOX 2: High-risk situations for pneumococcal disease/vaccine.

- Immunodeficiency (including congenital immunodeficiency)
- Immunosuppressive therapy
- *Splenic:* A splenemia, hyposplenemia, and autosplenectomy (sickle-cell disease)
- Chronic cardiac disease
- Chronic pulmonary disease (but not asthma unless on high dose steroids)
- Chronic liver disease
- *Chronic renal disease:* Nephrotic syndrome and chronic renal failure
- Diabetes insipidus
- *Miscellaneous:* Cerebrospinal fistula, cerebrospinal fluid rhinorrhea, and cochlear implants

- *Cautions:* Severe cardiopulmonary disease, acute febrile illness; reduced protection in immunocompromised subjects; monitor respiratory function, especially in preterm infants.
- *Storage:* 2–8°C/35–46°F.

PNEUMOCOCCAL CONJUGATE VACCINE

Brand names: Prevenar-7 and Prevenar-13

- *Available as:* Single dose 0.5 mL prefilled syringes.
- *Dose and schedule:* 0.5 mL (IM and SC) at 6, 10, and 14 weeks followed by a booster at 15–18 months.
- *AEFIs:* Local painful erythema and induration, fever, and malaise. It is quite safe unlike nonconjugate vaccine.
- *Contraindications:* Hypersensitivity to any component of the vaccine.
- *Storage:* 2–8°C/35–46°F. It must never be freezed.

TETANUS TOXOID

According to current recommendations, its better substitute is tetanus-reduced dose diphtheria toxoid (Td) or tetanus-reduced dose diphtheria and acellular pertussis vaccine (Tdap) which provides better and more comprehensive protection.

Brand names: Tetanus toxoid and BETT
- *Available as:* 0.5 mL ampule, 10 and 20 dose vials; 0.5 mL providing 40 Lf units (constituting one dose).
- *Indication:* Active immunization against tetanus.
- *Dose:* 0.5 mL (IM) every 10 years if already immunized, having completed primary and booster vaccination with triple vaccine (DTwP or DTaP).
- Each and every pregnant woman, not previously immunized, must receive two doses of TT (preferably Td) at an interval of 1 month, the second dose at least 2 weeks prior to delivery. For subsequent pregnancy within next 5 years, a single dose suffices.
- *AEFIs:* Mild local reaction with painful swelling at the injection site.
- *Contraindications:* Acute febrile illness, outbreak of poliomyelitis.
- *Storage:* 2–8°C/35–46°F.

TETANUS TOXOID-REDUCED DOSE DIPHTHERIA TOXOID

This is a preferred substitute for TT.
- *Available as:* 0.5 mL ampule, 10, and 20 dose vials; 0.5 mL providing 40 Lf units (constituting one dose).
- *Indication*: Active immunization against tetanus.

- *Dose:* 0.5 mL (IM) every 10 years if already immunized, having completed primary and booster vaccination with triple vaccine (DTwP or DTaP).
- Each and every pregnant woman, not previously immunized, must receive two doses of TT (preferably Td) at an interval of 1 month, the second dose at least 2 weeks prior to delivery. For subsequent pregnancy within next 5 years, a single dose suffices.
- *AEFIs:* Mild local reaction with painful swelling at the injection site.
- *Contraindications:* Acute febrile illness, outbreak of poliomyelitis.
- *Storage:* 2–8°C/35–46°F.

ROTAVIRUS VACCINE

Rotavirus has earned the designation "democratic virus" since it infects children globally regardless of the socioeconomic status of the country. Rotavirus vaccine is a live-attenuated vaccine. IAP recommends it after one-to-one discussion with parents at/or >6 weeks of age. Two types are available:
1. A monovalent-attenuated human rotavirus vaccine (Rotarix)
2. Human bovine reassortant vaccine (RotaTeq)
   Their efficacy and safety profiles are similar.

Brand names: Human—Rotarix; Bovine—RotaTeq
- *Indication:* Prevention of rotavirus diarrhea.
- *Available as:*
  - *Rotarix:* Lyophilized vaccine needing reconstitution with liquid diluents.
  - *RotaTeq:* Liquid virus mixed with buffer, needing no reconstitution.

Chapter 55: Conventional and New Vaccines for Routine Use

- *Dose:* Starting at >6 weeks, two to three doses (PO) depending on the brand (Rota: 2 and RotaTeq: 3). The gap between two doses should be about 4–8 weeks.
- *AEFIs:* Minor reactions, including pain and redness at the injection site.
- *Contraindications:* Severe immunocompromised state, previous history of intussusception.
- *Caution*: Avoid in an acute illness, especially diarrhea/gastroenteritis. Complete the schedule by 24 weeks, never administer it after 24 weeks of age.
- *Storage:* 2–8°C.
- *Special remarks:* The vaccine was temporarily withdrawn following alleged occurrence of intussusception following it.

RUBELLA VACCINE

A live-attenuated vaccine, derived from RA 27/3 strain grown in human diploid/chick-embryo cell cultures. It is usually recommended as a part of MMR vaccine which also provided measles and mumps vaccine, thereby providing triple protection.

Brand name: R-Vac

- *Available as:* Freeze-dried with sterile diluents for reconstitution. Needs to be used within 6 hours of reconstitution.
- *Indications*: Prevention of maternal rubella through active immunization against rubella (a potential cause of congenital rubella syndrome) in: (i) girls between 1 year and puberty, (ii) susceptible females of child-bearing age (seronegative) provided that they are not already pregnant and conception is unlikely in the subsequent 2 months.

- *Dose:* 0.5 mL (deep SC and IM) as a single administration. In 95% cases, it provides lifelong immunity.
- *AEFIs:* Local erythema and soreness at the injection site, mild rubella-like illness with skin rash, pharyngitis, pyrexia, lymphadenitis, arthralgia, and arthritis; rarely thrombocytopenia, neuropathy, and paresthesia; rarely encephalitis.
- *Drug interaction:* Live vaccines and tuberculin reaction.
- *Contraindications:* Severe immunocompromised states and pregnancy.
- *Cautions:*
  - Availability of epinephrine injection
  - Defer it for at least 3 months after blood transfusion/immune serum globulin.
  - Defer for at least 1 month before/after other live virus vaccines (except OPV, measles, and mumps).
  - Defer pregnancy for 3 months after the rubella vaccine.
- *Storage:* 2–8°C/35–46°F (preferably upper shelf of the refrigerator).

TYPHOID VACCINES

Vi Capsular Polysaccharide Typhoid Vaccine

Brand names: Typherix, Typhim Vi, Typhobar, and Biotyph

- *Indication:* Active immunization from 2 years onward. It is not immunogenic in <2 years of age.
- *Dose:* 0.5 mL (25 µg ViCPS antigen) administered as a single IM and SC dose; to be repeated every 3 years for continuity of protection.
- *AEFIs:* Mild local pain and swelling, pyrexia, and headache.
- *Contraindication:* Hypersensitivity and acute severe febrile illness.

- *Precaution*: Availability of facility to handle a severe anaphylactic reaction, i.e., epinephrine injection 1:1,000.
- *Storage*: 2–8°C/35–46°F (preferably middle shelf of refrigerator).

Vi Conjugate Typhoid Vaccine

Brand names: Peda-Typh, Typbar-TCV

- In this, vaccine conjugation is with protein carrier, tetanus toxoid, to induce T-cell dependent immune response and immunogenicity.
- *Available as:* Freeze-dried with sterile diluents for reconstitution. Needs to be used within 6 hours of reconstitution.
- *Indications:* Active immunization from 3 months onward.
- *Dose:* Primary at 9–12 months. Booster at 2 years. Additionally, polysaccharide vaccine should be given at every 3 years.
- *AEFIs*: Mild local pain, erythema, induration, and mild fever in first 48 hours.
- *Contraindication:* Hypersensitivity to any component
- *Caution:* Availability of facility to handle a severe anaphylactic reaction, i.e., epinephrine injection 1:1,000.
- *Storage*: 2–8°C/35–46°F (preferably middle shelf of refrigerator).

Oral Typhoid Vaccine

This is an oral live-attenuated Ty21a vaccine, recommended for children of 6 years of age and above. Now, it is not available in India. A liquid form of the vaccine is in pipeline.

Brand name: Typhoral

- *Indication:* Active immunization in subjects over 6 years of age.

- *Dose:* One capsule on day 1, 3, and 5 to be taken 1 hour before meal, and given every 3 years.
- *AEFIs:* Slight gastrointestinal upset, rash, and pyrexia.
- *Contraindication:* Acute febrile illness, gastrointestinal tract (GIT) infection, immunodeficiency, immunosuppressant drugs, antimitotics, certain antibiotics, and sulfa active against *Salmonella*; pregnancy.
- *Storage:* 2–8°C/35–46°F; protect from light.

TETANUS, LOW-DOSE DIPHTHERIA VACCINE

- *Indications:*
  - As a replacement for TT in all situations.
  - As a replacement for DPT/DT >7 years of age when catch-up vaccination is needed. DT/DTP must not be employed in children >7 years of age on account of reactogenicity to high dose of diphtheria and pertussis components.
- *Dose:* 0.5 mL (IM).
- *AEFIs:* Local injection site reactions.
- *Storage:* 2–8°C/35–46°F.
- *Remarks:* TDAP, though expensive, is a superior replacement for TD since it provides more comprehensive protection.

TETANUS, LOW-DOSE DIPHTHERIA AND PERTUSSIS VACCINE

Brand name: Boostrix

- *Indications:*
  - Children who have received all three primary and two booster doses of DTP, it may be given at 10–12 years of age.

Chapter 55: Conventional and New Vaccines for Routine Use

- Children >7 years of age who missed the second booster of DTP.
- Children >7 years who failed to complete primary immunization with DTP.
- As a better option to TT/TD in wound management >10 years.

- *Dose:* 0.5 mL (IM).
- *AEFIs:* Local injection site reactions; rarely fever, headache, and fatigue.
- *Contraindications:* Allergic reactions to its component(s), history of encephalopathy secondary to pertussis vaccine.
- *Storage:* 2–8°C/35–46°F.

VARICELLA VACCINE

A lyophilized vaccine providing live-attenuated Oka strains of *Varicella zoster* virus.

Brand names: Varilrix, Okavax, and Varipox

- *Available as:* Subcutaneous (SC) injection 0.5 mL vial (constituting one dose). The diluent supplied in a separate ampule has to be added to the vial to dissolve the somewhat pink-colored pellet. The entire contents of the vial constitute a single dose.
- *Indications:* Active immunization against chickenpox (varicella) in healthy subjects over 1 year of age; susceptible healthy contacts of chickenpox patients within 3 days of exposure; medical and paramedical personnel who are likely to be in close contact of chickenpox patients; high-risk groups **(Box 3)**.
- *Dose:* 0.5 mL (SC), lateral aspect of upper arm, at 15 months followed by a booster at 18-24 months.

BOX 3: High-risk groups needing chickenpox vaccine.

- Humoral immunodeficiencies
- HIV, provided CD4 counts are >15%
- Leukemia, provided in remission and off chemotherapy for a minimum of 3–6 months
- Long-term salicylate therapy
- Long-term steroid therapy
- Chronic lung/heart disease
- Adolescents who had not suffered from varicella in the past, provided that they are seronegative
- Adolescents who are seronegative and are inmates of or working in an institutional set-up
- Postexposure prophylaxis in susceptible healthy nonpregnant contacts, preferably within 3 days of exposure (efficiency 90%) and potentially up to 5 days of exposure (efficiency 70% and 100% against severe disease)

- *AEFIs:* Infrequently, anaphylaxis, local reactions at the injection site, headache, GI upset, pyrexia, fatigue, and paresthesia.
- *Drug interactions:* Other live vaccines, tuberculin skin test.
- *Contraindications:* Acute severe febrile illness, TLC <1,200/cumm, lymphocytopenia, blood dyscrasia, active untreated tuberculosis, and lactation. Poor cellular immune response, primary or acquired immunodeficiency, known systemic hypersensitivity to neomycin, and concurrent administration of pneumococcal vaccine.
- *Caution:* Make sure that alcohol or any other disinfecting agent is totally evaporated from the skin before the injection is actually given; never administer intradermally; do not give within 3 months of blood transfusion or immunoglobulin.

- *Storage:* 2–8°C/35–46°F (preferably, in lower shelf of refrigerator; protect from light).

VACCINES UNDER SPECIAL CIRCUMSTANCES

Cholera Vaccine

Two types of safe and effective oral cholera vaccines are available. Both are whole-cell killed vaccines, one with a recombinant B-subunit, the other without. Both have sustained protection of over 50% lasting for 2 years in endemic settings.

Brand names: Shanchol and Dukoral

- *Available as*: Dukoral is WHO prequalified and licensed in over 60 countries. Dukoral has been shown to provide short-term protection of 85–90% against *V. cholerae* O1 among all age groups at 4–6 months following immunization.
- Shanchol provides relatively long-term protection against *V. cholerae* O1 and O139 in children under 5 years of age. WHO prequalification is, however, pending for this vaccine.
- *Dose*: Both vaccines are administered in two doses given between 7 days and 6 weeks apart. The vaccine with the B-subunit (Dukoral) is given in 150 mL of safe water.
- *AEFIs:* None.
- *Special remarks:* According to the WHO recommendations, immunization with currently available cholera vaccines should be used in conjunction with the usually recommended control measures.
- In areas where cholera is endemic as well as in areas at risk of outbreaks.
- Vaccines provide a short-term protection. Long-term activities like improving water and sanitation have got to be put in place.

- Vaccination should target vulnerable populations living in high-risk areas and should not disrupt the provision of other interventions to control or prevent cholera epidemics. The WHO three-step decision-making tool aims at guiding health authorities in deciding whether to use cholera vaccines in complex emergency settings.

INFLUENZA VIRUS VACCINES

Trivalent Influenza Vaccine

A killed and split-product vaccine containing 15 µg each of the WHO-recommended two influenza A strains and one influenza B strain [the seasonal vaccine contains novel H1N1 strain (recent pandemic strain) rather than the old H1N1 strain] provides 80% efficacy; licensed for use >6 months of age.

Brand names: Vaxigrip, Influvac, Fluarix, and Agripaal

- *Available as:* Single dose vial, prefilled syringe or ampule; multidose vial.
- *Indications:* Protection against influenza virus infection, especially in subjects with underlying chronic cardiac or bronchopulmonary disease, immunocompromised state, diabetes, chronic renal insufficiency, or sickle-cell anemia.
- *Dose:* This is detailed in **Table 1**.
- *AEFIs:* Local pain, erythema and induration at the injection site, pyrexia, and malaise; rarely, anaphylaxis; and very rarely GBS.
- *Contraindication:* Hypersensitivity to its components.
- *Caution:* Avoid in children with history of GBS and severe egg allergy.
- *Storage:* 2–80°C (35–46°F).

TABLE 1: Dose of trivalent influenza vaccine (TIV) for protection against influenza.

Age group	Dose	Number of doses
6–35 months	0.25 mL (SC and IM)	1 or 2*
3–8 years	0.5 mL (SC and IM)	1 or 2*
≥9 years	0.5 mL (SC and IM)	1

*Second dose after 4–6 weeks is for subjects who have not received the vaccine earlier.
(IM: intramuscular; SC: subcutaneous)

Live-attenuated Influenza Vaccine

Live-attenuated reassortants of the three WHO-recommended strains (two influenza A and one influenza B); licensed for use after 2 years of age; superior efficacy than inactivated vaccine (TIV).

Brand name: FluMist

- *Available as:* Prefilled, single-use sprayer containing 0.2 mL of vaccine.
- *Dose:* As a nasal spray. Approximately, 0.1 mL (i.e., half of the total sprayer contents) is sprayed into one nostril while the recipient is in the upright position. An attached dose-divider clip is removed from the sprayer to administer the second half of the dose into the other nostril.
- *AEFIs:* Mild fever, rhinorrhea, nasal congestion, sore throat, etc., which perhaps result from effects of intranasal vaccine administration or local viral replication.
- *Contraindications:* Children <2 years of age.
- *Cautions:*
  - Avoid in children with history of hypersensitivity to egg and GBS.

- Vaccine prepared for a previous influenza season should not be administered to provide protection for any subsequent season.
- *Storage:* 2–8°C/35–46°F.

RABIES VACCINE

The earlier "nerve tissue vaccine" with poor efficacy and serious adverse (neuroparalytic) reactions are no longer in use. The modern tissue culture vaccines (MTCVs) include:

- *Purified chick embryo cell vaccine (PCECV):* Rabipur
- *Human diploid cell vaccine (HDCV):* Rabivax
- *Purified vero cell vaccine (PVRV):* Abhayrab
- *Purified duck embryo vaccine (PDEV):* Vaxirab

As a rule, all cases of rabies exposure belonging to Category III (transdermal bites, single or multiple, contamination of mucous membrane with saliva or exposure to a bat) need to be administered rabies immunoglobulin (RIG):

- Human rabies immunoglobulin (HRIG) which is slightly superior with least anaphylaxis risk but is expensive.
  Or
- Equine rabies immunoglobulin (ERIG) which is equally effective, less expensive but carries some risk of anaphylaxis.

Purified Chick Embryo Cell Vaccine

Brand name: Rabipur

- *Indications:* Protection against rabies in cases of bite by a dog suspected of suffering from rabies (postexposure) and prophylactic vaccination against rabies before exposure.
- *Dose:* For postexposure, full course of six injections (1 mL each), one each on 0 day (the day of first injection, not

necessarily the day of dog bite), 3rd day, 7th day, 14th day, 30th day, and 90th day (IM and SC). In case of antirabies treatment is started immediately with cleansing of bitten area with soap and water and administration of antirabies serum. Sixth injection may well be missed.

For prophylaxis, full course of three injections (1 mL each) on 0 (first) day, 28th day, and 56th day or 0 day, 7th day and 21st day in urgent situations (IM and SC).

- *AEFIs:* Gastrointestinal upset, painful injection site, and lymphadenopathy.
- *Contraindication:* Hypersensitivity.

Vero Cell Vaccine

Brand name: Verorab

See details provided for PCEC vaccine.

Human Diploid Cell Vaccine

Brand name: Rabivac

- *Indication:* Protection against rabies in cases of bite by a dog suspected of suffering from rabies (postexposure) and prophylactic vaccination against rabies before exposure.
- *Dose:* For postexposure, full course of six injections (1 mL each), one each on 0 day (the day of first injection, not necessarily the day of dog bite), 3rd day, 7th day, 14th day, 30th day, and 90th day (IM and SC). In case antirabies treatment is started immediately with cleansing of bitten area with soap and water and administration of antirabies serum. Sixth injection may well be missed.

For prophylaxis, full course of four injections (1 mL each) on 0, 7th, 21st, and 28th day (IM and SC).

- *AEFIs:* GI upset, painful injection site, and lymphadenopathy.
- *Contraindication:* Hypersensitivity.
- *Storage:* 2–8°C
- *Special remarks:* The active principle, efficacy, safety, and dosage of the three vaccines remain by and large same. Cost wise, however, whereas HDCV is priced around ₹ 950/dose, PCEC and Verorab are priced at ₹ 370/dose.

JAPANESE ENCEPHALITIS VACCINE

Brand name: JENVAC

- *Available as:*
  - Cell culture derived live SA-14-14-2 vaccine (most suitable in Indian settings)
  - Cell culture derived inactivated vaccine
  - Mouse brain-derived inactivated JE vaccine
- *Indication:* Single most important control measure against Japanese encephalitis in rural belts of endemic areas
- *Dose:*
  - *Live-attenuated vaccine:* 0.5 mL (SC) for all ages; two doses, 4 weeks apart.
  - *Formalin-inactivated mouse brain or hamster kidney vaccine*: Two doses, 1 mL each (0.5 mL for <3 years age) and administered at an interval of 7–14 days (SC). After 6–12 months, a third dose is given. Every 3–4 years, a booster is needed.
- *AEFIs:* No serious adverse effects.
- *Contraindications:* JE vaccine is contraindicated in high fever, diabetes mellitus, liver and heart disease, and immunodeficiency.
- *Storage:* 2–8°C/35–46°F.

- *Special remark:* JENVAC is India's first fully indigenous vaccine. It is based on Indian strain.

MENINGOCOCCAL VACCINE

Though both unconjugated and conjugated vaccines are available, conjugated vaccines should be preferred. These are either bivalent (A + C) or quadrivalent (A, C, Y, and W135).

Brand names: MPSV-A + C + Y + W135: Quadri Meningo (Biomed), Mencevax (GSK) A + C: Biomaigo (Biomed).

- *Available as*: Single dose (0.5 mL), 10 and 50 dose vials, providing 50 µg each of *N. meningitidis* group A and group C/unit (0.5 mL).
- *Indication:* Active immunization against *Neisseria meningitidis (group A and C)* infection which may cause serious illness like meningitis or septicemia. Precise indications as per IAP are listed in **Box 4**.

The Centers for Disease Control and Prevention (CDC) Advisory Committee on Immunization Practices (ACIP) has provided revised recommendations for conjugate meningococcal vaccine **(Box 5)**, approving two new recommendations, namely:

1. Routine vaccination of adolescents, preferably at age 11 or 12 years, with a booster dose at age 16 years.
2. A two-dose primary series administered 2 months apart for persons aged 2 through 54 years with persistent complement component deficiency (e.g., C5–C9, properdin, factor H, or factor D) and functional or anatomic asplenia, and for adolescents with human immunodeficiency virus (HIV) infection.
   - *Dose*: Dose: 0.5 mL (SC, IM) at 9 and 12 months.
   - *AEFIs:* Local redness and swelling, and pyrexia.

BOX 4: Indications of meningococcal vaccine.

- During disease outbreaks if caused by serogroups included in the vaccine. Mass chemoprophylaxis is generally not recommended for control of mass outbreaks due to cost, implementation problems, adverse reactions, and drug resistance
- Children with terminal complement component deficiencies
- Children with functional/anatomical asplenemia/hyposplenemia Ideally, vaccine should be given 2 weeks before splenectomy
- Laboratory personnel and healthcare workers who are exposed routinely to *N. meningitidis* in solutions that may be aerosolized should be considered for vaccination
- Haj pilgrims to Saudi Arabia. This is a mandatory vaccine for them
- Travelers to African meningitis belt, particularly between December and June and especially if there is an ongoing epidemic
- As an adjunct to chemoprophylaxis in close contacts of patients with meningococcal disease
- Students grouping for study abroad. It is mandatory for most universities in the United States

- *Contraindication:* Acute febrile illness and evolving disease
- *Caution*: Avoid in children <2 years.
- *Storage*: 2–8°C (35–46°F).

YELLOW FEVER VACCINE

A live-attenuated vaccine derived from 17D strain of the virus grown in chick embryo cells.

Brand name: Stamnil

- *Indication:* Prophylaxis against yellow fever, influenza-like or severe hepatitis-like illness, caused by the virus 17D with the vector, *Aedes aegypti,* endemic in African countries

BOX 5: New recommendation of Advisory Committee on Immunization Practices (ACIP) concerning meningococcal vaccine.

- Specific recommendations for meningococcal conjugate vaccine by risk group are as follows:
  - For persons 11–18 years old, the primary series should be one dose, preferably at age 11 or 12 years. The booster dose should be at the age of 16 years if the primary dose was at age 11 or 12 years, and at ages 16–18 years if the primary dose was at ages 13–15 years. If the primary dose was on or after age 16 years, no booster is needed
  - For HIV-infected persons of 11–18 years old, the primary series should be two doses, 2 months apart. The booster dose should be at the age of 16 years if the primary dose was at age 11 or 12 years, and at ages 16–18 years if the primary dose was at ages 13–15 years. If the primary dose was on or after age of 16 years, no booster is needed
  - For persons 2–55 years old with persistent complement component deficiency or functional or anatomic asplenia, the primary series should be two doses, 2 months apart, and the booster dose every 5 years. If a one-dose primary series was administered, the booster dose should be given at the earliest opportunity, then at every 5 years
  - For persons 2–55 years old with a prolonged increased risk for exposure, the primary series should be one dose. The booster dose should be given after 3 years for persons 2–6 years old, and after 5 years for persons 7 years or older, if the person remains at increased risk

(both sub-Saharan—33 and South American—11). Since this vector is common in India and travelers from endemic areas keep visiting India, possibility of its occurrence any time in future cannot be ruled out.
- International Health Regulations make it a mandatory vaccine for travelers to endemic areas.

- *Available as*: Freeze-dried, single, or multi-dose vials with sterilize saline as diluents. In India, it is available at select government-controlled centers.
- *Dose:* 0.5 mL (SC) over anterolateral aspect of thigh or lateral aspect of upper arm.
- *AEFIs:* Usually local injection site problems; rarely neuropathy (encephalitis, GBS, Bell palsy, and acute disseminated encephalomyelitis), yellow fever-associated viscerotropic disease (YEL-AVD).
- *Contraindications:* Age <6 months, thymus disease, severely immunocompromised state (say, HIV with CD4 count <15% of age-related cut-off), and serious egg allergy.
- *Caution:* Whereas it is contraindicated <6 months, it is best avoided in 6–9 months age group. Hence, minimal recommended age is 9 months.
- *Storage*: 2–8°C.

Chapter 56: Combination Vaccines

INTRODUCTION

A combination vaccine is defined as a vaccine that aims at providing protection against a number of infectious diseases through at least two antigens in a single preparation. Such a vaccine contains several immunogens in a single shot for protection against quite a few infectious diseases.

Understandably, its efficacy, immunogenicity, and safety profile should be comparable to the independently administered vaccines.

Usually, the term, combination vaccines, is employed for vaccines providing protection against multiple pathogens, e.g., diphtheria, tetanus, and pertussis (DTP) [both DTwP (diphtheria and tetanus toxoids and whole-cell pertussis) and DTaP (diphtheria, tetanus, and pertussis)], measles, mumps, and rubella (MMR), DTwP + *Haemophilus influenzae* type b (Hib), DTaP + Hib, DTwP + hepatitis B (Hep B), etc.

However, many consider single pathogen vaccines such as oral polio vaccine (OPV), inactivated polio vaccine (IPV), influenza, pneumococcal, etc. also combination vaccines since they contain various antigens or serotypes of pathogens.

The first combination vaccine was DTP that was developed as far back as 1943 and licensed in 1948. The triple influenza vaccine, developed in 1944, was licensed in 1945. Now, we have a number of combination vaccines. Some of these are listed in **Box 1**.

BOX 1: Some important combination vaccines.

- *DTP:* Diphtheria, tetanus, and pertussis
- *MMR:* Measles, mumps, and rubella
- *Pentavalent:* Diphtheria, pertussis, and tetanus (DPT) + *Haemophilus influenzae* type b (Hib) + inactivated polio virus (IPV)
- *Hexavalent:* Diphtheria, pertussis, tetanus (DPT) + Hep B + IPV + Hib

BENEFITS

Too many vaccines, predominantly injections, especially with inclusion of newer vaccines in the schedule, are a burden on the child and also the family. Too many individual vaccines also mean several visits. Any medical modality demanding several visits suffers from the malady of poor compliance and, at times, falls flat. This backdrop has led to the development of combination vaccines that reduce the number of pricks and the visits.

The earliest combination vaccine to become available was DPT/DTP in 1945 followed by MMR in 1971. Various tetravalent and pentavalent vaccines are built up around DTP.

Consumer-related Benefits

- Reduction in number of pricks
- Reduction in number of visits to the health center
- Reduction in cost of administering and stocking vaccines
- Improved compliance, resulting in fall in incidence of missed vaccinations
- Facilitation in the introduction of new vaccines in the immunization schedule

Health Department/Facility-related Benefits

- Reduction in pressure on cold chain

- Reduction in paperwork
- Enhanced compliance, contributing to success of immunization program
- Reduced vaccination visits
- Economic gains

Advantages of combination vaccines are overwhelming notwithstanding the slight hike in adverse events, justifying their enhanced use.

ADVERSE EVENTS

A marginal increase in incidence of minor adverse events following immunization (AEFI) may occur following a combination vaccine.

Adverse effects, if any, are on similar lines as in case of independently administered vaccines though with somewhat higher frequency than in case of the latter.

Adverse effects include febrile seizures the risk of seizures being higher on the day of vaccination.

Compared to an increase in adverse events, advantages of combination vaccines are overwhelming, overweighing the slight hike in adverse events, and justifying their enhanced use.

RECOMMENDATIONS IN INDIA

Available combination vaccines are at par with the independently administered vaccines as far as immunogenicity, efficacy, and safety profiles are concerned, except for a marginal increase in minor adverse effects. Vigilance and compliance to instructions with regard to mixing of different vaccines in the same syringe by the healthcare professionals in accordance with the manufacturer's instructions are warranted.

PRECAUTIONS AND WARNINGS

- Never prepare your own combination vaccine by mixing two or three vaccines. Mixing is permitted only in case of combination vaccines specifically packed for this purpose. Manufacturer's instructions for mixing need to be strictly followed.
- In the nomenclature, the hyphen (-) is intended to indicate that the antigens are mixed together by the manufacturer before the product is sold. The forward slash (/) indicates that the two products are to be reconstituted by the user in compliance with the manufacturer's instructions.

Immunization Schedules in India

INTRODUCTION

The Universal Immunization Program (UIP) has two huge achievements on the card in India, namely elimination of polio in 2014 and elimination of maternal and neonatal tetanus in 2015. Currently, we have two immunization schedules that are followed in India:
1. Indian Academy of Pediatrics (IAP) immunization schedule
2. National immunization schedule.

INDIAN ACADEMY OF PEDIATRICS IMMUNIZATION SCHEDULE

Tables 1 and 2 present the Indian Academy of Pediatrics (IAP) immunization schedule.
- HPV2 is no longer available in India.
- HPV4 available as Gardasil by MSD licensed for use only in females in India.
- HPV4 available as Cervavax by the Serum Institute of India (SII) licensed for use in females and males aged 9–26 years and as two doses 0–6 months for 9–14 years and three doses as 0-2-6 months for 15–26 years old.
- HPV-9 available as Gardasil-9 licensed for use in females aged 9–26 years and males aged 9–16 years and three doses 0–2–6 months at any age in India.

TABLE 1: Current Indian Academy of Pediatrics (IAP) immunization.

Vaccine	Birth	6 w	10 w	14 w	6 m	7 m	9 m	12 m	13 m	15 m	16–18 m	18–24 m	2–3 y	4–6 y	9–14 y	15–18 y
BCG	BCG															
Hepatitis B	HB-1[a]	HB-2	HB-3	HB-4[b]												
Polio	OPV	IPV-1[c]	IPV-2[c]	IPV-3[c]							IPV B1			IPV B$_2$		
DTwP/DTaP		DPT-1	DPT-2	DPT-3							DPT B1			DPT B$_2$		
Hib		Hib-1	Hib-2	Hib-3							Hib B1					
PCV		PCV-1	PCV-2	PCV-3						PCV B						
Rotavirus		RV-1	RV-2	RV-3[d]												
Influenza					Dose 1[e]	Dose 2				Annual vaccination						
MMR							Dose 1			Dose 2				Dose 3		
TCV								Dose 1				Dose 2[f]				
Hepatitis A								Dose 1				Dose 2[g]				
Varicella								Dose 1		Dose 1						
Tdap[h]/Td																
HPV															1 and 2[i]	1, 2, and 3[j]
Meningococcal[k]							Dose 1	Dose 2								
JE								Dose 1	Dose 2							
Cholera								Dose 1	Dose 2							

Contd...

Contd...

Vaccine	Birth	6w	10w	14w	6m	7m	9m	12m	13m	15m	16-18m	18-24m	2-3y	4-6y	9-14y	15-18y

Age in completed weeks/months/years

PPSV-23

Rabies

Yellow fever

☐ Recommended age ☐ Catch-up age range ☐ Vaccines in special situations

(BCG: Bacillus Calmette–Guérin; DTwP: diphtheria, tetanus, and whole cell pertussis; DTaP: diphtheria, tetanus, and pertussis; Hib: *Haemophilus influenzae* type b; HPV: human papillomavirus vaccines; IPV: injectable polio vaccine; JE: Japanese encephalitis; MMR: measles, mumps, and rubella; PCV: pneumococcal conjugate vaccines; PPSV-23: pneumococcal polysaccharide vaccine-23; TCV: typhoid conjugate vaccine; Tdap/Td: tetanus, diphtheria, and pertussis/tetanus and diphtheria)

Vaccine CME 2023, by IAP Mumbai.

[a] To be given within 24 hours after birth when this is missed, it can be administered at first contact with health facility;
[b] An extra dose of hepatitis B vaccine is permitted as part of a combination vaccine when use of this combination vaccine is necessary;
[c] IPV can be given as part of a combination vaccine.
[d] Third dose of Rota vaccine is not necessary for RV1; [e] Influenza vaccine should be started after 6 months of age. Two doses 4 weeks apart. usually in the premonsoon period. At other times of the year, the most recent available strain should be used. Annual influenza vaccination should be continued for all till 5 years of age. after the age of 3 years, this vaccine is recommended in the high-risk group only.
[f] Single dose is to be given for the live-attenuated hepatitis A vaccine. The inactivated vaccine needs two doses.
[g] Second dose of Varicella vaccine should be given 3–6 months of age after dose 1. However, it can be administered anytime 3 months after dose 1 or at 4-6 years.
[h] Tdap should not be administered as the second booster of DPT at 4–6 years. For delayed second booster, Tdap can be given after 7 years of age. A dose of Tdap is necessary at 10–12 years, irrespective of previous Tdap administration. If Tdap is unavailable/unaffordable, it can be substituted with Td;
[i] Before 14 completed years), HPV vaccines are recommended as a second-dose schedule, 6 months apart;
[j] From 15th year onward and the immunocompromised subjects at all ages. HPV vaccines are recommended as a third-dose schedule: 0–1–6 (HPV2) or 0–2–6 (HPV4).
[k] Menactra is approved in a second-dose schedule between 9 and 23 months. Minimum interval between two doses should be 3 months. Menveo is recommended as a single-dose schedule after 2 years of age.

TABLE 2: Indian Academy of Pediatrics (IAP) immunization timetable: IAP vaccines for routine recommended vaccines for routine use.

Age	Vaccine	Comments
Birth	BCG	BCG: Before discharge
	OPV	OPV: As soon as possible after birth
	Hepatitis B-I (BD)	Hepatitis B should be administered within 24 hours of birth
6 weeks	DTwP and DTaP-1 IPV-1 Hib-1 Hepatitis B-2 Rotavirus-1 PCV-1	• DTwP or DtaP may be administered in primary immunization • IPV: 6–10–14 weeks is the recommended schedule. If IPV, as part of a hexavalent combination vaccine is unaffordable, the infant should be sent to a government facility for primary immunization as per UIP schedule
10 weeks	DTwP and DTaP-2 IPV-2 Hib-2 Hepatitis B-3 Rotavirus-2 PCV-2	RV1: Two-dose schedule: All other rotavirus brands: three-dose schedule
14 weeks	DTwP and DTaP-3 IPV-3 Hib-3	An additional fourth dose of hepatitis B vaccine is safe and is permitted as a component of a combination vaccine
6 months	Hepatitis B-4 Rotavirus-3 PCV-3	

Contd...

Contd...

Age	Vaccine	Comments
	Influenza (IIV)-I	Uniform dose of 0.5 mL for DCGI approved brands
7 months	Influenza (IIV)-2	To be repeated every year in premonsoon period till 5 years of age
6–9 months	Typhoid conjugate vaccine	As of available data, there is no recommendation for a booster dose
9 months	MMR-1	
12 months	Hepatitis A	Single dose for live-attenuated vaccine
15 months	MMR-2, varicella-1, PCV booster	
16–18 months	DTwP/DTaP-B1, Hib-BI, and IPV-B1	
18–19 months	Hepatitis A-2, varicella-2	Only for inactivated hepatitis A vaccine
4–6 years	DTwP/DTaP-B2, IPV-B2, and MMR-3	

10–12 years	Tdap and HPV	Tdap is to be administered even if it has been administered earlier (as DTP-B2)
		• HPV:
		  – 9–14-year-old girls: 9vHPV and 4vHPV are recommended in two-dose series (0–6 m)
		  – 9–14-year-old boys: HPV9 is recommended in a two-dose schedule of 0–6 months

Contd...

Contd...

Age	Vaccine	Comments
		– 5–45 years: 4vHPV (0–2–6 m) is recommended in a three-dose series
		– 15–26 years: 9vHPV is recommended in a three-dose schedule of 0–2–6 months

(BCG: bacillus Calmette–Guérin; DCGI: Drugs Controller General of India; DPT: diphtheria, pertussis, and tetanus; DTap: diphtheria, tetanus, and pertussis; DTwP: diphtheria, tetanus, and whole cell pertussis; HPV: human papilloma virus; IPV: injectable polio vaccine; MMR: measles, mumps, and rubella; OPV: oral poliovirus vaccines; PCV: pneumococcal conjugate vaccine; Tdap: tetanus, diphtheria toxoids, and acellular pertussis; UIP: Universal Immunization Program)

India's National Immunization Schedule

Immunization is provided free of cost against 12 vaccines preventable diseases as follows:

- *Nationally against nine diseases:* Diphtheria, pertussis, tetanus, polio, measles, rubella, severe form of childhood tuberculosis, hepatitis b, meningitis, and pneumonia caused by *Haemophilus influenza* type B.
- *Subnationally against three diseases:* Rotavirus diarrhea, pneumococcal pneumonia, and Japanese encephalitis. Whereas, rotavirus vaccine and pneumococcal conjugate vaccine (PCV) are in process of expansion. Japanese encephalitis (JE) vaccine is available in endemic belts only.

Table 3 presents national immunization schedule.

TABLE 3: National immunization schedule.

Age	Vaccines given
Birth	Bacillus Calmette–Guérin (BCG), oral polio vaccine (OPV)-O dose, and hepatitis B birth dose
6 weeks	OPV-1, pentavalent-1, rotavirus vaccine (RVV)-I, fractional dose of inactivated polio vaccine (fIPV)-I, and pneumococcal conjugate vaccine (PCV)-I*
10 weeks	OPV-2, pentavalent-2, and RVV-2
14 weeks	OPV-3, pentavalent-3, fIPV-2, RVV-3, and PCV-2*
9–12 months	Measles and rubella (MR)-I, *JE-1,*** *PCV-booster**
16–24 months	MR-2, JE-2,** diphtheria, pertussis, and tetanus (DPT)-booster-1, OPV booster
5–6 years	DPT-booster-2
10 years	Tetanus and adult diphtheria (Td)
16 years	Td
Pregnant mother	*Td-1, Td-2, or Td-booster****

(JE: Japanese encephalitis)

*PCV in selected states/districts: Bihar, Himachal Pradesh, Madhya Pradesh, Uttar Pradesh (selected districts) and Rajasthan; in Haryana, as state initiative.
**JE in endemic districts only.
***One dose, if previously vaccinated within 3 years.

Chapter 58: Adverse Events Following Immunization

Sl. No.	Adverse events	Vaccine	Symptoms	Management
1.	Anaphylaxis	Any vaccine	• Within minutes • Acute decompensation of circulatory system • Hypovolemic shock • Laryngospasm/edema • Acute respiratory distress within 12 hours	• Adrenaline • Cardiopulmonary resuscitation • IV volume expanders or hydrocortisone • Dopamine/Dobutamine
2.	Hypotensive—hyporesponsive episode	DPT	• Acute paleness • Transient decreased level or loss of consciousness • Decrease or loss of muscle tone	• IV fluids • Dexamethasone • Oxygen
3.	Incessant cry	DPT	• Within 48–72 hours after DPT immunization • Excessive inconsolable crying	• Sedation with triclofos 50 mg/kg/24 h and give paracetamol (10–15 mg/kg/dose) • Feeding advice

Contd...

Contd...

Sl. No.	Adverse events	Vaccine	Symptoms	Management
4.	Toxic shock syndrome	Contamination of measles vaccine by *S. aureus*	• Within 30 minutes to few hours • Mounting fever • Vomiting • Diarrhea • Septic shock	• IV fluids • Antimicrobials • Cloxacillin 50–100 mg/kg/24 h • Steroids • Antipyretics • Supportive therapy
5.	Lymphadenitis	BCG	• Within 2–6 months • Firm to soft axillary lymphadenitis • 1.5–3 cm size with or without sinus	• If firm, no treatment • If soft and fluctuant HR 3, aspiration (if need be) • If sinus present, steroid therapy
6.	Bacterial abscess	Any vaccine	• Within 72 hours fluctuant or firm • Abscess with or without fever	• Antibiotics • Antipyretics • Drainage (if need be)
7.	Sterile abscess	DPT, DT, TT, typhoid, and HB	• By 72 hours • Minimum inflammation • No fever	Drainage (if need be)
8.	Moderate-to-severe local reaction	Any vaccine	Nonfluctuant swelling/redness 3–10 cm in size at the injection site	Paracetamol
9.	Seizure(s) with fever (rare)	DPT measles	Always generalized simple or complex	• Anticonvulsants • Antipyretics • IV fluids (if need be)

BCG: Bacillus Calmette–Guérin; DPT: diphtheria, pertussis, and tetanus toxoid; DT: diphtheria and tetanus; TT: tetanus toxoid)
Source: Gupte S. Instructive Case Studies in Pediatrics, 5th edition. New Delhi: Jaypee Brothers Medical Publishers, 2011.

Section 8

Drugs for Neutralizing Toxicity/Poisoning of Chemical Agents

59. Specific Antidotes

Specific Antidotes

Chapter 59

INTRODUCTION

Antidote (Latin *antidotum*, Greek *antidoton*—meaning "anti" and "to give") is defined as a chemical agent that counteracts or neutralizes the toxicity of a drug or poison. **Table 1** presents the salient features of antidotes against common toxic agents.

TABLE 1: Antidotes against common toxic agents.

Toxic agent	Antidote
• Amphetamine • Atropine/ Belladona/ Datura	*Chlorpromazine:* 1 mg/kg (IM and IV) *Physostigmine:* 0.5–2.0 mg (IM) *Stat:* to be repeated every half an hour, if needed. Or, *Pilocarpine:* 2–4 mg (PO); 0.25–0.5 mg (IM)
Arsenic	*BAL:* 2.5 mg/kg/dose (IM); first day six doses, second day four doses, and third day two doses; later a single daily dose for the next 10 days
Benzodiazepines	IV flumazenil (Romazicon) 0.1, 0.2, 0.3, 0.4, and 0.5 mg every alternate minute
β-blocker (Propranolol)	SC atropine, 0.01–0.02 mg/kg/dose until atropinization occurs (dry mouth, tachycardia, and dilated pupils)

Contd...

Contd...

Toxic agent	Antidote
Carbon monoxide	Oxygen (100%) inhalation for half an hour
Cyanide	*Amyl nitrite:* 0.3 mL (inhalation) for 15–30 seconds; repeat every minute *Sodium nitrite:* 5 mL (3.5% solution), intravenously every minute followed by sodium thiosulfate 2.5 mL (25% solution) every minute subject to a maximum of 50 mL
Heparin	*Protamine sulfate:* 2.5–5.0 mg/kg (IV); half of the dose needs to be repeated 4 hourly
INH (Isoniazid)	IV vitamin B6 for every 1 mg of INH
Iron	*Desferrioxamine:* 20 mg/kg/dose (IM) every 4–6 hourly until urine color returns to normal, i.e., 12–36 hours Alternatively, EDTA or BAL may be employed
Lead	*BAL:* See Arsenic *EDTA:* 50–75 mg/kg/day (IM and IV) in four divided doses *Penicillamine:* 20–40 mg/kg/day (PO)
Mercury	*BAL:* See Arsenic *Penicillamine:* See Lead
Opium, morphine, etc.	*Nalorphine (Naloxone):* 0.1 mg/kg (IV) stat; needs to be repeated after 15–30 minutes, if needed
Organic phosphates	*Atropine:* 0.03–0.04 mg/kg/(IV); half of this dose needs to be repeated every 15–30 minutes until pupils begin to dilate, mouth becomes dry, and tachycardia results (atropinization) + *Pyridoxine aldoxime methiodide (PAM):* 25–50 mg/kg (IV) slowly over 5 minutes period; repeat after 0.5 hour; may give maintenance dose

Contd...

Contd...

Toxic agent	Antidote
Paracetamol	*N-acetylcystein (NAC):* 150 mg/kg (IV) as infusion in 200 mL 5% dextrose in 15 minutes; then 50 mg/kg in 500 mL 5% dextrose in 4 hours
Phenothiazine	*Diphenylhydramine:* 1–2 mg/kg (IV) stat; repeat half hourly *Diazepam:* 0.3–0.5 mg/kg IV stat

[BAL: British anti-Lewisite (Dimercaprol); EDTA: ethylenediaminetetraacetic acid]

Section 9

Adverse Drug Reactions

60. Adverse Drug Reactions Specific to Certain Drugs

Chapter 60

Adverse Drug Reactions Specific to Certain Drugs

A

Abdominal Pain

- Tetracyclines
- Erythromycin
- Lincomycin
- Cephalosporins
- Ethionamide
- Para-aminosalicylic acid sodium (PAS)
- Rifampicin
- Trimethoprim
- Vincristine
- Azathioprine
- Corticosteroids
- Niclosamide
- Dichlorophen
- Amitriptyline
- Carbamazepine
- Chlordiazepoxide
- Ergotamine
- Gentian violet
- Iodides
- Iron
- Nystatin

- Diphenylhydantoin sodium
- Piperazine
- Primidone
- Troxidone
- Lead salts.

Arthritis/Arthralgia

- Corticosteroids (on discontinuation after prolonged course)
- Barbiturates
- Penicillin
- Carbamazepine
- Chlordiazepoxide
- Cimetidine
- Ethambutol
- Isoniazid

B

Behavior Problems like Aggressiveness and Temper Tantrums

- Phenobarbital
- Tricyclic antidepressants

Bone Marrow Depression

- Chloramphenicol
- Sulfonamides
- Diphenylhydantoin sodium
- Anticancer drugs
- Phenylbutazone
- Oxyphenbutazone

- Carbimazole
- Carbamazepine
- Rifampicin
- Pyrimethamine
- Trimethadione
- Ibuprofen
- Amphotericin B
- Analgin
- Griseofulvin
- Penicillin
- Antihistaminics
- Chlorothiazide
- Isonex
- Thiabendazole

Bullous or Vesicular Lesions

- Nalidixic acid
- Penicillamine
- Rifampicin
- Sulfas
- Antimetabolites
- Tricyclic antidepressants
- Thiazide diuretics
- Salicylates
- Acetazolamide
- Phenobarbital
- Bromides
- Chlordiazepoxide
- Clonidine
- Nitrazepam
- Diphenylhydantoin

C

Clumsiness/Ataxia
- Diphenylhydantoin sodium
- Phenobarbital
- Carbamazepine
- Valparin sodium
- Vincristine
- Antihistaminics
- Streptomycin
- Piperazine
- Chlordiazepoxide
- Diphenoxylate HCl
- Niclosamide
- Colistin sulfate
- Cyclopentolate
- Indomethacin
- Polymyxin
- Virtually all sedatives and tranquilizers

Color Vision
- Ethambutol
- Digoxin
- Barbiturates
- Sulfas
- Nalidixic acid
- Thiazide diuretics
- Streptomycin
- Troxidone

Coma
- Barbiturates
- Opiates

- Alcohol
- Carbon monoxide
- Kerosene oil
- Lead
- Haloperidol
- Diphenoxylate HCl
- Aspirin
- Amphetamines
- Antihistaminics
- Phenothiazines
- Organophosphates
- Piperazine
- Diphenylhydantoin sodium
- Solvent sniffing

Constipation
- Laxative abuse
- Purgative abuse
- Isoniazid
- Chlordiazepoxide
- Imipramine
- Amitriptyline
- Vincristine

Convulsions
- Phenothiazines
- Aminophylline
- Antihistaminics
- Acetazolamide
- Diphenoxylate HCl
- Strychnine
- Propoxyphenes

- Hexachlorophene
- Corticosteroids
- Amitriptyline
- Amphetamine
- Imipramine
- Pyrimethamine
- Chloroquine
- Carbamazepine
- Nalidixic acid
- Isoniazid
- Metoclopramide

Confusion, Delirium, or Hallucinations

- Cephalexin
- Cotrimoxazole
- Griseofulvin
- Nitrofurantoin
- Piperazine
- Alcohol
- Amitriptyline
- Diphenylhydantoin sodium
- Antihistaminics
- Amphetamine
- Mepacrine
- Bromides
- Carbamazepine
- Indomethacin
- Digoxin
- Ethionamide
- Chlordiazepoxide
- Ethosuximide
- Fenfluramine

Chapter 60: Adverse Drug Reactions Specific to Certain Drugs

- Cyclopentolate
- Diazepam
- Hyoscine
- Primidone
- Monoamine oxidase inhibitors
- Cannabis
- Lysergic acid diethylamide
- Solvent sniffing

D

Deafness
- Ampicillin
- Colistin sulfate
- Cotrimoxazole
- Gentamicin
- Framycetin
- Kanamycin
- Neomycin
- Streptomycin
- Tobramycin
- Rifampicin
- Vancomycin
- Vincristine
- Chloroquine
- Quinine
- Actinomycin
- Ethacrynic acid
- Frusemide
- Ibuprofen
- Indomethacin
- Propranolol

- Salicylates
- Medroxyprogesterone
- Nortriptyline

Diarrhea
- Ampicillin
- Iron
- PAS
- Phenothiazines
- Nalidixic acid
- Thiabendazole
- Carbamazepine
- Niclosamide
- Dichlorophen
- Thyroxine

Diplopia
- Vitamin A excess
- Chloroquine
- Quinine
- Antihistaminics
- Chlorpropamide
- Diazepam
- Carbamazepine
- Vincristine
- Sulfas
- Nalidixic acid
- Fenfluramine
- Imipramine
- Indomethacin
- Diphenylhydantoin sodium

Dryness of Mouth

- Isoniazid
- Amitriptyline
- Amphetamine
- Antihistaminics
- Anticholinergics
- Atropine
- Carbamazepine
- Codeine
- Clonidine
- Diazepam
- Fenfluramine
- Niclosamide
- Phenothiazines
- Vitamin A overdose
- Haloperidol
- Hyoscine
- Imipramine

Drowsiness

- Nalidixic acid
- Phenothiazines
- Tranquilizers
- Sedatives
- Antiepileptics
- Antihistaminics
- Diphenoxylate HCl
- Fenfluramine
- PAS
- Indomethacin

Dystonia

- Phenothiazines
- Metoclopramide
- Amitriptyline
- Amphetamines
- Antihistaminics
- Chloroquine
- Carbamazepine
- Cephalosporins
- Diazoxide
- Methaqualone
- Carbon monoxide
- Ethosuximide
- Haloperidol
- Imipramine
- Diphenylhydantoin

E

Eczema

- Kanamycin
- Penicillin
- Neomycin
- Sulfas
- Streptomycin
- Thiazide diuretics
- Amitriptyline
- Antihistaminics
- Iodides
- Phenothiazines
- Salicylates
- Quinine

Chapter 60: Adverse Drug Reactions Specific to Certain Drugs

Erythema Nodosum
- Phenobarbital
- Salicylates
- Sulfas
- Corticosteroids (on discontinuation)
- Bromides
- Iodides
- Penicillin
- Thiouracil

Excessive Drooling
- Clonazepam
- Nitrazepam
- Chlordiazepoxide
- Dicyclomine
- Ethionamide
- Haloperidol
- Organophosphates
- Anticholinesterase eye drops

Excessive Irritability
- Phenobarbital
- Primidone
- Acetazolamide
- Thyroxine
- Fenfluramine
- Antihistaminics
- Amidophylline
- Clonazepam
- Hyoscine
- Ethionamide
- Ephedrine

- Cyclopentolate
- Cycloserine
- Imipramine
- Amphetamine

Excessive Sweating

- Amitriptyline
- Phenothiazines
- Amphetamine
- Haloperidol
- Antihistaminics
- Ephedrine
- Imipramine
- Pethidine
- Thyroxine

F

Floppiness/Hypotonia

- Diazepam
- Tricyclic antidepressants
- Kanamycin
- Colistin sulfate
- Cycloserine
- Ethionamide
- Gentamicin
- Nitrofurantoin
- Neomycin
- Isoniazid
- Cyclophosphamide
- 6-mercaptopurine
- Lead
- Vincristine

Frequency of Micturition

- Demeclocycline
- Carbamazepine
- Hypervitaminosis D
- Antihistaminics
- Fenfluramine
- Loperamide

Polydipsia or Polyuria

- Clonazepam
- Vitamin D excess

G

Gastrointestinal Bleeding

- Aspirin
- Chlortetracycline
- Acetazolamide
- Thiazides
- Indomethacin
- Methotrexate
- Antimetabolites
- Iron

Gingivostomatitis

- Diphenylhydantoin sodium
- Sulfas
- Actinomycin D
- Methotrexate
- 6-mercaptopurine
- Vincristine
- Troxidone

- Tetracyclines
- Lincomycin
- Ethosuximide
- Griseofulvin
- Gold salts
- Niclosamide

Gynecomastia

- Cytotoxic drugs
- Vincristine
- Tricyclic antidepressants
- Phenothiazines
- Anabolic steroids
- Testosterone
- Amphetamine
- Cannabis
- Cimetidine
- Digitalis
- Gonadotropins
- Imipramine
- Reserpine
- Spironolactone
- Progesterone
- Metoclopramide

H

Headache

- Antihistaminics
- Acetazolamide
- Amitriptyline
- Diazepam

Chapter 60: Adverse Drug Reactions Specific to Certain Drugs

- Chlorpromazine
- Ephedrine
- Carbamazepine
- Vincristine
- Ethosuximide
- Ethambutol
- Troxidone
- Trimethoprim
- Tetracyclines
- Thiabendazole
- Griseofulvin
- Sulfas
- Valproate sodium
- Isoniazid
- Indomethacin
- Niclosamide
- Diphenylhydantoin sodium
- Nalidixic acid
- Nitrofurantoin

Hematuria

- Anticoagulants
- Aspirin
- Methicillin
- Thorazine
- Acetazolamide
- Cyclophosphamide
- Sulfas
- Diphenylhydantoin sodium
- Troxidone
- PAS

- Kanamycin
- Cephalosporins
- Bacitracin
- Aminophylline

Hepatotoxicity

- Mepacrine
- Chlorpromazine
- Rifampicin
- Tetracyclines
- Lignocaine
- Isonex
- Paracetamol
- Nalidixic acid
- Colistin sulfate
- Penicillamine
- Ethambutol
- Erythromycin estolate
- Griseofulvin

Hiccup

- Barbiturates (Short-acting)
- Ethosuximide
- Muscle relaxants (during recovery)
- Diazepam
- Minoxidil

Hyperactivity

- Phenobarbital
- Diphenylhydantoin sodium
- Primidone

- Chlordiazepoxide
- Tricyclic antidepressants
- Tartrazine (employed as food additive)

Hypothermia
- Phenothiazines
- Chlormethiazole

Hyperpyrexia
- Dantrolene (used for relief of spasticity)
- Tricyclic antidepressants
- Salicylate poisoning

Hypertrichosis
- Corticosteroids
- Anabolic steroids
- Diphenylhydantoin
- Diazoxide
- Penicillamine
- Streptomycin

I

Insomnia
- Griseofulvin
- Niclosamide
- Vincristine
- Antihistaminics
- Barbiturates
- Amphetamines
- Diphenoxylate HCl
- Ephedrine

- Fenfluramine
- Diazepam
- Imipramine
- Methylphenidate

L

Lacrimation/Epiphora

- Nitrazepam
- Bromides
- Mercury
- Arsenic

Lassitude

- Amitriptyline
- Chloroquine
- Nalidixic acid
- Clonazepam
- Corticosteroids
- Diuretics
- Streptomycin
- Ethosuximide
- β-blockers

Loss of Scalp Hair

- Ethambutol
- Ethionamide
- PAS
- Gentamicin
- Fenfluramine
- Amphetamines

- Anticoagulants
- Antimetabolites
- Mepacrine
- Nitrofurantoin
- Trimethoprim
- Troxidone
- Vitamin A excess
- Valproate sodium
- Carbamazepine
- Bismuth
- Carbimazole
- Gold
- Heparin
- Indomethacin
- Primidone
- Diphenylhydantoin
- Propylthiouracil

Lymphadenopathy

- Diphenylhydantoin sodium
- Cephaloridine
- Sulfas
- Carbamazepine
- Iron-dextran complex
- PAS
- Meprobamate
- Phensuximide
- Troxidone
- Phenylbutazone
- Bacillus Calmette–Guérin (BCG)

M

Mental Depression

- Amphetamine withdrawal
- Propranolol
- Phenothiazines
- Methyldopa
- Physostigmine
- Prednisolone
- Reserpine
- Clonidine
- Codeine
- Morphine
- Dextropropoxyphene
- Antihistaminics

Myopia

- Tetracyclines
- Sulfas
- Acetazolamide
- Corticosteroids

N

Nephrotoxicity

- Gentamicin
- Kanamycin
- Tetracyclines
- Cephaloridine
- Neomycin
- Nalidixic acid
- Penicillamine
- Colistin sulfate

- Rifampicin
- Propranolol
- Griseofulvin
- Amphotericin B
- Cycloserine
- Viomycin
- Mercurials
- Trimethadione

Neutropenia

Antimicrobials
- Chloramphenicol
- Sulfas
- Tetracyclines
- Streptomycin
- Isonex
- PAS
- Chloroquine and other antimalarials

Anticonvulsants
- Trimethadone
- Diphenylhydantoin sodium

Tranquillizers
- Chlorpromazine
- Promethazine

O

Overexcitment

- Phenobarbital
- Diazepam
- Nitrazepam
- Alcohol

- Antihistaminics
- Acetazolamide
- Nortriptyline
- Chlordiazepoxide
- Imipramine
- Mepacrine
- Solvent sniffing

P

Paresthesia

- Kanamycin
- Nalidixic acid
- Nitrofurantoin
- Streptomycin
- Polymyxin
- Trimethoprim
- Vincristine
- Thiabendazole
- Acetazolamide
- Amitriptyline
- Ergotamine
- Piperazine
- Niclosamide
- Imipramine
- Chlorothiazide

Photo Allergy

- Sulfonamides
- Tetracyclines
- Antihistaminics
- Neuroleptics
- Para-aminobenzoic acid (PABA)

- Fluoroquinolones
- Griseofulvin

Photophobia

- Amphetamines
- Atropine eye drops
- Cocaine
- Ethosuximide
- Idoxuridine
- Mercury
- Para-aminosalicylic acid sodium (PAS)
- Phenylephrine
- Tetracyclines (including doxycycline)
- Trioxidone
- Tropicamide

Phototoxicity

- Sulfonamides
- Tetracyclines
- Nalidixic acid
- Neuroleptics
- Promethazine
- Griseofulvin
- Coal-tar derivatives
- Antibacterial soaps

Pruritus/Urticaria

- Antibiotics
- Sulfas
- Diphenylhydantoin sodium
- Tetracyclines
- Tetanus toxoid

- Piperazine
- Amitriptyline
- Aminophylline
- Antihistaminics
- Antisera
- Aspirin
- Nalidixic acid
- Phenobarbital
- Carbamazepine
- Chloroquine
- Quinine
- Diphenoxylate HCl
- Indomethacin

Pseudotumor Cerebri
- Tetracyclines
- Vitamin A excess/deficiency
- Corticosteroids
- Nalidixic acid
- Nitrofurantoin
- Diphtheria, pertussis, and tetanus (DPT) vaccine

Ptosis
- Chloroquine
- Vincristine
- Sulthiame

S

Squint
- Tricyclic antidepressants
- Nalidixic acid

T

Trismus
- Tranquilizers
- Metoclopramide
- Antihistaminics
- Strychnine
- Anticonvulsants
- Trimethadione
- Diphenylhydantoin sodium

Tranquilizing States
- Chlorpromazine
- Promethazine

Antihistaminincs
- Promethazine
- Chlorpheniramine maleate

Antirheumatic
- Phenylbutazone
- Gold salts

Antithyroids
- Thiouracil
- Carbimazole

V

Vertigo
- Colistin sulfate
- Gentamicin

- Griseofulvin
- Isoniazid
- Kanamycin
- Minicycline
- Nalidixic acid
- Polymyxin
- Sulfas
- Trimethoprim
- Thiabendazole
- Thiazides
- Aspirin
- Clonidine
- Clonazepam
- Piperazine
- Acetazolamide
- Diphenylhydantoin sodium
- Phenothiazines
- Amitriptyline
- Antihistaminics
- Meprobamate
- Carbamazepine
- Diazepam
- Ethosuximide
- Dicyclomine
- Fenfluramine
- Imipramine
- Indomethacin
- Pethidine
- Primidone
- Solvent sniffing

APPENDICES

Useful Information Related to Pediatric Drug Therapy

Appendix 1: Principles of Drug Administration in Infants and Young Children
Appendix 2: Various Solutions Used in the Treatment of Dehydration and Dyselectrolytemia
Appendix 3: Drugs in Treatment/Prevention of Fetal Disease
Appendix 4: Therapeutic Range of Some Drugs
Appendix 5: Drugs Excreted into Breast Milk
Appendix 6: Drugs that Discolor the Stools
Appendix 7: Drugs that Discolor the Urine
Appendix 8: Drugs Likely to Cause Hemolysis in G6PD Deficiency
Appendix 9: Drugs that may Cause Peculiar Side Effects

Appendix 10: Drug Groups with Adverse Effects on Vitamin Status
Appendix 11: Potential Drug Interaction with Chemotherapy
Appendix 12: Banned Single-dose Drug Combinations (in India)
Appendix 13: Banned Fixed Dose Drug Combinations with Other Agents (in India)
Appendix 14: Nomogram for Estimation of Surface Area
Appendix 15: Weight to Surface Area Conversion Chart

Appendix 1

Principles of Drug Administration in Infants and Young Children

- Drugs that may Cause Specific Side Effects
- Use of calibrated devices provided with the product rather than the kitchen spoons should be encouraged.
- In order to circumvent difficulties in drug administration, advantage should be taken of special equipment such as measuring cups and spoons, oral syringes, oral droppers, cylindrical dosing spoons, etc.
- Until 5 years of age, liquid preparation. Beyond 5 years of age, it is good to give dispersible or chewable form of drug.
- Maximum volume allowed in parenteral administration is: subcutaneous = 0.5 mL, intradermal = 0.01-1 mL, intramuscular 0.5-1 mL, intravenous = use smallest recommended diluent for dilution.
- For IM prefer shorter (1.2-2.5 cm and smaller (23-30 G) needles.
- Prefer giving IV via pediatric drip set with microdrip chamber.
- For ID route, use 1 mL syringes calibrated in 0.01 mL units.

- For SC route, use 1 mL syringes calibrated in 40 or 80 units.
- Always compare the ordered dose with the recommended formulary dose based on a child's weight or body surface area (BSA).
- The ordered dose is safe if it is less than or equal to the recommended formulary dose.

Appendix 2

Various Solutions Used in the Treatment of Dehydration and Dyselectrolytemia

Solution	Ions (mEq/L)						
	Na^+	K^+	Ca^{++}	Cl^-	HCO_3^-	Lactate	NH_4
Isotonic saline	154	–	–	154	–	–	–
Half strength isotonic saline	77	–	–	77	–	–	–
Glucose saline (5%)	154	–	–	154	–	–	–
Hypertonic saline (5%)	855	–	–	855	–	–	–
Hypotonic saline (0.45%)	77	–	–	77	–	–	–
Ringer solution	147	4	4	155	–	–	–
Ringer lactate solution	130	4	4	111	–	28	–
1/6th molar sodium lactate	167	–	–	–	–	167	–
Potassium (1.5 g)	–	20	–	20	–	–	–
Chloride (2.2 g)		30		30			
Sodium (1.5%)	178	–	–	–	178	–	–
Ammonium chloride (0.9%) Isotonic	–	–	–	168	–	–	168
Darrow solution	122	35	–	104	–	53	–
Plasma	143	5	–	103	–	–	–
Blood	80	4	–	32	–	–	–

Appendix 3: Drugs in Treatment/Prevention of Fetal Disease

Fetal disease	Treatment/Prevention
Hypothyroidism	Thyroid hormone
Erythroblastosis fetalis	Rh (D) immune globulin
	Intrauterine blood transfusion
Galactosemia	Galactose-free diet. Tocolytic agents
Asphyxia/distress	• High concentration of oxygen to the mother • Positioning the uterus to avoid vascular compression • Operative delivery before severe fetal trauma occurs.
Hyaline membrane disease	Steroids to mother to facilitate fetal lung maturation
Prematurity	Tocolytic agents
Adrenogenital syndrome	Steroids
Pulmonary immaturity	Steroids
Diabetes mellitus	Good insulin control
Syphilis	Penicillin
Tuberculosis	Antituberculous therapy
Toxoplasmosis	Spiramycin
Paroxysmal tachycardia	Digoxin, quinidine, and propranolol
Withdrawal syndrome	Methadone

Appendix 4: Therapeutic Range of Some Drugs

Drugs	Serum concentration (mg)
Antibiotics	
Isoniazid	2–10
Chloramphenicol	10–25
Gentamicin	4–10
Amikacin	15–25
Kanamycin	15–25
Carbenicillin	90–110
Tobramycin	4–10
Antipyretic/analgesic/anti-inflammatory	
Paracetamol	50–100
Aspirin	50–150 (Short-term antipyretic therapy)
	100–300 (Long-term antiarthritic therapy)
Anticonvulsants	
Phenobarbital	10–40
Carbamazepine	4–12
Diphenylhydantoin	10–20

Contd...

Contd...

Valproate	50–150
Clonazepam	0.02–0.07
Ethosuximide	40–100
Tridione	6–40
Diazepam	0.15–0.06
Antiarrhythmic	
Digoxin	0.0008–0.0025 (0–12 months)
	0.0008–0.0016 (Above 1 year)
Quinidine	1–5
Propranolol	0.02–0.2
Miscellaneous	
Chloral hydrate	5–10
Chlorpromazine	0.04–0.3
Imipramine	0.05–0.16
Theophylline	10–20

Appendix 5

Drugs Excreted into Breast Milk

VITAMINS

Practically all.

TRANQUILIZERS

- Chlorpromazine (Largactil)
- Reserpine

AMPHETAMINES

- Dextroamphetamine (Dexedrine)
- Amphetamine sulfate

ANALGESICS

Narcotics

- Morphine
- Codeine
- Heroin

Nonnarcotics

- Aspirin
- Acetaminophen
- Dextropropoxyphene
- Phenacetin

ANTIBIOTICS

- Chloramphenicol
- Erythromycin
- Isonex
- Neomycin
- Para-amino-salicylic (PAS) acid
- Streptomycin
- Cycloserine
- Penicillin (Benzyl-G)
- Sulfonamides
- Tetracyclines

ANTIHISTAMINICS

Diphenhydramine (Benadryl) and most others

BARBITURATES

Phenobarbital (Luminal and gardenal) and most others

LAXATIVES AND CATHARTICS

- Mercurous chloride (Calomel)
- Rhubarb
- Senna
- Cascara

METALS AND ALLIED AGENTS

Lead	Iodide
Arsenic	Phosphate
Mercury	Potassium
Magnesium	Sodium
Calcium chloride	Sulfur

SEDATIVES

- Chloral hydrate
- Barbiturates
- Bromides

MISCELLANEOUS

Reserpine
Quinine
Pseudoephedrine
Diphenylhydantoin
Phenylbutazone
Oxyphenbutazone
Nicotine
Imipramine HCl
Mandelic acid
Estrogens
Corticosteroids

Alcohol
Allergens
Aminophylline
Chloroform
Ether
Caffeine
Oral contraceptives
DDT
Ephedrine
Bromides
Cyclophosphamide

Appendix 6

Drugs that Discolor the Stools

- Iron*
- Bismuth
- Lead
- Aspirin
- Activated charcoal
- Anticoagulants
- Aluminum hydroxide
- Pyrvinium (Vanquin)
- Dithiazanine (Delvex)
- Added color or flavor to make a "preparation" more pleasing
- Carmine dye
- Phenazopyridine (Pyridium)

---

*Iron causes discoloration of stools by (a) formation of sulfide or tannate and (b) production of gastrointestinal bleeding.

Appendix 7

Drugs that Discolor the Urine

YELLOW OR GREEN DISCOLORATION
- Vitamin B-complex
- Vitamin C
- Methylene blue

RUST YELLOW OR BROWNISH
- Furazolidone
- Nitrofurantoin
- Chloroquine
- Primaquine
- Mepacrine
- Sulfonamides
- Chloral hydrate
- Alcohol
- Bismuth
- Mercury
- Arsenicals
- Naphthalene

PINK TO RED BROWN
- Phenothiazine
- Hemolysis-producing drugs

- Hematuria-producing drugs
- Diphenylhydantoin sodium
- Desferrioxamine

MAGENTA TO PURPLE ORANGE

Phenolphthalein

GREEN

- Methylene blue
- Resorcinol

BROWN TO BLACK DISCOLORATION

- Resorcinol
- Methylene blue
- Quinine
- Furazolidone (Furoxone)
- Nitrofurantoin (Furadantin)
- Naphthalene
- Iron sorbitol (Jectofer)
- Aniline dyes

BLUE DISCOLORATION

Methylene blue

Drugs Likely to Cause Hemolysis in G6PD Deficiency

SULFONAMIDES
- Sulfacetamide
- Sulfamethoxypyridazine
- Sulfisoxazole
- Acetylsulfanilamide
- Salicylazosulfapyridine

NITROFURANS
- Nitrofurantoin
- Furazolidone
- Nitrofurazone

SULFONES
- Diaminodiphenyl sulfone (DDS)
- Sulfoxone
- Thiazolsulfone

VITAMINS
Vitamin K (water-soluble analogs)

MISCELLANEOUS

- Dimercaprol/BAL (British anti-Lewsite)
- Methylene blue
- Tolbutamide
- Quinidine
- Probenecid
- Fava bean (broad beans)
- Naphthalene (mothballs)

ANTIMALARIALS

- Primaquine
- Pamaquine
- Pentaquine
- Mepacrine
- Quinine

ANTIPYRETICS/ANALGESICS

- Aspirin
- Phenacetin
- Acetanilid
- Phenazone
- Amidopyrine

ANTIBIOTICS

- Chloramphenicol
- Novobiocin
- Gentamicin
- Kanamycin
- Cloxacillin
- Paraaminosalicylic acid

Appendix 9

Drugs that may Cause Peculiar Side Effects

Drugs that may cause specific adverse drug reactions:
- *Acetylsalicylic acid (Aspirin):* Reye syndrome (hepatic encephalopathy from aspirin in children suffering from an exanthemata-like varicella or influenza)
- *Anabolic steroids/Glucocorticoids (chronic therapy):* Stunting
- *Aminoglycosides:* Enhanced nephrotoxicity and ototoxicity (especially tinnitus)
- *Chloramphenicol:* Gray baby syndrome
- *Fluoroquinolones:* Arthropathy
- *Furosemide/Frusemide:* Nephrocalcinosis
- *Indomethacin:* Intestinal perforation and nephrotoxicity
- *Imipramine:* Enhanced anticholinergic effects
- *Phenobarbital:* Paradoxical hyperactivity
- *Phenytoin:* Coarse facies, thickened skull, atrophied nails
- *Phenothiazines:* Dystonias (extrapyramidal reactions)
- *Sulfas:* Kernicterus
- *Tetracyclines:* Staining of teeth, defective dental enamel, and growth retardation
- *Verapamil:* Conduction defects
- *Propylene glycol:* *Hyperosmolarity (in infants)
- *Benzyl alcohol:* *Metabolic acidosis, gasping, seizures, and cardiovascular collapse.

---
*Employed as a preservative in several injectable medications.

10

Appendix

Drug Groups with Adverse Effects on Vitamin Status

Vitamin	Thia-mine	Ribo-flavin	Pyri-doxine	Vitamin B_{12}	Folic acid	Ascorbic acid	Vitamin A	Vitamin D	Vitamin E	Vitamin K
Analgesics and antirheumatics		×				×				×
Anorectics					×					
Antacids and other gastric agents	×					×				
Antibiotics	×	×	×	×	×	×	×	×		×
Anticholinergics		×			×					
Antidiabetics (Oral)				×						

Contd...

Contd...

Vitamin	Thia-mine	Ribo-flavin	Pyri-doxine	Vitamin B_{12}	Folic acid	Ascorbic acid	Vitamin A	Vitamin D	Vitamin E	Vitamin K
Antihypertensives			×	×						
Anticonvulsants			×	×	×	×		×		×
Contraceptives (Oral)	×	×	×	×	×	×	×		×	
Digitalis-based glycosides										
Diuretics					×					
Glucocorticoids			×		×			×		
Hypnotics					×	×		×		
Laxatives							×	×	×	×
Lipid-lowering agents				×	×		×	×	×	×
Psychotropic agents								×		
Neuroleptics					×					
Sulfonamides	×	×	×	×	×	×				
Tuberculostatics			×	×	×					
Uricosurics/uricostatics		×		×		×				

Appendix 11

Potential Drug Interaction with Chemotherapy

Chemotherapeutic drug	Interacting drug	Effect of combined action
Aminoglycosides	• Amphotericin B, cyclosporine, cisplatin, and NSAIDs vancomycin • Penicillins (in patients with renal failure) Ethacrynic acid, and furosemide	• Increased nephrotoxicity • Decreased efficacy of parenteral aminoglycosides • Enhanced potential for ototoxicity
Amoxicillin and ampicillin	• Allopurinol • Oral β-blockers	• Increased frequency of rash • Decreased β-blocker absorption
Clindamycin	Kaolin	Decreased absorption of clindamycin
Macrolides (erythromycin and clarithromycin)	Carbamazepine • Corticosteroids • Theophylline • Warfarin sodium • Digoxin • Ergot alkaloids • Nonsedating antihistamines (terfenadine and astemizole)	Increased toxicity risk for carbamazepine • Increased effects of steroids • Theophylline-induced toxicity • Increased risk of bleeding • Digoxin toxicity • Ergot toxicity • Ventricular arrhythmias

Chemotherapeutic drug	Interacting drug	Effect of combined action
Fluoroquinolones All	Cimetidine, aluminum, calcium, iron, magnesium, zinc, antacids, and sucralfate	• Increased quinolone levels • Decreased absorption of quinolones • Decreased quinolone levels
Enoxacin	Fenbufen and theophylline	Seizures, increased theophylline levels
Norfloxacin	Theophylline	Increased theophylline levels
Ciprofloxacin	Theophylline	Increased theophylline levels
Nitrofurantoin	Magnesium antacids	• Decreased nitrofurantoin • Absorption
Metronidazole	• Warfarin sodium • Alcohol	• Increased risk of bleeding • Disulfiram-like reaction
Sulfonamides	• Oral anticoagulants • Cyclosporine • Methotrexate • Phenytoin • Sulfonylureas	• Increased hypoprothrombinemia • Decreased cyclosporine levels • Methotrexate toxicity • Phenytoin toxicity • Increased hypoglycemic risk
Tetracyclines	• Aluminum, bismuth, and iron • Barbiturates and carbamazepine • Phenytoin and digoxin	• Decreased tetracycline absorption • Decreased tetracycline effect • Increased digoxin toxicity
Trimethoprim-sulfamethoxazole	• Oral anticoagulants • Cyclosporine • Phenytoin • Glipizide • Methotrexate	• Increased anticoagulant effect • Nephrotoxicity • Phenytoin toxicity • Increased risk of hypoglycemia • Bone marrow suppression

Appendix 12

Banned Single-dose Drug Combinations (in India)

1. Penicillin with sulfonamides.
2. Tetracyclines with vitamin C.
3. Antitubercular drugs with vitamins [exception is isoniazid with pyridoxine (vitamin B_6)]
4. Vitamins with analgesics/anti-inflammatory drugs.
5. Vitamins with tranquilzers.
6. Atropine in analgesic and antipyretics.
7. Yohimbine and strychnine with testosterone and vitamins.
8. Strychnine and caffeine in tonics.
9. Iron with strychnine, arsenic, and yohimbine.
10. Antihistaminics with antidiarrheals.
11. More than one antihistamine in the same preparation.
12. Sedatives/hypnotics/anxiolytics with analgesic-antipyretics.
13. H_2-receptor antagonists with antacids (with exception of those approved by the Drug Controller of India).
14. Anthelmintics (with exception of piperazine) with cathartic/purgative.
15. Bronchodilators, including salbutamol, with centrally-acting antitussive and/or antihistamine.
16. Centrally-acting antitussives with antihistamines having high atropine-like activity in expectorants.

17. Centrally-acting antitussives and/or antihistamines in preparations for cough associated with asthma.
18. Laxatives and/or antispasmodics in enzyme preparations.
19. Glycophosphates and/or other phosphates and/or CNS stimulant in liquid oral tonics.
20. Estrogen and progestin (with exception of oral contraceptives) containing per tablet estrogen >50 mg ethinyl estradiol (or equivalent) and progestin >3 mg of norethisterone acetate (or equivalent) and all fixed dose combination injectable preparations.
21. Ethambutol with isoniazid except in the following daily doses:
    Isoniazid 200 mg + Ethambutol 600 mg
    or
    Isoniazid 300 mg + Ethambutol 800 mg.
22. Pyrazinamide with other antitubercular drugs except those which provide the following daily doses:
    - Rifampicin 450–600 mg
    - Isoniazid 300–400 mg
    - Pyrazinamide 1,000–1,500 mg.
23. Essential oils with alcohol having percentage higher than 20% proof (with the exception of preparations given in IP).
24. Liquid oral tonic preparations containing alcohol 30%.
25. Analgin (Metamizol) with antispasmodics and other drugs.
26. Antidiarrheals containing adsorbents such as kaolin, pectin, attapulgite, activated charcoal, etc.
27. Antidiarrheals containing phthalylsulfathiazole, succinyl sulfathiazole, sulfaguanidine, neomycin, streptomycin, and dihydrostreptomycin.

28. Antidiarrheal formulations for pediatric use containing diphenoxylate, loperamide, atropine, hyoscyamine, halogenated hydroxyquinolines.
29. Antidiarrheals with electrolytes.
30. Fixed dose combinations of hemoglobin in any form.
31. Pancreatin or pancrelipase containing amylase, protease, and lipase with any other enzyme.

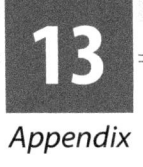

Appendix

Banned Fixed Dose Drug Combinations with Other Agents (in India)

1. Corticosteroids with any other drug meant for internal use.
2. Chloramphenicol with any other drug for internal use.
3. Sodium bromide/chloral hydrate with other drugs.
4. Ergot with any other drug, except preparations containing ergotamine, caffeine, analgesics, and antihistamines for treatment of migraine.
5. Anabolic steroids with other drugs.
6. Metoclopramide with other drugs, except aspirin/paracetamol.
7. Pectin and/or kaolin with any drug that is systemically absorbed from the gut.
8. Hydroxyquinolines with any other drug, except in preparations for external use.
9. Oxyphenbutazone or phenylbutazone with other drugs.
10. Dextropropoxyphene with any drug except antispasmodic and/or nonsteroidal anti-inflammatory drugs (NSAIDs).

Appendix 14

Nomogram for Estimation of Surface Area

The surface area is indicated where a straight line connecting the height and weight levels intersects the surface area column; or if the patient is roughly of average size, from the weight alone (enclosed area).

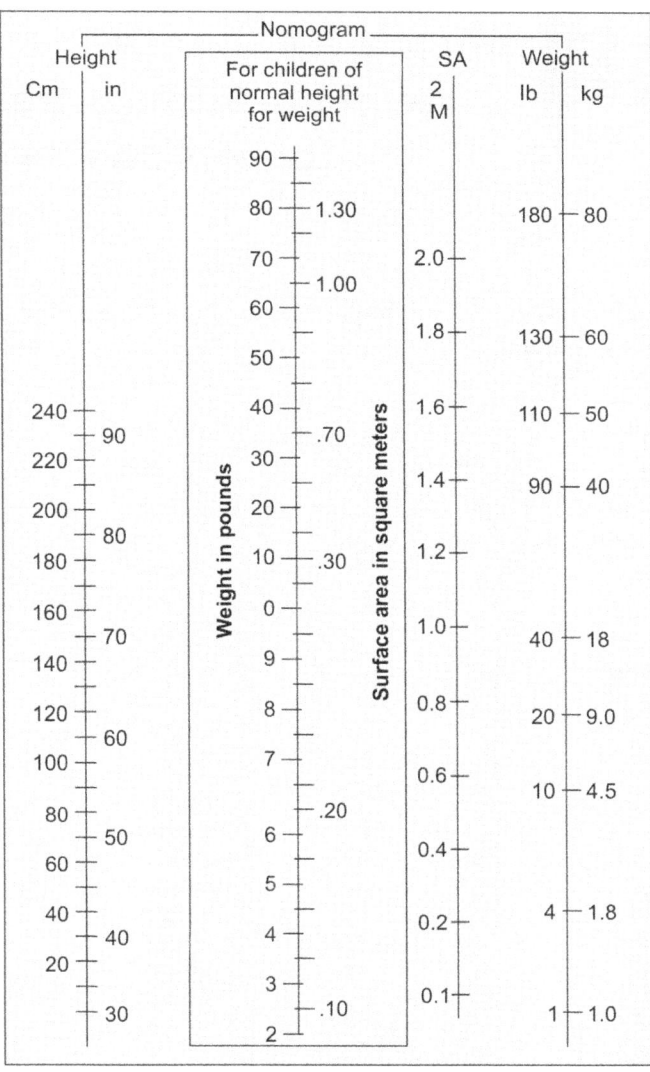

Appendix 15

Weight to Surface Area Conversion Chart

Age	Weight (kg)	Surface area (m²)
Weeks (gestation)		
26	0.9–1.0	1.0
30	1.3–1.5	0.12
32	1.6–2.0	0.15
38	2.9–3	0.2
40 (full-term at birth)		
Months		
3	5	0.29
6	7	0.38
9	8	0.42
Years		
1	10	0.49
2	12	0.55
3	15	0.64
4	17	0.74
5	18	0.76
6	20	0.82
7	23	0.90
8	25	0.95
9	28	1.06
10	33	1.18
11	35	1.23
12	40	1.34

Note: Surface area in an adult is around 1.73 m².

Index

Page numbers followed by '*b*' refer to box and '*t*' refer to table.

A

Abacavir 337
Abdominal
    cramps 91
    discomfort 39, 106
    distension 92, 135
    pain 62, 91, 117, 121, 513
Acellular triple vaccine 463
Acemiz 108
Acenocoumarol 68
Acetamide 171
Acetaminophen 33, 41, 407
Acetazolamide 171, 407, 515, 517, 523, 525-527, 532, 534, 538
Acetein 121
Acetylsalicylic acid 34
Acid reflux, symptoms of 44
Acid-resistant penicillin 260
Acitrom 69
Acquired immunodeficiency syndrome 334
Acthib 463
Actinomycin 519, 525
Acute radiation syndrome 170
Acyclovir 332-335, 423
Adapalene 46
Addison's disease 88, 120, 174
Adefovir dipivoxil 349
Adenine arabinoside 333
Adenosine 100, 407
Adrenal corticosteroid 190
Adrenal hyperplasia, congenital 412
Adrenal insufficiency 412
Adrenaline 49, 157, 411
Adrenals-related drugs 190
Adrenergic receptor antagonist 121
Adrenocorticotropic hormone 87, 185
Adrenogenital syndrome 19
Adriamycin 63
Advisory Committee on Immunization Practices 489*b*
Aggressiveness 514
AGGSall scorpion stings 153
Agiepril 121
Airways to intrinsic, hyper-reactivity of 48
Albendazole 359, 365
Albumin 232, 408
Albuterol 408
Alcohol 517, 518, 533
Aldosterone-receptor blocker 123
Alidac 364
Allegra 112
Allergens 549
Allergic
    bronchial asthma for prophylaxis 113
    conjunctivitis 113
    rhinitis 113
Allergies, types of 193
Allopurinol 198
Allylamines 356
Alopecia 62
Alprostadil 408
Aluminum hydroxide 44
Alum-precipitated dual antigen 462
Amantadine 345
Amantrel 345
Ambistryn-S 256, 318
Ambroxol 156
Amicar 182
Amicin 252, 324
Amicline 360
Amicor 158
Amikacin 252, 324, 415
Amiloride 119
Aminocaproic acid 182

Aminoglycoside 26, 251, 252
   antibiotic 363, 370
   first semisynthetic 252, 324
Aminohexanoic acid 182
Aminophylline 49, 181, 408, 517, 523, 528, 536, 549
Amiodarone hydrochloride 101
Amitriptyline 513, 517, 518, 521, 522, 524, 526, 530, 534, 536, 538
Amitriptyline hydrochloride 141
Amitru 120
Amlodipine 120
Amodiaquine hydrochloride 374
Amoxicillin 415
Amoxicillin-Clavulanate 416
Amphetamines 177, 517, 518, 521, 522, 524, 526, 529, 530, 535, 547
Amphetamines withdrawal 532
Amphotericin B 352, 384, 515, 533
Ampicillin 519, 520
Amrinone lactate 158, 408
Anabolic steroids 195, 526, 529
Analgesics 33, 547, 554
Analgin 515
Anaphylaxis 437
Anesthal 88
Angiotensin-converting enzyme inhibitors 119
Angiotensin-II receptor blockers 119
Angizem 123
Antacids 44, 45, 113, 117, 135-137, 140, 188, 222, 236, 271
Antepar 371
Anthelmintics 365
Anthranilic acid derivative 39
Anti-acne drugs 46
Antiallergic 110, 194
   symptomatic treatment of 109
Antianxiety property 81
Antiarrhythmics 26
Antiasthma drugs 48
Antibacterial
   drugs 251, 310
   soaps 535
Antibiotics 251, 415, 535, 548, 554
   associated diarrhea 438
   therapy 60, 439, 450b, 514
Anticholinergic antihistamine 118
Anticholinergics 521
Anticholinesterase eye drops 523
Anticoagulants 68, 527, 531
   therapeutic effect of 68
Anticonvulsants 26, 73, 537
   drugs, standard 74
Antidepressants 27
   high-dose 115
Antidiarrheal drugs 89
Antidotes against common toxic agents 507t
Antiemetic drugs 73, 95, 135
Antiepileptics 521
Antifibrillatory drugs 100, 184
Antifilarial drugs 383
Antiflatulence drugs 146
Antiflatulent 146
Antiflu 345
Antifungal drugs 352, 423
   types of 352
Antigen-antibody reaction 17
Antihemophilic factor 183, 408
Antihistamines 108
Antihistaminic agents 108
Antihistaminics 515-518, 520-526, 529, 532, 534, 536-538, 548
Antihistaminics drugs 108
Antihypertensive agent 119, 172, 174
Anti-inflammatory agent 49, 190
Anti-influenza virus drugs 345
Antileishmania drugs 384
Antileprosy drugs 328
Antimalarials agent 374, 533, 554
Antimetabolites 515, 525, 531
Antimicrobial drugs 415
Antimyasthenic drugs 132
Antimyasthenics 132

Antimycobacterial drugs 314
Antineoplastic drugs 60
Antinontuberculous mycobacterial drugs 325
Antiparasitic drugs 359, 373
   broad-spectrum 366
Antipediculosis drugs 387
Antiprotozoal drugs 359, 365
Antipseudomonas 265
Antipsychotic drugs 141
Antipyretics 33, 554
Antireflux drugs 135
Antiretroviral drugs 337
Anti-Rh immunoglobulin 209
Antirheumatic 537
Antiscabies 387
Anti-schistosomiasis drugs 388
Antiscorpion venom 153
Antisecretory drugs like proton pump inhibitors 44
Antiseizure drugs 73
Antisera 536
Antisnake venom 151, 210
Antispasmodics 146
Antispasticity agent 224
Antithyroids 537
Antitoxins 151
Anti-toxoplasmosis drugs 385
Antituberculous drugs 314
   categories of 315*b*, 316*b*
Antitumor agents 63
Antitussives 154, 155
Antivenom sera derived 151
Antivenom serum desensitization, steps of 453*b*
Antiviral drugs 332, 344, 345, 349, 423
Antrenyl 148
Apnea 81
Arachidonic acid 230
Arkamin 122
Arovit 241
Arrhythmia 100
Arsenic 530

Arsenic phosphate 548
Artagen 41
Artamin 166
Artemether 374
Arterial lines 70
Artery walls 119
Artesunate 375
Arthralgia 514
Arthritis 514
Ascapil 366
Ascorbic acid 245
Aspirin 34, 517, 525, 527, 536, 538
Astelong 108
Astemizole 108
Asthafree 50
Asthalin 53
Asthma
   acute severe 436
   mild 56, 57
   moderate 56, 57
   severe 56, 57
   triggers 48
Atabrine 368
Atarax 113
Ataxia 102, 516
Atenolol 121
Atherosclerosis 119
Atocor 391
Atomoxetine 142, 179
Atorlip 391
Atorva 391
Atorvastatin 391
Atovaquone 391
Atrioventricular block, second and third degree 101
Atropine 521
   eye drops 535
Atropine sulfate 102, 146, 408
Atropinism, signs of 141
Attention-deficit disorder 122
Attention-deficit hyperactivity disorder 142, 177, 244
Attentrol 142

Auranofin 35
Autoimmune disease 191
Autoimmune disorders 193, 400
Avas 391
Axepta 142
Azatadine maleate 109
Azathioprine 513
Azderm 46
Azelaic acid 46
Azenam 281
Azithral 326
Azithromycin 284, 325, 416
Aziwok 326
Azoles 354
Azolin 270
Aztreonam 281, 417

B

Bacillary dysentery, acute 438
Bacillus Calmette-Guérin 460, 497,
    500, 503, 531
Bacitracin 528
Baclofen 224
Bacterial meningitis 439
Bambudil 50
Bambuterol hydrochloride 50
Banocide 383
Barbiturates 62, 514, 516, 528,
    529, 548
Beclate inhaler 55
Beclate nasal spray 55
Beclomethasone 190
Beclomethasone dipropionate 55
Behavior problems 514
Behavioral disorders 399
Benadon 244
Benadryl 112
Benalgis 242
Beneuron 242
Benign microorganisms 398
Benzac AC 47
Benzathine 421
Benzene hexachloride 388

Benzodiazepine possessing
    sedative 81
Benzothiadiazine derivative 122
Benzoyl peroxide 47
Benzyl benzoate 387
Beparine 69
Berin 242
Berirab 212
Beta-blocker 121, 530
Betaday 50
Betahistine dihydrochloride 201
Beta-lactams 258
    group 258, 266, 281
Betamethasone 190
Bevidox 244
Bharglob 210
Biduret 120
Biliary excretion 9
Biliary function 11
Biltricide 371
Biochemical changes 73
Bioclox 260
Biodoxi 296, 378
Biopolio 470
Biotin 241
Biotrexate 64
Bipolar disorder, treatment of 73
Birthweight, low 19
Bisacodyl 235
Bismuth 531
Bisolvon 156
Bladder hemorrhage 62
Bleeding diathesis 70
Bleeding disorder 35, 43, 182,
    230, 233
Blood coagulation disorders 37
Blood disorder 365
Blood glucose
    levels, increasing 162
    metabolism of 221
Blood pressure 119
    increasing 162
Blood thinners 68

Bloody diarrhea 438
Bludrox 269
Bodyweight method 14
Bone marrow depression 60, 62, 63, 514
Boostrix 478
Borderline personality disorder 73
    treatment of 73
Botox 225
Botulinum toxin 225
Brain
    calcium-channel plus sodium-channel locker in 394
    electrical activity 73
    growth and development, essential for 230
Breast milk 547
    excretion in 9
Breastfeeding 19, 20
Breath and cough, shortness of 48
Brethmol 53
Bricanyl 54
Bricanyl nebulizing solution 58
British anti-Lewisite 166, 509
Bromhexine 156
Bromides 470, 515, 518, 523, 530
Bronchiolitis, acute 432
Bronchodilator 48, 49
Bronchospasm 48, 54
Broncordil 54
Bronkine 54
Bronkosyrup 53
Bronkotab 53
Brufen 38
Budesonide 56
Bullous lesions 515
Bumet 172
Bumetanide 172, 408
Bumex 172
Burning feet syndrome 244
Buscopan 148
Busulfan 60

C

Cadigran 96
Cafcit 181
Caffeine 549
Caffeine citrate 180, 409
Cafirate 181
Calcigard retard 127
Calcitriol 409
Calcium-channel blockers 119
Calcium chloride 217
Calcium chloride sulfur 548
Calcium gluconate 217
Calcium phosphate 218
Calcium salts 409
Calmpose 75
Calpan 244
Calpol 33
Camoquin 374
Cancers 193
Candistat 354
Cannabis 519, 526
Capnea 181
Capreo 319
Capreomycin 319
Captopril 121, 238, 409
Carbamazepine 74, 513-516, 518, 520-522, 525, 527, 531, 536, 538
    ketoderivative of 82
Carbapenem group 283
Carbatol 74
Carbelin 265
Carbenicillin 417
Carbimazole 189, 515, 531, 537
Carbon monoxide 517, 522
Cardace 130
Cardcap 239
Cardiac conduction disorders 380
Cardiopril 130
Cardiotonic drugs 157
Cardiotoxicity 63
Cardiovascular disease 111, 117, 186
Cardiovascular disorders 144

Index

Cardiovascular system 19
Cardizem 123
Carnitine 229, 409
Castor 391
Catabolism-mediating corticosteroid
 receptors 195
Catapres 122
Cefaclor 266, 417
Cefadrox 269
Cefadroxil 269, 417
Cefadur 269
Cefazolin 418
Cefazolin sodium 270
Cefizox 277
Cefoperazone 273, 417
Cefotaxime 417
Ceftazidime 418
Ceftobiprole 275
Ceftriaxone 418
Cefuroxime 418
 oral prodrug of 280
Central nervous system 33
 depressants 109
 likelihood of 23
 stimulant 180, 395
Central nervous system
 disorder 283, 325, 363
Cephalexin 418, 518
Cephaloridine 531, 532
Cephalosporins 266, 513, 522, 528
 adverse reactions of 268b
 extended-spectrum
  semisynthetic 271
 fifth generation 267b, 269, 277, 281
 second generation 280
 semisynthetic broad-spectrum
  second generation 266
 third generation 272-274, 279
Cerebral disease 224
Cerebrospinal fluid 6
Cervarix 467
Cetirizine 114
Cetirizine dihydrochloride 109

Chédiak-Higashi syndrome 246
Chelating agents 164
Chemical agents, poisoning of 505
Chemotherapy 558
Chickenpox vaccine, high-risk
 groups needing 480b
Child's dose 14
Chloral hydrate 142, 409
Chlorambucil 61
Chloramphenicol 310, 418, 514, 533
Chlordiazepoxide 143, 513-518,
 523, 529, 534
Chlormethiazole 529
Chloroquine 446, 518-520, 522, 530,
 533, 536
Chloroquine sulfate 376
Chloroquine-resistant *Plasmodium
 falciparum* malaria 446
Chlorothiazide 173, 409, 515, 534
Chlorpheniramine maleate 110, 537
Chlorpromazine 95, 527, 528, 533, 537
Chlorpromazine hydrochloride 142
Chlorpropamide 520
Chlortetracycline 525
Chlorthalidone 173
Chlorzoxazone 226
Cholecalciferol 246
Cholera vaccine 481
Cholesterol in body,
 production of 391
Cholestyramine 392
Chromium 221
Cidofovir 334
Cifran 322
Cilamin 166
Cilanem-500 282, 325
Cilastatin 282, 325, 419
Cimetidine 136, 409, 514, 526
Cinirone 201
Cinnarizine 201
Ciplactin 110
Ciplar 129
Ciplox 322

Index

Ciprofloxacin 291, 322
Ciproval 110
Circulatory volume, restoration of 393
Cisapride 410
Citrate solutions 410
Claribid 285, 326
Clarithromycin 285, 326
Clark's rule 13, 14
Clemastine fumarate 110
Clerkin 388
Clexane 70
Clindamycin 290, 418
Cloba 74
Clobazam 74
Clofazimine 329
Clonazepam 27, 75, 523, 525, 530, 538
Cloneon 122
Clonid 122
Clonidine 179, 410, 515, 521, 532, 538
Clonidine hydrochloride 122
Clotrin 75
Clozam 74
Coagulation, acting via inhibition of 68
Coal-tar derivatives 535
Coamoxiclav 416
Cobalamin 207, 244
Cocaine 535
Codeine 36, 521, 532
Codeine linctus 36
Codokuff 36
Colchicine 199
Colimex 147
Colistin sulfate 89, 516, 519, 524, 528, 532, 537
Colloids 232
Colonic motility disorders 148
Colony-stimulating factors 168
Color vision 516
Coma 516
Combutol 317
Complamina 72
Confusion 518
Congestive cardiac failure 87, 440, 441t
Constipation 517
Convulsion 73, 517
Copper 164, 221
Copper chelator 166
Cordarone X 101
Coronary artery disease 54, 105
Coronary heart disease 19, 129
Corticosteroids 192t, 513, 514, 518, 523, 529, 530, 532, 536, 549
Cortin 191
Cortisone acetate 191
Cotrimoxazole 327, 391, 518, 519
Cough expectorants 154
Coumadin 71
Cremalax 237
Crocin 33
Cromoglycate disodium 56
Crotamiton 387
Crotorax 387
Crystalloids 231
Cubicin 303
Cuprimine 166
Cushing disease 87, 88, 186
Cushing syndrome 186, 193
Cyclic adenosine monophosphate, increases cellular levels of 158
Cyclopan 147
Cyclopentolate 516, 519, 524
Cyclophosphamide 61, 524, 527, 549
Cyclorine 320
Cycloserine 320, 524, 533
Cycloxan 61
Cylert 178
Cynocobalamine 207, 244
Cynomycin 298
Cyproheptadine HCl 110
Cytoblastin 66
Cytocristine 67
Cytotoxic drugs 526

D

Daktarin 355
Dalacin 290
Dalbavancin 302
Dalcap 290
Dalfopristin 306
Dantrium 225
Dantrolene 225, 529
Dapsone 329-331
Daptomycin 302
Daraprim 385
Daunorubicin 62
Deafness 519
Decongestant 116
    quick-acting 118
Deferasirox 164
Deferiprone 165
Deferoxamine 165
Defrijet 164
Dehydration 432
    treatment of 543
Delirium 102, 518
Delisprin 34
Demeclocycline 525
Demerol 42
Depin 127
Deriphyllin 54
Desferal 165
Desferrioxamine 165
Desloratadine 111
Desmopressin acetate 186
Dexamethasone 190, 410
Dexedrine 177
Dextran 233, 392, 393
Dextromethorphan
    hydrochloride 155
Dextropropoxyphene 532
Dextropropoxyphene
    hydrochloride 36
Dextrose 94, 232
Diabetic ketoacidosis 441
Diaminodiphenyl sulfone 329

Diamox 171
Dianabol 195
Diarrhea 520
    acute 432
Diazepam 75, 519-521, 524, 526,
    528, 530, 533, 538
Diazoxide 122, 238, 522, 529
Dibenzyline 128
Dichlorophen 513, 520
Diclofenac sodium 36
Diclomax 36
Dicyclomine 147, 523, 538
Didanosine 338
Dideoxycytidine 344
Diethylcarbamazine 383
Digitalis 526
Digitalis glycoside 159
Digoxin 62, 159, 410, 516, 518
    total digitalizing dose of 159
Dihydrotachysterol 410
Dilantin 84
Dilosyn 115
Diloxanide furoate 360
Diltiazem 123
Dimenhydrinate 95
Dimercaprol 166, 509
Dimethindene maleate 111
Dimethylpolysiloxane 147
Dimol 147
Dindevan 71
Dinex 338
Diphenhydramine 548
Diphenhydramine hydrochloride 112
Diphenoxylate HCl 517
Diphenoxylate hydrochloride 90,
    516, 517, 521, 529, 536
Diphenylhydantoin 515, 522, 529, 531
Diphenylhydantoin chloroform 549
Diphenylhydantoin sodium 84, 104,
    514, 516-518, 520, 525,
    527, 528, 531, 533, 535,
    537, 538
Diphtheria antitoxin 152, 210

Diphtheria, pertussis, and tetanus 461, 462, 463, 497, 500, 503, 536
Diplopia 520
Dipyridamole 70
Diseases, peculiar pathophysiology of 16
Disopyramide phosphate 102
Disprin 34
Distamin 166
Ditide 176
Diurem 175
Diuretics 171, 530
Dizikind 201
Dizzigo 201
DNA technology in cell culture 168
Dobucin 160
Dobustat 160
Dobutam 160
Dobutamine 410
Dobutamine hydrochloride 160
Dobutrex 160
Docosahexaenoic acid 230
Dolonex 42
Domperidone 95, 135
Dopamine 160, 410
Dopinga 160
Dorzox eye drops 171
Doxapram 411
Doxofylline 50
Doxorubicin 63
Doxycycline 296, 378, 535
Doxypal 296, 378
D-penicillamine 166
Dramamine 95
Drooling, excess 523
Drotaverine HCl 148
Drowsiness 521
Drowsiness, syndrome of 75
Droxyl 269
Drug
    absorption 6
    administration, principles of 541
    benzimidazole group of 359
    commonly needing therapeutic monitoring 26t
    concentration time curve 6
    dosage 13, 407
    drug interaction 9
        types of 9b
    emergency 424, 424b, 429
    for apnea of prematurity 180
    for attention-deficit hyperactivity disorder 177
    for bleeding control 182
    for endocrinal disorders 185
    for gout 198
    for infectious diseases 249
    for neutralizing toxicity 505
    for vertigo 201
    groups 556
    injectable 49
    metabolism, major site of 7
    oral absorption of 11t
    plasma protein-binding of 8
    safe therapy, seven rights of 4
    therapy 405
    wrong choice of 21
Duolin metered-dose inhaler 57
Durabolin 195
Duragesic 37
Dye, triple 402
Dyselectrolytemia, treatment of 543
Dyspepsia 44
Dystonia 522
Dystonic reaction 98

E

Ecosprin 34
Eczema 522
Edecrin 173
Edrophonium 132
Efavirenz 339
Electrical energy, sudden burst of 73
Electrobion 92
Emergency allergic disorders 115

Empirical antimicrobial selection 23
Enalapril 123
Enalapril maleate 123
Encephabol 144, 399
Endocrinal disorders 185
Endogenous immunomodulatory protein 349
Endoxan-N 61
End-stage renal disease 169
Enoxaparin 70
Ensamycin 256
Enterobacter 24
Enzyme deficiency 198
Enzyme induction 7
Enzymes 185
Eperenone 123
Ephedrine 523, 524, 527, 529
Ephedrine 549
Ephentine 161
Epiglottitis, acute 433
Epileptin 84
Epinephrine 49, 157, 411
Epiphora 530
Epithelial sodium channel 119
Eplecard 123
Eplerenone 123
Epoetin 169, 411
Epox 169
Eprex 169
Epsolin 84
Eptoin 84
Eptus 123
Equibrom 143
Ergotamine 513, 534
Erythema nodosum 523
Erythromycin 286, 419, 513
Erythromycin estolate 528
Erythromycin, methoxy derivative of 326
Erythropoietin 168, 411
Escherichia coli 23
Esidrix 175
Esomac 138

Esomeprazole 138
Esotrax 138
Estrogens bromides 549
Ethacrynic acid 173, 519
Ethambutol 317, 514, 516, 527, 528, 530
Ethamsylate 183
Ether 549
Ethionamide 319, 513, 518, 523, 524, 530
Ethosuximide 78, 518, 522, 526-528, 530, 535, 538
Ethylenediaminetetraacetic acid 509
Ethylestrenol 197
Etophylate 54
Eudemine 122
Euphoria 87
Eurythmic 101
Exifine 356
Expectorants 155
Extraintestinal drugs 373
Extraintestinal parasitic infections 373
Extrapyramidal syndrome 99, 340

F

Facid 137
Falciparum malaria 446
Famciclovir 334
Famocid 137
Famont 137
Famotidine 137
Famowal 137
Famtac 137
Famtrex 334
Fasigyn 364
Fatigue, syndrome of 75
Fenfluramine 518, 520, 521, 523, 525, 530, 538
Fentanar 128
Fentanyl citrate 37
Ferrous sulfate 203
Fersolate 203

Fetal disease
    prevention of 544
    treatment of 544
Fexofenadine 112
Fibrillations 100
Fibrinil 33
Flaccidity, causing 225
Flagyl 311
Floppiness 524
Fluconazole 353
Fluid
    absorption of 94
    retention 62
Flumadine 348
Flumist 483
Flunarizine 394
Fluorinated quinolone 294
Fluoroquinolones 291, 535
Fluticasone propionate 57
Fluvir 345
Folic acid 203, 411
    bacterial synthesis of 329
Foracort inhaler 58
Foracort rotacap 58
Forcan 353
Foristal 111
Formoterol 58
Fortum 276
Fortwin 41
Foscarnet 335
Foscavir 335
Fosolin 79
Fosphen 79
Fosphenytoin 79
Framycetin 519
Fred's rule 14
Frisium 74
Frusemide 174, 253, 254, 255, 257, 280, 519
Fudone 137
Fulsed 82
Funazole 355
Fungal infections, superadded 87
Fungiver 355
Fungizone 352
Furamide 360
Furazolidone 89, 361
Furomet 51
Furosemide 120, 172, 174
Furoxone 89, 361

G

Gabapentin 79
Gamafine 210
Gamma protect hepatitis 211
Gammalin 210
Ganciclovir 335
    product of 337
Gantrisin 309
Garamycin Genta
Gardasil 467
Gardenal 548
Gas gangrene antitoxin 153, 210
Gastric acid secretion 11
Gastric emptying time 11
Gastric motility disorders 95
Gastric ulcer 70
Gastroesophageal reflux disease 44, 136, 137
Gastrointestinal bleeding 525, 550
Gastrointestinal disorders 37
Gastrointestinal motility 11
Gastrointestinal tract upset 89
Gastrointestinal upset 62
Gelatin 234
Generalized anxiety disorder 380
Genetically engineered monoclonal antibodies 400
Genotropin 187
Gentamicin 419, 519, 524, 530, 532, 537
Gentamicin sulfate 252
Genticare 253
Genticyn 253
Gilles de la Tourette syndrome, attacks of 179

Gingivostomatitis 525
Glaucoma, narrow-angle 112, 141
Globunal 210
Glomerular filtration rate 8
Glomerulonephritis, acute 434
Glucagon 394, 411
Glucagon novo 394
Glucose 232
Glucose, types of 232
Glucose-6-phosphate dehydrogenase 17
Glycopeptide
   antibiotics 300
      newer first-generation 301
   first-generation 302
   inhibiting synthesis 300
Glycoprotein antibiotic, first generation complex 300
Gold salts 526, 537
Gonadotropins 526
Gout 198, 208, 317
   acute 199
   treat 199
Gram-negative organisms 252
Gram-positive bacteria 300
   infections 304
Grandem 96
Granicap 96
Granisetron 96
Granulocyte colony-stimulating factor 169, 411
Granulocyte macrophage colony-stimulating factor 170
Granulocyte precursors 61
Gray baby syndrome
   preterm newborns causes of 310
   risk of developing 310
Grisactin forte 357
Griseofulvin 357, 515, 518, 526-529, 533, 535, 538
Gromane 126
Group A streptococcus 24
Group B streptococcus 23

Growth hormone 187
Guaifenesin 155
Guanethidine sulfate 124
Guillain–Barré syndrome 209, 471
Gynecomastia 526

H

H_2-antagonists 136
Haemaccel 234
Haemophilus influenzae type B 23, 24, 459, 497
   conjugate vaccine 463
Half-life, elimination 23
Hallucinations 518
Haloperidol 143, 517, 521-524
Hansepran 329
Headache 526
Heart block 102
Heart disease 117
   congenital 213
   severe 141
Heart muscle fibers 100
Heartburn 44
Heat stroke 442
Hematemesis 443
Hematinics 203
Hematologic disorders 311
Hematopoietin 168
Hematuria 527
Hemolytic-uremic syndrome 215, 383
Hemostat 182
Hepabig 211
Hepaglob 211
Heparin 69, 531
Heparne 69
Hepatic disease 15, 156
Hepatic insufficiency 36
Hepatitis A 465*b*
   vaccine 464
   virus 465
Hepatitis B
   immunoglobulin 211
   vaccine 466

Index

Hepatotoxicity 528
Hetrazan 383
Hexachlorophene 518
Hiberix 463
Hibpro 463
Hiccup 528
Histamine antagonists 108
HIV/AIDS wasting syndrome 197
Hodgkin's disease 61
Homocodine 155
Hormones 185
Hostacycline 298
Human diploid cell vaccine 485
Human hepatitis B specific
　　　　globulin 211
Human normal immunoglobulin 210
Human papilloma virus 500
　vaccines 467, 497
Human polymerase 342
Human rabies specific
　　　　immunoglobulin 212, 213
Humatin 363, 370
Hyaline membrane disease 451
Hydralazine 411
Hydralazine hydrochloride 124, 238
Hydrazide 173
Hydrochlorothiazide 175, 411
Hydrocortisone 192, 412
Hydroxyzine hydrochloride 113
Hyoscine 519, 521, 523
Hyoscine butylbromide 148
Hyperactivity disorder 122
Hypercyanotic spell 444
Hyperpyrexia 529
Hypersensitivity syndrome 306
Hyperstat 122
Hypertension 119
Hypertensive crisis 444
Hypertrichosis 529
Hypervitaminosis D 525
Hypothermia 529
Hypotonia 524
Hythalton 173

I

Ibucon 38
Ibugesic 38
Ibuprofen 38, 515, 519
Ibusynth 38
Ibutab 38
Idiopathic apnea of prematurity 445
Idoxuridine 336, 535
Imferon 205
Imipenem 282, 325, 419
Imipramine 143, 517, 518, 520-522,
　　　　524, 526, 530, 534, 538
Immunization 457, 500, 502
　schedules 495
Immunodeficiency disorders 211
Immunoglobulins 209
　intravenous 212, 215, 412
Immunosuppressant
　　　　glucocorticoid 194
Immunosuppression 87
Imogam rabies 212
Imorab 212
Inactivated polio vaccine 469
Inderal 129
India's National Immunization
　　　　Schedule 500
Indian Academy of Pediatrics
　　　　Immunization
　current 496*t*
　schedule 495
　timetable 498*t*
Indigestion 44
Indocin 38
Indomethacin 38, 412, 516, 518-521,
　　　　525, 527, 531, 536, 538
Infanrix 463
Infantile myoclonic seizures 86, 87
Infantile spasms 86
Infantile tremor syndrome 105, 129,
　　　　207, 222, 245
Infection 73
　life-threatening 278
　medical devices-associated 24

Infective endocarditis 70
Inflammation 73
Inflammatory and allergic disorders, treatment of 193
Inflammatory bowel disease 92
Influenza
    prophylaxis of 346
    virus vaccines 482
Ingredients like aluminum 44
Inhalation therapy 55
Inhaler hygiene 58
Inhibit platelet aggregation 68
Initiation complex, freezing of 252
Inosiplex 336
Inotrope 158
    drugs 162
Insomnia 529
Insulin 188, 412
    resistance, regulation of 221
Intestinal drugs 359
Intramuscular route 11
Intrauterine growth restriction 19
Iodides 513, 522, 523
Ipcazide 315
Ipratropium bromide 57
Iron 164, 204, 222, 513, 520, 525
    chelator, injectable 165
    content 205t
    dextran complex 11, 205, 531
    salts, oral 205t
    sorbitol 206
    sucrose complex 206
Irritability, excess 523
Irritable bowel syndrome 92, 147, 398
Irritating substances 11
Ischemic heart disease 49, 105, 130, 158
Ismelin 124
Isokin 315
Isonex 315, 515, 528, 533
Isoniazid 315, 514, 517, 518, 521, 524, 527, 538
Isonicotinic acid 315
Isoprinosine 336
Isoptin 106, 131
Isopto 102
Isosorbide dinitrate 239
Isoxsuprine hydrochloride 239
Itraconazole 354
Ivermectin 366, 388

J

Japanese encephalitis 497, 501
    vaccine 486
Jectofer 206
Jenvac 486
Juvenile gout 198
Juvenile idiopathic arthritis 42

K

Kanamycin 320, 519, 522, 524, 528, 532, 534, 538
    derivative of 252, 324
Kanamycin sulfate 253
Kancin 253, 320
Kapilin 248
Kawasaki disease 35, 209, 215
Kaypen 260
Keflor 266
Kelfer 165
Kenadon 248
Kepra 81
Kerosene oil 517
    poisoning 445
Ketasma 113
Ketek 288
Ketoconazole 355
Ketorolac 70
Ketotifen 113
Kidney disease 88, 171, 222
Kidney disorders 150
Kidney dysfunction, cause 44
Kidney injury, acute 435
Klebsiella 270, 281
Klebsiella pneumoniae 24
Knee-chest position, child in 444

L

Labetalol 125
Lacasa 80
Lacosam 80
Lacosamide 80
Lacoset 80
Lacrimation 530
Lactated ringer solution 2
Lactobacillus based super ors 94
Lactulose 236
Lametec 80
Lamitor 80
Lamivudine 339, 423
Lamotrigine 80
Lanoxin 159
Lansoprazole 138
Largactil 95, 142
Laridox 382
L-asparaginase 63
Lasride 120
Lassitude 530
Lastuss 155
Laxative abuse 517
Laxicon 236
Lead 164, 517, 524
Lead iodide 548
Lead salts 514
Leeflox 323
Left heart syndrome 399
Legionella pneumophila 288
Lennox-Gastaut syndrome 74, 85, 86
Leprosy 328
Lesch-Nyhan syndrome 198
Lethargy, syndrome of 75
Leukemia 61, 63
    acute 64
    lymphoma, acute 63
Leukeran 61
Leukine 170
Leukopenia 62
Levamisole 366
Levetiracetam 81
Levilex 81

Levocetirizine 114
Levoflox 323
Levofloxacin 292, 323
Levolin 51
Levosalbutamol 48, 51
Levothyroxine 412
Levroxa 81
Librium 143
Lidocaine hydrochloride 103
Lignocaine 528
Lignocaine hydrochloride 103
Lincomycin 513, 526
    hydrochloride 289
    semisynthetic derivative of 290
Lincosamides 289
Lincotuss 36
Linezolid 304
Linox 305
Lipicure 391
Lipids, metabolism of 221
Lipitor 391
Lipobal 243
Liponorm 391
Lipoprotein cholesterol, low-density 119
Lippan 139
Liquid hydrocarbons, mixture of 237
Liquid paraffin 237
Listeria monocytogenes 23
Live-attenuated influenza vaccine 483, 497
Live-attenuated Ty21a vaccine, oral 477
Liver disease 37, 50, 74, 88, 171
    advanced 75
Liver disorder 207, 245, 248
Lobazam 74
Lomflox 292, 323
Lomicid 139
Lomodex-40 233, 393
Lomodex-70 233, 393
Lomorest 91
Lomotil 90

Longacillin 259
Loniten 126
Loop diuretic 172
Loperamide 525
Loperamide hydrochloride 90
Lopinavir 340
Loratadine 114
Lorazepam 81, 412
Lorfast 114
Loridin 114
Lorin 114
Low molecular weight dextran 392
Low molecular weight heparin 70
Low osmolarity oral rehydration salt 93*t*
  composition of 396*t*
Lumefantrine 378
Luminal 548
Lupenox 70
Lupus-like syndrome 239
Lymphadenopathy 531
Lymphoblastic leukemia, chronic 61
Lynx 289
Lysergic acid diethylamide 519
Lysozymes, changes pH of 345

M

M2-inhibitor antiviral 345
Macrolide 284, 325
Macrominerals 217
Magnamycin 273
Magnesia, milk of 45
Magnesium
  act 44
  content 218*t*
Magnesium hydroxide 44, 45
Magnesium sodium 548
Magnesium sulfate 52, 218, 413
Magnex 273, 279
Malaria 446
Malignancy 61
Malignant lymphoma, acute 63
Malocide 382

Mandelic acid 549
Mannitol 175
Manocalm 98
Maternal medication 17, 19
Maxepa 230, 395
Maxiguard 230, 395
Mazetol 74
Measles, mumps, and rubella 469, 497, 500
Mebendazole 367
Meconium aspiration syndrome, severe 401
Medroxyprogesterone 520
Mefenamic acid 39
Mefloquine 379
Meflotas 379
Meftal 39
Mega-3 230, 395
Megatil 95
Mejoral 34
Melphalan 64
Memtiz 175
Menadione sulfate 248
Ménière's disease 201
Meningococcal vaccine 487, 489*b*
  indications of 488*b*
Meningococcus 23, 24
Meningoencephalitis 447
Mental depression 532
Mepacrine 368, 518, 528, 531, 534
Meperidine 42
Mephentermine sulfate 161
Mephentine 161
Meprobamate 531, 538
Mepron 392
Mercaptopurine 64, 524, 525
Mercurials 533
Mercury 164, 530, 535, 548
Meropenem 283
Merotrol 283
Meroza 283
Metabolism 7
Metacin 33

Metakelfin 381
Metapro 126
Metasafe 51
Metatop 51
Methadone 413
Methandienone 195
Methaqualone 522
Methdilazine hydrochloride 115
Methicillin 419, 527
Methocarbamol 226
Methotrexate 64, 525
Methyldopa 125, 532
Methylene blue 552
Methylphenidate 178, 530
Methylprednisolone 194
Metiz 175
Metoclopramide 136, 413, 518, 522, 526, 537
Metoclopramide hydrochloride 96
Metolazone 175
Metoprolol 126
Metrogyl 311
Metronidazole 311, 361, 420
Mezlocillin 420
Mezolam 82
Micogel 355
Miconazole 355, 423
Microbial flora 11
Micronutrients 221
Micropyrin 34
Micturition, frequency of 525
Midamor 120
Midazolam 82, 413
Mikacin 252
Mikastar 252
Mikicin 324
Milicor 162
Milrinone 162
Minicycline 538
Minipress 129
Minipril 123
Minocycline 298
Minoxidil 126, 239, 528

Mitomycin C 65
Modafinil 395
Modalert 395
Mometasone sodium 51
Monoamine oxidase inhibitors 519
Montair 52
Montelukast 52
Moraxella catarrhalis 24, 288
Morocrit 283
Morphine 413, 532
Morphine sulfate 39
Mouth, dryness of 521
Movement disorder 179, 202, 245
Movement, sudden change in 73
Mucaine gel 44
Mucolite 156
Mucolytic agent 156
Mucosal inflammation 48
Muscle relaxants 224, 528
Mustargen 66
Mustine hydrochloride 66
Mutamycin 65
Myasthenia gravis 132
Mycobacterium genus 314
Mycobacterium leprae 328
Mycoplasma pneumoniae 24, 288
Myeloblastic leukemia, acute 62
Myelodysplastic syndromes 164
Myelofibrosis 60
Myeloid
 elements, alkylating agent for 61
 leukemia, chronic 60
Myocardial depressant 106
Myocardial disease 53
Myopia 532

N

Nafcillin 420
Nalidixic acid 293, 515, 516, 518, 520, 521, 527, 528, 530, 532, 534-536, 538
Naloxone 413
Nandrolone 195

Naproxen 41
Nariz 394
Nasal decongestants 227
Nasal spray 56
National Immunization Schedule 501*t*
Nebulization 59
Nebulizing solution 59
Nelfinavir 341, 423
Neocalm 98
Neomycin 254, 519, 522, 524, 532
Neonatal apnea 49
Neonatal disorder 15
Neonatal intensive care unit 15, 424
Neonatal medicinal development, regulatory framework for model-based 16
Neonatal pharmacotherapy 13
   robust information on 16
Neonatal seizures 447
Neoplastic disease 214
Neoplastic disorder 190
Neostigmine 6, 133
Nephrotic syndrome 61, 65, 79, 87, 121, 174, 190, 191, 193, 222, 233, 471, 472
Nephrotoxicity 532
Nerve tissue vaccine 484
Netilmicin 255
Netromycin 255
Neupogen 169
Neuraminidase
   glycoprotein 348
   inhibitor 345, 348
   natural substrate of 348
Neurobion 244
Neurodevelopmental disorders 177
   incriminated for causing 469
Neuroleptics 534, 535
Neurologic disorder 363, 365
   risk of 230, 395
Neuromuscular blockers act 224
Neuromuscular disease, chronic 132
Neuromuscular disorder 256

Neurons 73
   excessive rapid firing of 73
Neuropathic pain, treatment of 73
Neuropsychiatric drugs 141
Neutropenia 533
Nevirapine 342
Nexpro 138
Niacin 243
Niclosamide 369, 513, 516, 520, 521, 526, 527, 529, 534
Nicotinic acid 243
Nifedipine 127, 239
Nimesulide 40
Nitazoxanide 362, 370
Nitrazepam 82, 515, 523, 530, 533
Nitrofurans 553
Nitrofurantoin 518, 524, 527, 531, 534, 536
Nitroglycerine 239
Nitroprusside 127
Nitroxazepine hydrochloride 144
Nomigrain 394
Nomogram 14
Noncephalosporin beta-lactams 281
non-Hodgkin's lymphomas 61
Nonnucleoside reverse transcriptase inhibitor 342
Nonpenicillin 281
Nonselective antiviral drugs 349
Nonsteroidal anti-inflammatory drug 33, 137, 147
Nonstimulants 179
Nonvariceal bleed 448
Nonvariceal hematemesis 448*b*
Noradrenaline 162
Norditropin 187
Norepinephrine 162
   immediate precursor of 160
Norfloxacin 293
Nortriptyline 520, 534
Nose, stuffy 58
Nucleoside antiviral drug, semisynthetic 350

Index

Nutritional supplements 229
Nystatin 357, 423, 513

O

Obstructive gastrointestinal disease 147
Ocular tension 76
Odoxil 269
Ofloxacin 294
Ofloxacin, levo isomer of 323
Omega-3 fatty acids 230, 395
Omeprazole 44, 139
Omnikacin 252
Ondansetron hydrochloride 97
Opiates 516
Oral rehydration salt 92, 93*t*, 396
    standard 93*t*
    super 94
Orciprenaline sulfate 53
Organophosphate 517, 523
    poisoning 449
Oritavancin 304
Ornidazole 363
Oseltamivir 345
Otitis media, acute 435
Overexcitment 533
Oxacillin 421
Oxazolidinone antibiotics 304
Oxcarbazepine 82
Oxymetazoline hydrochloride 228
Oxymetholone 197
Oxyphenbutazone 514, 549
Oxyphenonium bromide 148
Oxytetracycline 297

P

Palonosetron 97
Palpitations 102
Pancreas-related drugs 188
Pancreatic disorders 185
Pancreatin 188
Pancuronium bromide 397
Pantaprazole 139
Pantocid 139
Pantop 139
Pantoprazole 44
    intravenous dose of 448*b*
Pantothenic acid 244
Para-aminobenzoic acid 534
    structural analog of 321
Para-aminosalicylic acid 321
Para-aminosalicylic acid sodium 513, 535
Paracetamol 33, 41, 147, 528
Paraldehyde 83
Parenteral nutrition, energy component of 232
Paresthesia 534
Paromomycin 363, 370
Partial seizure 73
Pediatric
    age groups, pharmacokinetics of 3
    cancer, cytotoxic drugs for 60
    dose
        calculation of 14*b*
        therapy 539
            golden rules of safe 28
    emergencies, pharmacotherapy of 427, 432
    oncology armamentarium, growing 60
    population, age-based grouping of 3*b*
Pefloxacin 295
Pemoline 178
Penamine 166
Pendramine 166
Penicillamine 166, 515, 528, 529, 532
Penicillin 265, 514, 515, 522, 523
    extended-spectrum 261, 264
    G 258, 421, 422
    semisynthetic 260
Penicillinase
    resistant penicillins 260
    sensitive penicillins 258

Index

Penidure LA-6, 12, and 24 259
Penivoral 260
Pentamidine isethionate 384
Pentavalent antimony 385
Pentazocine hydrochloride 41
Pentothal 88
Peptic ulcer 87, 193, 200
Periactin 110
Periodontal disorders 351
Peripheral arterial disease 121
Peritol 110
Permard 388
Permethrin 388
Permisol 388
Permite 388
Pethidine 524, 538
Pethidine hydrochloride 42
Petit mal 73, 78
Petroleum product 237
Pharmacotherapy, basics of 1
Phenergan 98, 116
Phenindione 71
Pheniramine maleate 115
Phenobarbital 413-516, 523, 528, 533, 536
Phenobarbital sodium 83
Phenolphthalein 552
Phenothiazines 517, 520-522, 524, 526, 529, 532, 538
Phenoxybenzamine 128, 240
Phensuximide 531
Phentolamine 128
Phenylbutazone 514, 531, 537, 549
   depress enzyme induction 8
Phenylephrine 535
Phenylpropanolamine 227
Phenytoin 414
Phenytoin sodium 84, 104
Pholcodine 155
Photo allergy 534
Photophobia 535
Phototoxicity 535
Physostigmine 532

Pipenzolate methylbromide 149
Piperacillin 422
Piperazine 371, 514, 516-518, 534, 536, 538
Piracetam 397
Piroxicam 42
Pituitary diseases 185
Pituitary-related drugs 185
Plasma expanders 231
Plasma volume expanders 231, 393
Plasmodium falciparum,
   erythrocytic stages
   of 378
Pneumococcal conjugate vaccine 459, 472, 497, 500
Pneumococcal disease 472b
Pneumococcal polysaccharide vaccine 471, 497
Pneumococcal vaccine 472b
Pneumococcus 23
Pneumocystis carinii 391
Pneumonia 450, 450b
Polio vaccine, injectable 497, 500
Poliovirus vaccines, oral 500
Polycythemia vera 60
Polydipsia 525
Polyenes 352
Polymyxin 516, 534, 538
Polyunsaturated fatty acids 230
   long-chain
Polyuria 525
Potassium 548
Potassium chloride 219
Potassium-sparing 119
Practin 110
Praziquantel 371
Prazopress 129
Prazosin 240
Prazosin hydrochloride 129
Prednisolone 63, 87, 193, 532
Pregnancy 18t
   first trimester of 17
Primacor 162

Primaquine phosphate 380
Primicef 181
Primidone 85, 414, 514, 519, 523, 528, 531, 538
Probenecid 200
Probiotics 91, 398
Procainamide 104
Procaine 422
Prochlorperazine 98
Progesterone 526
Prokinetics 135
Promegapoietin 170
Promethazine 533, 535, 537
Promethazine hydrochloride 98, 116
Propantheline bromide 149
Propoxyphene 517
Propranolol 129, 414, 519, 532, 533
　hydrochloride 105
Propylthiouracil 531
Prostaglandin 408
Prostaglandin E1 398
Protamine sulfate 184
Proteus 270, 281
Prothionamide 321
Proton pump inhibitors 136, 138
Pruritus 535
Pseudoephedrine 116, 227, 549
　hydrochloride 228
Pseudomonas 270, 278
　aeruginosa 24
Pseudotumor cerebri 536
Psychiatric conditions like bipolar disorder 221
Psychiatric disorders 39
Psychosis 87
　acute 87
Psychosomatic disorders 143
Ptosis 536
Pulmicort inhaler 56
Pulmonary 13
　embolism 68, 69
　excretion 9
　fibrosis 61
　reactions 17
　status 65
Punarjal 92
Purely luminal amebicide 360
Purgative abuse 517
Purified chick embryo cell vaccine 484
Pyrantel pamoate 369
Pyrazinamide 317
Pyridostigmine 134
Pyridoxine 88, 244
　deficiency causing neuritis 88
　dependent seizures 88
　disulfide 399
Pyrimethamine 381, 382, 385, 515, 518
Pyrithioxine 144, 399
Pyritinol 144, 399

Q

Quinacrine 368
Quinidine 106
　sulfate 106
Quinine 519, 520, 522, 536, 549
　sulfate 382
Quinolones 291
Quinupristin 306

R

Rabies
　specific immunoglobulins 212
　vaccine 484
Racecadotril 91
Racotil 91
Radiation therapy 60
Ramihart 130
Ramipres 130
Ramipril 130
Ranbiotic 253
Ranitidine 137, 414
Rash lupus-like syndrome 383
Rational drug therapy 21
Rational drug therapy program 21

Rectal diazepam, administration of 78
Rectal route 12
Red man syndrome 301
Refractory partial seizures 86
Regitine 128
Renal and hepatic failure 62
Renal disease 15, 37, 74, 174, 175
 dose in 134
Renal excretion 8
Renal failure, acute 435
Renal impairment 71
Reserpine 130, 526, 532
Respiratory distress syndrome 240, 401, 451
 rescue therapy in 401
Respiratory syncytial virus 212
Resteclin 298
Rett syndrome 80, 247
Reye syndrome 35
Rheumatoid and lupus-like syndromes 124
Ribavirin 350
Riboflavin 243
Rifampicin 312, 317, 331, 513, 515, 519, 528, 533
Rifamycin 312
Rimantadine 348
Ringer solution 232
Rituximab 400
Rofecoxib 42
Rota vaccine, dose of 497
Rotavirus 474
 vaccine 474
Rovamycin 287
Rowezy 326
Roxithromycin 287
Rubella syndrome, congenital potential cause of 475
Rubella vaccine 475

S

Sabin strain type 470
Sabril 86
Safe drug therapy, seven "rights" of 28
Saizen 187
Salaam seizures 86
Salaam seizures syndrome 85, 87
Salazopyrin 309
Salbetol 53
Salbutamol 48, 53
 levoversion of 51
Salicylates 515, 520, 522, 523
 poisoning 529
Salmeterol 58
Scabies and pediculosis, first-line drug for 388
Scabitol-P 388
Scalp hair, loss of 530
Scorpion
 antivenom 153
 sting 451
  antitoxin 216
  manifestations of 451
 venom antitoxin 153
Secnidazole 364
Secrotolytic agent 156
Sedatives 521, 549
Seizure 73
 absence 78
 acute 453
 control 87
 disorder 74, 284, 293, 296, 371, 469
 focal onset 73
 generalized tonic-clonic 82
 partial
Sensorium 73
Sepsis 92, 136, 170, 180, 215, 277, 283, 401
 neonatal 320
 postoperative 324
 prevention of 291, 322
Serum sickness syndrome 17
Shigellosis 438
Shock 412
 syndrome 160

Sibelium 394
Sick sinus syndrome 101, 122
Sickle cell disease 164
Sildenafil 400
Simethicone 149
Singular leukotriene receptor blocker 51
Sinus bradycardia 102
Siozide 315
Siquil 98
Sisomicin sulfate 256
Sisomin 256
Sisonest 256
Sisoptin 256
Sisowill 256
Skin disorder, common 46
Sleep disorder 81, 375, 376
Snakebite 452
Sneezing 58
Sodium bicarbonate 219
 chloride 220
 excess 73
 nitroprusside 130, 240
 picosulfate 237
 stibogluconate 385
Sodium-channel blocker 102, 105, 119
Sodium-channel protein inhibitor 104
Solitary drug therapy 328
Solonex 315
Solvent sniffing 517, 519, 534, 538
Somatostatin 187
Somatropin 187
Somicin 256
Somnolence, syndrome of 75
Sorbtrate 239
Sparfloxacin 295
Spastic cerebral palsy 224
Spinal disease 224
Spiramycin 287
Spironolactone 176, 414, 526
Squint 536

Staphylococcus
 aureus 24, 270, 275
 infections 258
Status asthmaticus 436
 epilepticus 453
Stavudine 342
Stemiz 108
Steven–Johnson syndrome 65, 198, 258–260, 269, 291, 296, 307, 309, 322, 326, 339, 342, 357, 378, 382, 383, 386
Stomach, acidity in 44
Stool softeners 235
Streptococcus pneumoniae 24
 pyogenes 288
Streptokinase 70
Streptomycin 6, 318, 516, 519, 522, 529, 530, 533, 534
 sulfate 256
Stress ulcers, prevention of 136
Strictly speaking 141
Strychnine 517, 537
Sublimaze 37
Sucralfate 139
Sudafed 116, 228
Sudden infant death syndrome 19
Sulbacef 279
Sulbacin 263
Sulbactam 263
Sulfadiazine 307, 386, 422
Sulfadoxine 382
Sulfamethoxazole 308
Sulfamethoxypyrazine 381
Sulfas 515, 516, 520, 522, 523, 525, 527, 531–533, 535, 538
Sulfasalazine 309
Sulfide, formation of 550
Sulfisoxazole 309
Sulfonamide 307, 514, 534, 535, 553
Sulfonamide loop diuretic 174
Sulfone 553
Sulfone antimicrobial resembling sulfonamides 329

Sulfone syndrome 330
Sulthiame 536
Suppressa 155
Supraventricular arrhythmias 441*t*
Sweating, excessive 524
Sympathomimetic amine vasopressor 160
Synthetic lipid-lowering agent 391
Syphilis 258
Systemic lupus erythematosus-like syndrome 104

T

Tachycardia 102
Tagamet 136
Tailoring research tools 16
Tamiflu 345
Tannate, formation of 550
Tartrazine 529
Teicoplanin 301
Telithromycin 288
Tendon disorder 292
Tenofovir 343
Terbinafine 356
Terbutaline 48
    sulfate 54
Terfenadine 117
Testosterone 526
Tetanus
    antitoxin 152, 215
    low-dose diphtheria and pertussis vaccine 478
    toxoid 461, 473, 503, 535
Tetanus, diphtheria toxoids, and acellular pertussis 500
Tetracycline 296, 513, 526-528, 532-536
    hydrochloride 298
Thalizide 173
Theophylline 54, 414
Therapeutic drug monitoring 10, 25
Thiabendazole 515, 520, 527, 534, 538

Thiamine 242
Thiazide 525, 538
    diuretics 119, 515, 516, 522
Thioamide derivative 321
Thiopental 88
Thiouracil 523, 537
Thorazine 527
Thrombocytopenia 62
Thyroid 188, 189
    disorder 88, 351
    function tests 101
Thyroxine 188, 520, 523, 524
Ticarcillin 422
Tigecycline 299
Tiniba 364
Tinidazole 364
Tissue culture vaccines, modern 484
Tobramycin 252, 324, 422, 519
    sulfate 257
Tocoferol 247
Tolazoline 414
    hydrochloride 240
Tolmetin 43
Tomoxetin 142, 179
Tonsillitis, acute severe 437
Topcid 137
Topiramate 85
Total parenteral nutrition 223*t*
Toxic shock syndrome 468, 503
Toxicity, clinical signs and symptoms of 101
Tramadol 43
Tranexamic acid 184
Tranquilizers 521, 533, 537, 547
Tranquilizing states 537
Trazine 98
Tretinoin 47
Triamcinolone 194
Triamterene 176
Triazole
    first generation 354
    second generation 355

Index

Tricyclic amine 345
    antidepressants 514, 515, 524, 526, 529, 536
Trifluoperazine 98
Trifluridine 336
Trimethadione 515, 533, 537
Trimethoprim 308, 327, 513, 527, 531, 534, 538
Trioxidone 535
Tripacel 463
Triprolidine hydrochloride 118
Trismus 537
Trivalent influenza vaccine 482
    dose of 483t
Tromethamine 415
Tropicamide 535
Troxidone 514, 516, 525, 527, 531
Turner syndrome 187
Tylenol 33
Typhoid conjugate vaccine 497
Typhoid vaccine 476
    oral 477
    Vi capsular polysaccharide 476
    Vi conjugate 477

U

Universal Immunization Program 495, 500
Ursodeoxycholic acid 402, 415
Urticaria 535

V

Vaccines 457, 481, 497
Vagal activation, effects of excessive 102
Valethamate bromide 150
Valganciclovir 337
Valium 75
Valparin sodium 516
Valproate 27
    sodium 86, 527, 531
Valproic acid 415
Valupenem 283
Vancomycin 300, 423, 519
Variceal bleed 443
Varicella vaccine 479
    dose of 497
Varicella zoster immunoglobulin 213
Vasodilation 238
Vasodilator 158, 238
    drug 162
Vasopressin 163, 187
    analog 186
Ventolin 58
Ventricular tachycardia, treatment of 102
Veramil 106, 131
Verapamil 106, 131
Veritek 355
Veritop 355
Verkab 355
Vero cell vaccine 485
Vertigo 201, 537
Vertigon 201
Verz 355
Vesicular lesions 515
Vestibular disorder 298
Vidarabine 423
Vigabatrin 86
Vigilance disorders 295
Vinblastine 66
Vincristine 63, 67, 513, 516, 517, 519, 520, 524-527, 529, 534, 536
Viomycin 533
Vision disorders 351
Vitamins 241-248, 547, 553
    A 11, 241
        deficiency 536
        excess 520, 531, 536
        overdose 521
    B complex (water-soluble) 207, 244
    B_1 207, 242
    B_2 243
    B_3 243

B_5 244
B_6 88, 244
   seminatural analog of 399
B_{12} 169, 203, 204, 207, 218, 244
C 245
D 246
   analog 409
   excess 525
E 230, 247, 415
K 71, 248
   antagonist 68
   deficiency 71
   high content 72
   water-soluble analogs 553
   quantity of 241
Vomiting 95
von Willebrand disease 186
Vorage 355
Voraprin 131
Voratril 106, 131
Voriconazole 355

W

Walavin-250, 357
Walyte 92
Warfarin 71
Water in urine, excretion of 171
West syndrome 85–87, 185
Willebrand's disease 183
Wilson disease 166

X

Xantinol nicotinate 72
Xerophthalmia, treatment schedule of 242t
Xylometazoline hydrochloride 228

Y

Yellow fever vaccine 488
Young's rule 14

Z

Zafirlukast 55
Zalcitabine 344
Zanamivir 348
Zidovudine 344, 423
Zinc 94, 222
   supplements 223t
Zinepress 124
Zocef 279
Zolamide 171
Zonisamide 86
Zycolchin 199
Zytanix 175